Food Allergens
Analysis Instrumentation and Methods

Food Allergens
Analysis Instrumentation and Methods

Edited by
Leo M.L. Nollet and Arjon J. van Hengel

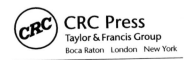

CRC Press
Taylor & Francis Group
Boca Raton London New York

CRC Press is an imprint of the
Taylor & Francis Group, an **informa** business

CRC Press
Taylor & Francis Group
6000 Broken Sound Parkway NW, Suite 300
Boca Raton, FL 33487-2742

© 2011 by Taylor and Francis Group, LLC
CRC Press is an imprint of Taylor & Francis Group, an Informa business

International Standard Book Number: 978-1-4398-1503-8 (Hardback)

This book contains information obtained from authentic and highly regarded sources. Reasonable efforts have been made to publish reliable data and information, but the author and publisher cannot assume responsibility for the validity of all materials or the consequences of their use. The authors and publishers have attempted to trace the copyright holders of all material reproduced in this publication and apologize to copyright holders if permission to publish in this form has not been obtained. If any copyright material has not been acknowledged please write and let us know so we may rectify in any future reprint.

Except as permitted under U.S. Copyright Law, no part of this book may be reprinted, reproduced, transmitted, or utilized in any form by any electronic, mechanical, or other means, now known or hereafter invented, including photocopying, microfilming, and recording, or in any information storage or retrieval system, without written permission from the publishers.

For permission to photocopy or use material electronically from this work, please access www.copyright.com (http://www.copyright.com/) or contact the Copyright Clearance Center, Inc. (CCC), 222 Rosewood Drive, Danvers, MA 01923, 978-750-8400. CCC is a not-for-profit organization that provides licenses and registration for a variety of users. For organizations that have been granted a photocopy license by the CCC, a separate system of payment has been arranged.

Trademark Notice: Product or corporate names may be trademarks or registered trademarks, and are used only for identification and explanation without intent to infringe.

Library of Congress Cataloging-in-Publication Data

Food allergens : analysis instrumentation and methods / Leo M.L. Nollet, Arjon J. van Hengel, (eds.).
    p. ; cm.
Includes bibliographical references and index.
Summary: "Covering all of the major recognized food allergens in the US and EU, this comprehensive work begins with an introduction to the problem and prevalence of food allergens. It discusses health issues and the presence of allergens in various food products, examines methodologies for analysis and detection, and details specific methods for each food type. Maintaining a consistent structure and format throughout, each chapter describes the properties of the allergen, and demonstrates the appropriate sample extraction and clean-up, separation and analysis, and detection and quantification techniques"--Provided by publisher.
    ISBN 978-1-4398-1503-8 (hardcover : alk. paper)
    1. Food allergy. 2. Allergens--Analysis. I. Nollet, Leo M. L., 1948- II. Hengel, Arjon J. van.
    [DNLM: 1. Allergens--immunology. 2. Food Hypersensitivity--immunology. 3. Allergens--analysis. WD 310]
    RC596.F637 2011
    616.97'5--dc22   2010027442

Visit the Taylor & Francis Web site at
http://www.taylorandfrancis.com

and the CRC Press Web site at
http://www.crcpress.com

Contents

Preface vii
About the Editors ix
Contributors xi

Chapter 1
Introduction 1

Arjon J. van Hengel

Chapter 2
Detection of Allergens in Foods 13

Phil E. Johnson, Ana I. Sancho, Rene W. R. Crevel, and E. N. Clare Mills

Chapter 3
Allergens in Peanut, Soybean, and Lupin 29

Christiane K. Fæste

Chapter 4
Allergens in Tree Nuts, Sesame Seeds, Mustard, and Celery 77

Thomas Holzhauser and Martin Röder

Chapter 5
Allergens in Milk and Eggs 129

Mirva Steinhoff and Angelika Paschke-Kratzin

Chapter 6
Detection of Allergens in Cereals 153

Dimosthenis Kizis and George Siragakis

Chapter 7
Fish, Crustaceans, and Mollusks 177

Poi-Wah Lee and Steve L. Taylor

Index 207

Preface

Food allergies represent an important health problem in industrialized countries. Allergens in food products pose a major risk for sensitized persons. Detection and quantification methods are necessary to comply with food labeling and to improve consumer protection.

The book contains seven chapters. The introduction provides an insight into the extent of the problem caused by food allergens. Health implications and the presence of plant food and animal-derived allergens in different foodstuffs are discussed.

In Chapter 2, methodologies for the analysis and detection of allergens are examined.

In Chapters 3 to 7, analysis and detection methods of allergens of different foodstuffs are detailed. The author of Chapter 3 deals with allergens in peanut, soybean, and lupin. In the next chapter, a discussion follows on allergens in tree nuts, sesame seeds, mustard, and celery. Allergens in milk and egg are detailed in Chapter 5. Chapter 6 provides an in-depth discussion of allergens in cereals. The book ends with a chapter on allergens in fish, crustaceans, and mollusks.

In the chapters on allergens in different foodstuffs (Chapters 3–7), first allergen properties are briefly discussed. Next, after sample extraction and cleanup, separation and analysis methods are specified. Finally, detection and quantification techniques are enumerated.

This book is intended to be concise, compact, and inexpensive; even so, it provides in-depth information.

For all their excellent efforts, we thank the authors of the different chapters.

Arjon J. van Hengel
Leo M. L. Nollet

By perseverance the snail reached the ark.

C. H. Spurgeon

About the Editors

Arjon J. van Hengel studied biology (Utrecht, NL) and received his PhD in molecular biology in 1998 (Wageningen, NL). He worked as a research scientist from 1998 to 2004 at the John Innes Centre (Norwich, UK). In January 2005, he began working for the Joint Research Centre of the European Commission at the Institute for Reference Materials and Measurements (Geel, Belgium), where he leads the allergen research group.

The work of the allergen research group focuses on the validation of allergen detection methods, the optimization of such methods, the development of novel methods, and the generation of allergen reference materials.

Leo M. L. Nollet is the editor and associate editor of numerous books. He edited for Marcel Dekker, New York (now CRC Press of the Taylor & Francis Group), the first and second editions of *Food Analysis by HPLC* (2000) and *Handbook of Food Analysis* (2004). The last edition is a three-volume book. He also edited *Handbook of Water Analysis, Chromatographic Analysis of the Environment*, third edition (CRC Press, 2005), and the second edition of *Handbook of Water Analysis* (CRC Press, 2007). He coedited two books with Fidel Toldra, *Advanced Technologies for Meat Processing* (CRC Press, 2006) and *Advances in Food Diagnostics* (Blackwell, 2007). With Michael Pöschl, he coedited *Radionuclide Concentrations in Foods and the Environment* (CRC Press, 2006).

He has coedited several books with Y. H. Hui and other colleagues: *Handbook of Food Product Manufacturing* (Wiley, 2007); *Handbook of Food Science, Technology, and Engineering* (CRC Press, 2005); *Food Biochemistry and Food Processing* (Blackwell, 2005); and *Handbook of Flavors from Fruits and Vegetables* (Wiley, 2010).

Finally, he edited the *Handbook of Meat, Poultry and Seafood Quality* (Blackwell, 2007) and *Analysis of Endocrine Compounds in Foods* (Blackwell-Wiley, 2010).

With Fidel Toldra, he prepared or is preparing six books on meat analysis methodologies:

- *Handbook of Muscle Foods Analysis*
- *Handbook of Processed Meats and Poultry Analysis*
- *Handbook of Seafood and Seafood Products Analysis*
- *Handbook of Dairy Foods Analysis*
- *Handbook of Analysis of Edible Animal By-Products*
- *Handbook of Analysis of Active Compounds in Functional Foods*

With Hamir Rathore, he worked or is working on two books related to pesticide analysis: *Handbook of Pesticides: Methods of Pesticides Residues Analysis* and *Pesticides: Evaluation of Environmental Pollution*.

Contributors

Rene W. R. Crevel
Institute of Food Research
Colney, Norwich, UK

Christiane K. Fæste
Department of Food and Food Safety
National Veterinary Institute
Oslo, Norway

Thomas Holzhauser
Paul-Ehrlich-Institut, Division of
 Allergology
Langen, Germany

Phil E. Johnson
Institute of Food Research
Colney, Norwich, UK

Dimosthenis Kizis
Food Allergens Laboratory
North Heraklio, Greece

Poi-Wah Lee
Food Allergy Research and Resource
 Program
University of Nebraska, Department of
 Food Science and Technology
Lincoln, Nebraska, USA

E. N. Clare Mills
Institute of Food Research
Colney, Norwich, UK

Angelika Paschke-Kratzin
University of Hamburg, Institute of
 Biochemistry and Food Chemistry
Hamburg, Germany

Martin Röder
Paul-Ehrlich-Institut, Division of
 Allergology
Langen, Germany

Ana I. Sancho
Institute of Food Research
Colney, Norwich, UK

George Siragakis
Food Allergens Laboratory
North Heraklio, Greece

Mirva Steinhoff
Institute of Biochemistry and Food
 Chemistry
University of Hamburg
Hamburg, Germany

Steve L. Taylor
Food Allergy Research and Resource
 Program
University of Nebraska, Department of
 Food Science and Technology
Lincoln, Nebraska, USA

CHAPTER 1

Introduction

Arjon J. van Hengel

CONTENTS

Food Allergy: A Problem on the Rise 1
Managing Allergenic Foods: The Efforts to Protect Allergic Consumers 3
Allergenic Foods and Food Allergens: The Culprits 4
Analytical Methods and Instrumentation: The Tools that Are Needed 5
Method Performance: The Tools and Their Requirements 8
The Allergenic Foods and Their Detection Methods 8
References 10

FOOD ALLERGY: A PROBLEM ON THE RISE

Food allergy has evolved from being a problem for the food-allergic individual to one of significant public health importance.[1] The increased awareness of food-allergic disorders has resulted from better understanding and improved diagnosis. It has been estimated that currently as much as 4% of the total population is affected by food-allergic disorders, while the frequency is even higher for infants and children, with prevalence levels reaching 8%.[2–4] Despite the numerous advances in medicine and modern health care that have led to many improvements of the general heath of the population, no reduction in the frequency of allergic disorders like food allergy has been achieved. In contrast, there are unfortunately clear indications that the problem of food allergy shows a contrasting trend, and that the prevalence of food allergy has risen in recent years. This was confirmed in a study that found a doubling of the prevalence of peanut allergy over a period of only 5 years.[5] Not only the prevalence levels are high and on the rise, but also the awareness among the general population is high, with 25% of parents believing that their children suffer from a food allergy.[6]

This recognition of the importance of food allergy has led to a multitude of research initiatives that have clearly increased our understanding of food-based allergic disorders. The causative factors for food-allergic reactions are proteins that are termed *allergens*. Such allergens are components that are present in foods that are part of our normal human diet. They are found in many basic foods consumed on a daily basis. Allergenic proteins usually have high nutritional value for the major part of the population but threaten the health of a subset, the food-allergic consumers. Investigations of allergenic food proteins and the immunologic responses that they can trigger in susceptible individuals have now moved to the molecular level. This has led to the identification of a large number of allergenic proteins that are known to be able to trigger the production of specific immunoglobulin E (IgE) antibodies, which can lead to sensitization to a particular food. When a food product containing the allergenic protein that caused the sensitization is consumed again, the renewed contact with the allergen allows the IgE antibodies to bind to allergen molecules; this can then trigger an allergic reaction. It has to be noted that two different types of abnormal immune responses can occur: immediate hypersensitivity and delayed hypersensitivity reactions.[7] Immediate hypersensitivity reactions involve abnormal responses of the immune system mediated by the allergen-specific (IgE) antibodies.[8] These reactions are referred to as immediate hypersensitivity reactions because symptoms ensue within minutes to a few hours after ingestion of the offending food. In contrast, symptoms develop more slowly, after 24 hours or more following ingestion of the offending food in delayed hypersensitivity reactions. Delayed hypersensitivity reactions involve cell-mediated, typically T-cell-mediated, immune reactions.[7] With the exception of celiac disease, which involves an abnormal response to wheat, rye, barley, and related grains, the role of delayed hypersensitivity in adverse reactions to foods remains poorly understood.

The severity of allergic reactions varies from mild urticaria to potentially fatal anaphylactic shocks. It has been estimated that in the United States alone around 30,000 anaphylactic reactions to food are treated in emergency departments, and that food allergy results in 150–200 deaths each year.[9]

Food allergy is not a static condition; sometimes it can develop later in life, or it can resolve naturally over time. For milk allergy, it has been reported that the condition can be outgrown in many cases, while other food allergies, like peanut or fish allergy, are rarely resolved over time.[10–12] Unfortunately, in many cases the condition is typically lifelong. The reactivity toward an allergenic food varies per patient, and sometimes minute amounts are capable of triggering a serious allergic reaction.

Despite the severity, the prevalence, and the impact that food allergy has on daily life, a patient diagnosed with this condition unfortunately cannot as yet be cured. At the moment, the only proven therapy for food allergy is a strict avoidance diet and a treatment of allergic reactions after accidental exposure to the offending food. This implies that people with a food allergy need to know whether the food products they purchase are indeed free from the ingredient that can trigger an allergic reaction in their body. Their health depends on the purchase and consumption of "safe" food products that do not endanger their health.

MANAGING ALLERGENIC FOODS: THE EFFORTS TO PROTECT ALLERGIC CONSUMERS

During the purchase of food products, food-allergic consumers, or the people who care for them, need to be able to make informed choices to identify products that do not contain certain allergenic ingredients so that they can protect their health by adhering to an avoidance diet. Identifying foods that are safe to eat requires a high level of vigilance and experience. Therefore, living with a food allergy clearly has a negative impact on the quality of life and puts pressure on the social networks of allergic consumers. Although the amount of objective data on this topic is still scarce, studies have demonstrated that food-allergic children are at risk of considerable negative emotional experiences that can have a direct impact on their psychosocial development in a disease-specific manner.[13] Food allergy affects not only people with this condition but also many people in their environment. Particularly, parents caring for children with a food allergy often experience high levels of stress and anxiety. The constant pressure on providing safe food and the feeling of guilt when a child suffers from a reaction to a food can have an enormous impact on their life. Preadolescence can be an extra difficult period. When children gain more autonomy and want to demonstrate their control on events in their own life, they often adopt a more risk-taking behavior, which increases the likelihood of experiencing allergic reactions.

Transferring the information on the presence of allergenic ingredients in food products to the consumer is crucial to allow the consumer to identify food products that are potentially harmful and to make an informed choice of products they want to purchase. Allergic consumers and parents of allergic children want to control the food that comes into their homes, and this very much restricts the choice of food products that they can purchase. Currently, the complexity of food products and the number of ingredients used by the food industry is enormous. The launch of new products, especially the changes in production and composition of known products, creates many difficulties for food-allergic consumers (Figure 1.1).

Labeling allows the food producer to communicate information on the quality and especially the content of their product directly to the consumer. This information plays a crucial role in enabling the consumer to identify allergenic ingredients in food products. Labeling has the potential not only to identify foods that are unsafe for allergic consumers but also to increase the choice of safe food products.

Legislators and regulatory agencies have recognized the importance of labeling with regard to protecting the allergic consumer. As a result of this, in many jurisdictions in different parts of the world new legislation specifically aimed at the protection of allergic consumers has been put in place. Examples of this are Directive 2003/89/EC and Directive 2007/68/EC, issued by the European Commission.[14,15] This legislation has resulted in a mandatory labeling of the 13 most commonly allergenic foods (plus sulfites) as well as ingredients derived from those foods (a few derivatives are exempt from labeling as stated in the latter directive). A similar labeling approach is mandated in the United States with the enactment in 2004

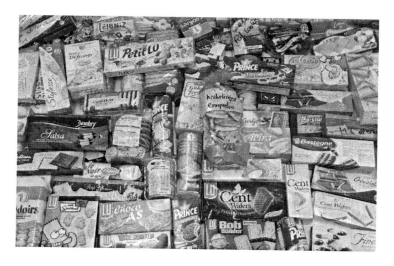

Figure 1.1 The enormous variety and complexity of food products available to the consumer makes the identification of foods that are safe for allergic consumers a daunting task.

of the Food Allergen Labeling and Consumer Protection Act.[16] This demand for a declaration of allergenic ingredients has led to a variety of different types of labels appearing on food products. Such labels can declare the presence of allergenic ingredients; alternatively, they can indicate that, although the allergenic food has not been used as an ingredient, there is a chance that the food product contains the allergenic food unintentionally. The last type of labeling is generally referred to as *precautionary labeling*.

ALLERGENIC FOODS AND FOOD ALLERGENS: THE CULPRITS

Over the last two decades, a vast number of allergens have been identified; now, almost 1,500 allergenic structures are known.[17] The collection of data on allergenic structures and the establishment of databases containing allergenic molecules together with information on their physicochemical properties and their allergenic relevance have provided us with a wealth of information.[18] This improved knowledge of food allergens is likely to improve diagnostics and is important to assess the risk of cross-reactivity. In some cases, IgE molecules of an allergic patient that were raised after sensitization with one particular allergenic food can also bind to allergens from a different, sometimes unrelated, food. This is due to cross-reactivity between allergens from different food sources. Such cross-reactivity can be explained either by phylogenetic relationships or by a structural relationship between allergens from different foods. Although the number of known allergens is high, bioinformatic analysis has shown that they belong to only a small minority of the known protein families.[19,20] An allergenic food, however, can contain many different

INTRODUCTION

allergens, which sometimes belong to different protein families. Allergic patients can react to one or more allergens of a particular food. Patients with an allergy to a food containing many different allergens, like peanut or milk, can therefore differ in the allergenic proteins that are recognized by the IgE present in their bodies.

Despite the existence of so many allergens and the fact the diversity of the human diet is enormous, it has to be recognized that there are only a few foods that account for the majority of allergic reactions.[21] This has been taken into account by regulatory authorities, which have issued legislation that aims to protect allergic consumers by introducing a mandatory declaration of only the most relevant allergenic ingredients on the label of food products.

In 1993, the Codex Alimentarius Commission adopted recommendations made by the Codex Committee on Food Labeling. This formed the basis of using science-based criteria to determine which foods should be placed on a priority list of foods that should always be declared in the list of ingredients. In the United States on January 1, 2006, the Food Allergen Labeling and Consumer Protection Act of 2004 (FALCPA) became effective.[16] It requires all packaged foods to declare the presence of "major food allergens" or their protein derivatives. The major food allergens covered by this piece of legislation include milk, egg, fish, crustacean shellfish, tree nuts, wheat, peanuts, and soy. In Europe, in 2003 the European Commission amended the food labeling Directive 2000/13/EC[22] by issuing Directive 2003/89/EC.[14] The latter directive contains a list (in Annex IIIa) of allergenic foodstuffs that require mandatory labeling when they are used as ingredients in food products. The allergenic foodstuffs (and most of their derivatives) that are listed in Annex IIIa include the major allergenic ingredients mentioned regarding FALCPA and celery, mustard, sesame seeds, and sulfites in addition. Directive 2007/68/EC[15] was issued that amended the labeling directive. The updated Annex IIIa now contains a listing of 14 (groups of) allergenic foodstuffs that require a mandatory declaration. Besides this, it mentions which derivatives are exempt from the ingredient declaration.

Table 1.1 gives an overview of allergenic food ingredients whose presence in food products needs to be declared in different parts of the world. It is apparent from this table that the lists of allergenic foods are often similar. Despite the similarities, some interesting differences can be observed. For example, in Canada a regulatory proposal requires the declaration of any gluten sources on the food label.[23]

ANALYTICAL METHODS AND INSTRUMENTATION: THE TOOLS THAT ARE NEEDED

Since proteins are the causative factors in triggering allergic reactions, analytical techniques that are aimed at the characterization and identification of proteins like allergens are important tools to improve our understanding of food allergy. A systematic approach to diagnosis of a food allergy includes a careful analysis of the history of adverse reactions, followed by laboratory studies, elimination diets, and often food challenges to confirm a diagnosis. The molecular characterization of many food allergens has increased our understanding of the immunopathogenesis

Table 1.1 Allergenic Ingredients that Require a Mandatory Declaration on the Label of Food Products According to Legislation in Different Parts of the World

Allergenic Food	Codex Alimentarius	EU	United States	Japan	Canada	Australia & New Zealand
Cereals	√	√	√	√	√	√
Crustaceans	√	√	√	√	√	√
Egg	√	√	√	√	√	√
Fish	√	√	√		√	√
Milk	√	√	√	√	√	√
Peanut	√	√	√	√	√	√
Soybean	√	√	√		√	√
Tree nuts	√	√	√		√	√
Sesame seeds		√			√	√
Mustard		√			√	
Celery		√				
Lupin		√				
Mollusks		√				√
Buckwheat				√		
Sulfur dioxide and sulfites		√			√	

of food allergy and might soon lead to novel diagnostic and therapeutic approaches. The analytical detection of IgE in the serum of individuals is used as a diagnostic tool. The development of such diagnostic tests has subsequently led to the development of tests that employ human IgE to detect the presence of allergenic ingredients in food products.[24] Although using human IgE allows the detection of allergenic proteins in food matrices, the limited availability and the individual differences prevent, respectively, the use of IgE on a large scale and the standardization of methods employing IgE. Over the last decades, many efforts have been made to develop a variety of analytical methods suitable for the detection of allergenic ingredients in food products. This type of analytical methodology is key to enable the management of food allergens in the food production environment and to enforce legislation in this area (Figure 1.2). In Chapter 2, an overview of the various types of currently available methods is presented.

The complexity of food production systems stresses the importance of good manufacturing practices (GMPs), which are an important tool for the food industry to produce products that are safe for the consumer. The management of allergenic ingredients, especially the possibility of cross-contamination during industrial production, poses a problem for the food industry and constitutes a threat to the allergic consumer.[25] Analytical tools are needed that allow food companies to determine that incoming raw materials do not contain detectable residues of undeclared allergenic foods. Furthermore, such tools are required to put a sanitation program aimed at removing allergenic ingredients from shared production equipment into place. The introduction of legislation specifically aimed at the protection of allergic consumers also implies that analytical methods to detect undeclared allergenic ingredients in

INTRODUCTION

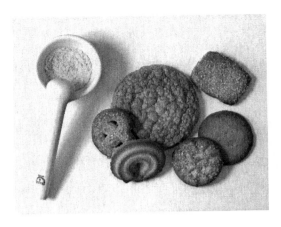

Figure 1.2 The analysis of food products aimed at the detection of allergenic ingredients requires extraction of the analytical targets. Solid food products need to be ground, after which the resulting powder has to be incubated with a suitable extraction buffer to solubilize the target molecules. Such targets can subsequently be detected using analytical tools.

food products are required to enforce this type of legislation. Public health authorities need these tools to assess the safety of food products and to follow up consumer complaints resulting from allergic reactions that might have been caused by undeclared allergens. The Rapid Alert System for Food and Feed (RASFF) of the European Union plays an important role in assessing the safety of food products destined for the European market. Between 2005 and 2008, the number of alerts related to allergens increased considerably (http://ec.europa.eu/food/food/rapidalert/rasff_portal_database_en.htm). This is a result of due diligence of the food industry in combination with an increase in testing for undeclared allergens by food control authorities. The presence of undeclared allergens can render a food unsafe for a particular group of consumers, namely, allergic consumers. When an undeclared allergen (one that requires a mandatory declaration) is a known ingredient of the food product, the producer is in breach of the law. When such an allergen is present but does not constitute an ingredient (e.g., it entered the food product as a result of poor sanitation of production lines), product liability and product safety legislation might be relevant. European legislation as well as national legislation can be applicable, and in some jurisdictions (e.g., the United Kingdom) an injury or death resulting from failures in the food safety management can lead to indictment under health and safety at work or corporate manslaughter legislation.[26] Pele et al.[27] analyzed hundreds of cookies and chocolates that did not declare the presence of the allergenic commodities peanut or hazelnut on their labels. The results of this study showed that the majority of chocolates and almost half the cookies that did not declare peanut or hazelnut as an ingredient tested positive and therefore posed a risk to allergic consumers. Market surveys like this stress the need to implement allergen management systems and to control adherence to the legislation that aims to protect the allergic consumer.

METHOD PERFORMANCE: THE TOOLS AND THEIR REQUIREMENTS

Although the need for analytical methods capable of detecting allergenic residues in food products is apparent, the development of such analytical tests faces many challenges.[28] These tests are expected to be highly specific, they should be sensitive and reliable, and they should be able to perform well on extracts of food products that can contain a large number of different ingredients that might have undergone a variety of food-processing conditions. On top of that, ease of use and low-cost tests are preferred. Chapter 2 presents a comprehensive overview of the methodology and the instrumentation that is currently employed for the detection of allergenic ingredients in food products.

Another important aspect is the validation of analytical methods. The validation of food allergen detection methods faces several specific areas of concern that need to be addressed. Among those are the lack of reference materials, the diversity of spiking methods, the choice of food matrices for validation studies, and the limited availability of proficiency tests. Abbott et al.[29] published a guidance document for the validation of enzyme-linked immunosorbent assay (ELISA) methods for the detection of food allergens. The guidance and best practices described in this document were developed with inputs from a wide range of experts working under the auspices of the AOAC Presidential Task Force on Food Allergens and address many of the problematic areas mentioned.

Food processing is of particular concern since it can have dramatic effects on the integrity of the analytical target molecules; in addition, it can severely decrease the solubility, and therefore the extractability, of these target analytes.[30,31] To take such negative effects of food processing into account, the use of incurred samples or naturally incurred samples for validation of allergen detection methods is strongly recommended. Such samples have undergone food processing in a manner that is similar to "real-world" food processing and therefore can reveal limitations of the analytical methods.[32]

Proficiency testing allows investigation of the quality of analytical results and can be of high value for laboratories carrying out such analysis. Proficiency tests for quality assurance of allergen detection methods have revealed that when different (commercial) analytical tests are employed, the quantitative result is often dependent on the brand of the assay kit.[33] The reliability of analytical results that can be obtained with the currently available analytical methods can be investigated by assessing the quality of the method as well as the quality of the method performer. Method validation and proficiency testing are playing crucial roles in this.

THE ALLERGENIC FOODS AND THEIR DETECTION METHODS

The scientific community faces the challenge to develop analytical methods that are capable of detecting all the allergenic foods that are listed in legislation. The fact that some of those foods are actually groups of sometimes quite diverse species (e.g., fish, crustaceans, tree nuts, mollusks, and gluten-containing cereals)

INTRODUCTION

poses a major problem. Methods that would work well for one species of such a group might not work, or perform poorly, when used for the detection of another member of the same group. Legislation that requires a declaration of the source of the allergenic ingredient, as proposed in Canada for gluten-containing cereals, implies that methods capable of differentiating between different (gluten) sources are needed. Many of the currently available methods were developed for the detection of components of single species of allergenic foods. It was shown that a method based on the immunological detection of lupin showed a 10-fold difference in its capacity to detect two closely related lupin species.[34] This illustrates the fact that many methods need to be developed to reliably detect all allergenic ingredients that require a mandatory declaration. Methods that are capable of detecting multiple allergens in a single analysis are likely to be needed to tackle this problem. Furthermore, the reliability of the methods needs to be investigated. Validation studies and proficiency testing are absolutely required. Guidance on the organization of validation studies as well as proficiency testing rounds is forthcoming, but currently only methods for a limited number of allergenic foods have been used in validation studies and proficiency test rounds.

This book provides an overview of the currently available methods and instrumentation that allows the detection of allergenic ingredients in food products. Often, the allergens and the target for the analytical methods are present in trace amounts; therefore, their detection is not evident. For the purpose of this book, we present the different types of methods that have been developed and that are currently being developed (Chapter 2), and we have focused on the characteristics and the detection of the major allergenic foods. All the allergenic foods that are subject to a mandatory declaration in the European Union as well as their detection methods are presented in Chapters 3–7. As is apparent from Table 1.1, the allergens dealt with here are not specific to the European legislation, but they cover almost all of the allergenic foods that require mandatory declaration in other parts of the world.

Chapter 3 presents the allergens of and detection methods for peanut, soybean, and lupin. These three commodities are all edible plant seeds. Furthermore, they are all phylogenetically related since they belong to the family Leguminosae. Chapter 4 presents the allergens of and detection methods for another group of foods of vegetable origin, namely, tree nuts, sesame seeds, mustard, and celery. These foods belong to different plant families, but except for celery, the consumed part of the plants again concerns the seeds. Chapter 5 presents the allergens of and detection methods for allergens of animal origin: milk and egg. Whereas plant seeds are nutritious since they contain proteins that are intended to nourish young plants, the allergenic proteins of milk and egg are in the first instance destined for the developing and growing offspring of cows and chicken. Chapter 6 presents the allergens of and detection methods for cereals. In contrast to the foods in Chapters 3 and 4, cereals are plants that are monocots. The distant evolutionary relationship between monocots and dicots lies at the basis of clear differences in the proteome. Gluten belongs to the proteomic components of cereals but is absent in dicots. Finally, Chapter 7 presents the allergens of and detection methods for fish, crustaceans, and mollusks, almost all of which are aquatic organisms.

REFERENCES

1. Crevel RW, Ballmer-Weber BK, Holzhauser T, Hourihane JO, Knulst AC, Mackie AR, Timmermans F, and Taylor SL. 2008. Thresholds for food allergens and their value to different stakeholders. *Allergy* 63:597–609.
2. Helm RM and Burks AW. 2000. Mechanisms of food allergy. *Curr Opin Immunol* 12:647–653.
3. Sicherer SH, Muñoz-Furlong A, and Sampson HA. 2004. Prevalence of seafood allergy in the United States determined by a random telephone survey. *J Allergy Clin Immunol* 114:159–165.
4. Sicherer SH and Sampson HA. 2010. Food allergy. *J Allergy Clin Immunol* 125:S116–S125.
5. Grundy J, Matthews S, Bateman B, Dean T, and Arshad SH. 2002. Rising prevalence of allergy to peanut in children: data from two sequential cohorts. *J Allergy Clin Immunol* 110:784–789.
6. Sampson HA. 2005. Food allergy: accurately identifying clinical reactivity. *Allergy* 60:19–24.
7. Taylor SL and Hefle SL. 2001. Food allergies and other food sensitivities. *Food Technol* 55:68.
8. Taylor SL and Hefle SL. 2002. Allergic reactions and food intolerances, In: *Nutritional Toxicology*, 2nd ed., ed. FN Kotsonis and M Mackey, Taylor & Francis, London, p. 93.
9. Sampson HA. 2003. Anaphylaxis and emergency treatment. *Pediatrics* 111:1601–1608.
10. Dannaeus A and Inganäs M. 1981. A follow-up study of children with food allergy. Clinical course in relation to serum IgE- and IgG-antibody levels to milk, egg and fish. *Clin Allergy* 11:533–539.
11. Bock SA. 1982. The natural history of food hypersensitivity. *J Allergy Clin Immunol* 69:173–177.
12. Priftis KN, Mermeri D, Papadopoulou A, Papadopoulos M, Fretzayas A, and Lagona E. 2008. Asthma symptoms and brochial reactivity in school children sensitized to food allergens in infancy. *J Asthma* 45:590–595.
13. DunnGalvin A, Dubois AEJ, de Blok BMJ, and Hourihane J'OB. 2007. Child versus maternal perception of HRQoL in food allergy: developmental trajectories and evolution of risk behaviour. *Allergy* 62:70–166.
14. European Parliament and Council. 2003. Directive 2003/89/EC. *Official J EU* L308:15–18.
15. European Parliament and Council. 2007. Directive 2003/68/EC. *Official J EU* L310:11–14.
16. U.S. Food and Drug Administration. 2004. *Food Allergen Labeling and Consumer Protection Act of 2004 (FALCPA)*. Public Law 108-282.
17. Mari A, Rasi C, Palazzo P, and Scala E. 2009. Allergen databases: current status and perspectives. *Curr Allergy Asthma Rep* 9:376–383.
18. Hoffmann-Sommergruber K and Mills EN. 2009. Food allergen protein families and their structural characteristics and application in component-resolved diagnosis: new data from the EuroPrevall project. *Anal Bioanal Chem* 395:25–35.
19. Jenkins JA, Griffiths-Jones S, Shewry PR, Breiteneder H, and Mills EN. 2005. Structural relatedness of plant food allergens with specific reference to cross-reactive allergens: an in silico analysis. *J Allergy Clin Immunol* 115:163–170.

20. Jenkins JA, Breiteneder H, and Mills EN. 2007. Evolutionary distance from human homologs reflects allergenicity of animal food proteins. *J Allergy Clin Immunol* 120:1399–1405.
21. Sampson HA. 2004. Update on food allergy. *J Allergy Clin Immunol* 113:805–819.
22. European Parliament and Council. 2000. Directive 2000/13/EC. *Official J EU* L109:29–42.
23. Weber D, Cléroux C, and Benrejeb Godefroy S. 2009. Emerging analytical methods to determine gluten markers in processed foods—method development in support of standard setting. *Anal Bioanal Chem* 395:111–117.
24. Nordlee JA, Taylor SL, Jones RT, and Yunginger JW. 1981. Allergenicity of various peanut products as determined by RAST inhibition. *J Allergy Clin Immunol* 68:376–382.
25. Röder M, Vieths S, and Holzhauser T. 2009. Commercial lateral flow devices for rapid detection of peanut (*Arachis hypogaea*) and hazelnut (*Corylus avellana*) cross-contamination in the industrial production of cookies. *Anal Bioanal Chem* 395:103–109.
26. Kerbach S, Alldrick AJ, Crevel R, Dömötör L, DunnGalvin A, Mills ENC, Pfaff S, Poms RE, Popping B, and Tömösközi S. 2009. Managing food allergens in the food supply chain—viewed from different stakeholder perspectives. *Qual Assur Safety Crops Foods* 1:50–60.
27. Pele M, Brohée M, Anklam E, and van Hengel AJ. 2007. Peanut and hazelnut traces in cookies and chocolates: relationship between analytical results and declaration of food allergens on product labels. *Food Addit Contam* 24:1334–44.
28. van Hengel AJ. 2007. Food allergen detection methods and the challenge to protect food-allergic consumers. *Anal Bioanal Chem* 389:111–118.
29. Abbott M, Hayward S, Ross W, Benrejeb Godefroy S, Ulberth F, van Hengel AJ, Roberts J, Akiyama H, Popping B, Yeung J, Wheling P, Taylor S, Poms RE, and Delahaut P. 2010. Validation procedures for quantitative food allergen ELISA methods: community guidance and best practises. *J AOAC Int* 93:442–450.
30. Scaravelli E, Brohée M, Marchelli R, and van Hengel AJ. 2009. The effect of heat treatment on the detection of peanut allergens as determined by ELISA and real-time PCR. *Anal Bioanal Chem* 395:127–137.
31. Schmitt DA, Nesbit JB, Hurlburt BK, Cheng H, and Maleki SJ. 2010. Processing can alter the properties of peanut extract preparations. *J Agric Food Chem* 58:1138–1143.
32. Taylor SL, Nordlee JA, Niemann LM, and Lambrecht DM. 2009. Allergen immunoassays—considerations for use of naturally incurred standards. *Anal Bioanal Chem* 395:83–92.
33. Owen L and Gilbert J. 2009. Proficiency testing for quality assurance of allergens methods. *Anal Bioanal Chem* 395:147–153.
34. Gomez Galan AM, Brohée M, Scaravelli E, van Hengel AJ, and Chassaigne H. 2010. Development of real-time PCR assays for the detection of lupin residues in food products. *Eur Food Res Technol* 230:597–608.

CHAPTER 2

Detection of Allergens in Foods

Phil E. Johnson, Ana I. Sancho, Rene W. R. Crevel, and E. N. Clare Mills

CONTENTS

Why Test for Allergens in Foods? 13
Labeling Food Allergens: Legal Requirements 14
What Needs to Be Managed? 17
How Much Causes a Problem? 18
Managing Allergens in Food Production 19
Methods: Past, Present, and Future 20
  DNA Methods 21
  Immunoassay Methods 22
  Mass Spectrometry 22
Method Application, Validation, and Standardization 23
References 24

WHY TEST FOR ALLERGENS IN FOODS?

A number of reproducible adverse reactions to foods have been described and include conditions such as lactose intolerance, resulting from the lack of the digestive enzyme lactase; pharmacological reactions to histamine-containing foods; as well as reactions involving the immune system, such as food allergies mediated by immunoglobulin E (IgE) and celiac disease.[1] In the absence of therapies for both these conditions, individuals suffering from them have to practice food avoidance, but the accidental consumption of "problem" food by celiac sufferers and those with IgE-mediated allergies has different consequences. Thus, for celiac sufferers the consumption of small quantities of gluten in foods can cause symptoms in a matter of hours; although unpleasant, these symptoms are seldom life threatening. In contrast, IgE-mediated allergic responses are more immediate in nature, happening within minutes and hours of ingesting a problem food. Symptoms from such reactions are diverse and can affect the skin (including rashes such as urticaria) and gastrointestinal (vomiting, diarrhea) and respiratory (obstruction of airways, asthma) systems. In rare cases, life-threatening anaphylactic reactions can be experienced by some individuals; these reactions are characterized by a rapid drop in blood pressure, together with other symptoms. There are records in the literature of the ability of small amounts of allergenic foods to trigger an allergic reaction in sensitive individuals such that an allergic individual can react to being kissed by someone who has been eating their problem food.[2].

Meta-analysis suggested that there is considerable heterogeneity in the prevalence of perceived and confirmed allergic reactions, as well as sensitization to food, in population-based studies, with rates ranging from 3% to 30%. It remains unclear whether the variation observed is related to genuine differences in study designs or a consequence of different methodologies.[3,4] It is generally thought that the prevalence of food allergy is higher in infants and young children, with allergies to foods such as cow's milk around 2.2–2.3% in Denmark and the Netherlands,[5,6] while hen's egg allergy is high (1.7%) in Danish children.[7] As a consequence of the prevalence of celiac diseases and IgE-mediated food allergies, and the fact both conditions have to be treated by food avoidance, there have been international efforts to ensure major allergenic foods are labeled when added as ingredients to prepackaged foods to allow allergic consumers to avoid their problem foods more effectively.[8,9]

LABELING FOOD ALLERGENS: LEGAL REQUIREMENTS

Following the publication of the Codex guidelines[8,9] new regulations have been put in place across the world, often with local adaptation of the original list of foods (and derived ingredients, including even highly refined and processed products) that required labeling regardless of the level at which they are included in prepackaged foods. The countries where such labeling is required are the European Union (EU; European Community), the United States, Canada, Australia, New Zealand, Hong Kong, and Japan (Table 2.1). There are adaptations of the lists across the different countries, and a limited number of allergenic ingredients or substances have been granted derogations (exceptions) in the European Union following submission of dossiers demonstrating the lack of allergenicity of these ingredients to the European Food Safety Authority (EFSA); although the facility for such derogations exists in the United States in the Food Allergen Labeling and Consumer Protection Act,[10] none have been granted so far. The Codex standard with regard to gluten-free foods has been developed[9] and has also been adopted in many countries. Thus, *gluten free* is now defined as foods or food ingredients that contain no more than 20 mg/kg gluten; in the European Union, foods that are prepared for a particular nutritional purpose (PARNUTS or dietetic foods) that contain gluten up to 100 mg/kg can be described as "very low gluten." This has been a practical option because complete removal of gluten from cereals (in particular wheat) is technically difficult and economically expensive.

At present, the legislation in general does not cover loose foods, foods sold in restaurants and other catering outlets, although forthcoming regulations on the provision

DETECTION OF ALLERGENS IN FOODS

Table 2.1 Allergen Labeling Requirements for Prepackaged Food across the World

Codex List	Country-Specific Adaptations	EU Derogations
Cereals containing gluten (i.e., wheat, rye, barley, oats, spelt, or their hybridized strains)	None	Wheat-based glucose syrups, including dextrose; wheat-based maltodextrins; glucose syrups based on barley; cereals used for making distillates or ethyl alcohol of agricultural origin for spirit drinks and other alcoholic beverages
Crustaceans	Specified, for example, as crab, lobster, shrimp in the United States and crabs, shrimp/prawn in Japan	None
Egg	None	None
Fish	Specified, for example, as bass, flounder, cod in the United States and salmon, salmon roe (ikura), mackerel, in Japan	Fish gelatin used as a carrier for vitamin or carotenoid preparations; fish gelatin or Isinglass used as fining agent in beer and wine
Peanuts	None	None
Soybeans		Fully refined soybean oil and fat, including interesterified and partially hydrogenated soybean oil and fat; natural mixed tocopherols (E306), natural D-alpha tocopherol; natural D-alpha tocopherol acetate, natural D-alpha tocopherol succinate from soybean sources; vegetable oil-derived phytosterols and phytosterol esters from soybean sources; plant stanol ester produced from vegetable oil sterols from soybean sources
Milk	None	Whey used for making distillates or ethyl alcohol of agricultural origin for spirit drinks and other alcoholic beverages; lactitol

Continued

Table 2.1 (Continued) Allergen Labeling Requirements for Prepackaged Food across the World

Codex List	Country-Specific Adaptations	EU Derogations
Tree nuts	Specified in the European Union as almond (*Amygdalus communis* L.), hazelnut (*Corylus avellana*), walnut (*Juglans regia*), cashew (*Anacardium occidentale*), pecan nut (*Carya illinoiesis*), Brazil nut (*Bertholletia excelsa*), pistachio (*Pistacia vera*), macadamia (Queensland) nut (*Macadamia ternifolia*). Canadian specifications are identical with the addition of pine nuts; in the United States, they are specified, for example, as almonds, walnuts, pecans, while in Japan the specification relates to walnut.	Nuts used for making distillates or ethyl alcohol of agricultural origin for spirit drinks and other alcoholic beverages.
None	Sesame seeds in the European Union and Australia/New Zealand	None
	Shellfish in the European Union and Canada; specified as abalone and squid in Japan	None
	Celery in the European Union only	None
	Mustard in the European Union and Canada	None
	Lupine in the European Union only	None
	Buckwheat; fruit as oranges, peach, kiwi fruit, apples; meat products as beef, pork, chicken; matsutake mushroom; yams; gelatin; in Japan only	Not applicable
Sulfites at concentrations of 10 mg/kg or higher	None	None

of information to consumers will address this issue. The inadvertent inclusion of allergenic foods in nonallergenic foods, often known as cross-contact, is also not specifically addressed. Such cross-contact issues can be especially problematic when different food products are manufactured within the same processing facility, sometimes using common processing lines for related food products (e.g., ice cream and sorbet or confectionary items prepared with differing ingredients, some containing peanuts or tree nuts, others not containing them). This can be covered by the general food safety legislation, which seeks to enshrine the rights of consumers to safe food, placing the onus on those manufacturing and placing such foods on the market, and EU Regulation 178/2002/EC[11] (the General Food Law) explicitly mentions the sensitivities of specific consumer groups. At present, two countries have regulations that specifically address cross-contact issues. One is Japan, where the legislation covers both deliberately added allergenic ingredients and "cross-contact" allergens (specifically cereals, eggs, peanuts, milk, and buckwheat). A second country is Switzerland, where a food or ingredient on the allergen labeling list present in a food at levels exceeding 1 g/kg because of cross-contact must be labeled as an ingredient.

Such issues mean that food manufacturers need to implement risk assessment and management procedures to minimize the presence of such cross-contact allergens. This is especially important when avoiding accidental inclusion of traces of allergenic ingredients in foods that are otherwise free from them. Some local regulators have developed guidelines for managing allergens in such foods, such as the U.K. Food Standards Agency.[12] Together with industry-led initiatives such as Vital[13] and the British Retail Consortium Guidelines,[14] there is better guidance on such issues, although there is still a need to develop more harmonized approaches to allergen risk assessment and management across the food chain and around the world.

WHAT NEEDS TO BE MANAGED?

As food allergies emerged as a public health issue, a landmark review by Bush and Hefle[15] identified only a limited number of foods as causing the majority of food allergies. This gave rise to the concept of the "big 8," which includes a number of foods of plant origin, such as peanuts, tree nuts, wheat, and soya, together with allergens of animal origin: cow's milk, egg, fish, and shellfish. Subsequent research has identified other foods as problematic in different geographic regions of the world, with foods such as buckwheat and bird's nest soup identified as important food allergens in the Far East.[16,17] Other foods appear relevant in others, with sesame described as an important allergenic food in countries such as Israel and Japan,[16,18] while root celery (celeriac) is widely acknowledged as a problem food in central Europe.[19] Such knowledge is undoubtedly giving rise to the need to tailor regulations and allergen management strategies to local issues, but this is difficult in the absence of cohesive studies to define the patterns of allergies in unselected populations, although relevant data are likely to emerge in the coming years.[20]

The components in foods that are responsible for triggering food allergies are proteins, which are also known as allergens.[21] In general, proteins (or polypeptide fragments) need to be several thousands of daltons in size to stimulate an IgE response in a process known as *sensitization*. In the second phase, when re-exposure to an allergen occurs, an allergic reaction takes place when IgE binds the target allergen molecules, triggering the release of histamine and other inflammatory mediators. It is these that cause the physiological changes that are manifested as allergic reactions. Multivalency is essential for an allergen to trigger release of histamine and other inflammatory mediators, and it is thought that although carbohydrate determinants are widely found on allergen molecules and can elicit IgE responses, they are largely monovalent and hence are generally unable to trigger histamine release.[22]

In terms of allergenicity, there is a view that "no protein" means no problem, and certainly the labeling derogations accepted by the EFSA largely relate to ingredients that contain little or no protein (Table 2.1). Thus, in managing allergens in the food chain and the factory environment, there is a need to focus on the proteinaceous allergen molecules and hence analytical methodology that is focused on measuring allergens in foods. However, in some instances when such methodology has been lacking, analysts have had to resort to methods based on detecting substances, such as DNA, indicative of the presence of material from an allergenic food species, or derived ingredient, rather than the molecules (allergens) that actually trigger food allergies.

HOW MUCH CAUSES A PROBLEM?

The precise amount that triggers an allergic reaction varies from individual to individual and may vary depending on time of day and other factors, such as infections, exercise, and even stress.[23] To establish how much of an allergen can cause a problem, studies are being undertaken with panels of allergic individuals, who are given increasing doses of a problem food in a blinded challenge procedure known as a double-blind, placebo-controlled food challenge (DBPCFC). The lowest observed adverse effect level (LOAEL) of a food that can elicit mild, objective symptoms in highly sensitive individuals is often known as its *threshold*, while a dose for which no symptoms are observed is referred to as the no observed adverse effect level (NOAEL). However, individuals can vary widely in their degree of sensitivity to specific allergenic foods, with as little as 1 mg eliciting an allergic reaction in some individuals.[23,24]

Although it is widely accepted that individual threshold doses below which a food-allergic consumer will not experience a reaction can be defined,[24] there remains a need to establish such thresholds at a population level while taking into account the distribution of individual threshold doses within that population. Probabilistic risk assessment models are seen to have many advantages in this regard[25] but require data on prevalence of food allergies in the population, intake of allergens by allergic consumers (a function of the likelihood of their eating allergen-containing foods and how much allergen is ingested) and the distribution of minimum eliciting doses (MEDs).[25,26] Other approaches, such as the benchmark dose (BMD) and margin of exposure (MoE) method, also require input data on clinical threshold doses to provide the BMD, with the MoE calculated on the basis of food intake and exposure.[23,25] Thus, two key requirements for effective allergen risk assessment are accurate data on clinical threshold doses and allergen intake, which relies in part on accurate analysis of levels of allergens in foods.

Estimation of a general threshold dose is rather difficult partly because studies have not always used the same challenge protocols; in some cases, blinding of the top dose of foods has not been completely effective, and there are issues that the most reactive food-allergic individuals have often not been included in these studies for ethical reasons (e.g., individuals with a history of anaphylaxis are usually excluded). More data are needed on low-dose challenges of individuals with specific food allergies using a consistently applied clinical protocol to obtain better estimates of threshold doses for various foods, including all those listed in the labeling regulations. In addition, extrinsic factors may affect threshold doses, such as exercise, consumption of alcohol, and stress.[25] For these reasons, some advisory bodies, such as the EFSA, have decided that no lower limit on allergens can currently be set. This is a major issue for the industrial management of allergens in foods. In addition to being vital to develop effective risk assessment processes, such thresholds are important in setting performance parameters for analytical methods.

MANAGING ALLERGENS IN FOOD PRODUCTION

At the start of developing a food product, checks need to be made regarding whether allergenic ingredients or derivatives are included and if they need to be declared on the label. Large companies may be able to have their own in-house databases of ingredients to assist in this, but this is not so for small and medium enterprises (SMEs). However, if such a database is going to play a core role in managing allergens in foods, it needs to be set up and maintained in a credible fashion. Some consideration then needs to be paid regarding whether the allergenic ingredient is essential in a given food formulation or if a nonallergenic substitute can be used. If the allergenic ingredient is necessary for product quality and attributes and must be included, its relevance to the target market around the world needs to be assessed (e.g., buckwheat might be more important for foods exported to Asia than the United States). Formulation also needs to take into account the manufacturing environment since it might be undesirable to introduce a new allergenic ingredient into a factory with all the follow-on consequences for potential cross-contact with foods that had hitherto been completely allergen free.

Management of allergenic foods and ingredients down the supply chain depends greatly on managing communications down the chain, which may also involve working across national boundaries with all the difficulties regarding language and culture that this entails. To facilitate the process, manufacturers need to be proactive in obtaining information from ingredient suppliers about allergenic foods and ingredients in their products. There is also a need for ingredients suppliers to be aware about which allergenic ingredients they market and how they are handled within the sites of suppliers. One aspect that is particularly important is that ingredient suppliers have a responsibility to inform their customers promptly of changes in formulation and how this affects the allergen status.

Systems need to be put in place to allow effective segregation of raw materials and protocols put in place to handle cleanup of any accidental ingredient spills to minimize the opportunity for cross-contact to occur. There is also a need for dedicated utensils, separated for different allergens. The big challenge facing manufacturers is when common processing lines are used for different foods, only some of which contain allergens, or adjacent processing lines that are prone to contamination in the air from dust. There are opportunities for allergenic ingredients to be inadvertently included in nonallergenic products. A particular issue is experienced in powdered food factories because of the difficulties that can be encountered in rigorously controlling contamination by dusts and powders in the air. It also relates to other types of low-water processing, such as chocolate manufacture, by which dark chocolate can become contaminated with milk proteins when the same line is first used to manufacture milk chocolate and then followed by dark chocolate. This is compounded by the need to avoid wet-based cleaning procedures in such manufacturing environments as they compromise the microbiological status; this has resulted in recourse to other approaches, such as using salt to provide some type of abrasive means of removing allergenic ingredients. Last, rework of materials needs to be explicitly managed as it increases the chances of inadvertent inclusion of allergens, often in significant amounts. These issues are much reduced in wet-processing lines, such as sauce manufacture, since wet cleaning procedures can be used without compromising the microbiological status of products or the plant.

In the past, managing allergens in a food production line was not a consideration, and hence many lines are not optimal for minimizing the possibilities of allergens entering foods through cross-contact. This situation is changing, with an increasing need for new processing plants to be designed in such a way that they minimize cross-contact and ease cleaning. An important tool for manufacturers in managing allergens in ingredients along the supply chain and the manufacturing process within factory environments, as well as finished products, are effective analytical tools to measure allergens. These are required to validate the approaches and subsequently monitor their implementation in a factory environment, for example, monitoring cross-contact allergens in ingredients, carryover of allergens on common processing lines and cleaning of equipment during runs, to mention but a few..[27,28]

METHODS: PAST, PRESENT, AND FUTURE

In general, until the recent past, analysis of allergens in foods has been dominated by two analytical methodologies: polymerase chain reaction (PCR) methods, based on detecting the presence of DNA from allergenic ingredients, and immunoassays, which use antibody reagents developed to either specific allergens or protein fractions from allergenic foods. A third technique has been applied to analysis of allergens in foods using quantitative mass spectrometric (MS) methods.

DNA Methods

PCR is the dominant DNA-based technique used for the detection of allergenic foodstuffs and the only DNA-based method for which commercial test kits are available. The reaction allows for the amplification of specific DNA sequences present in a sample, with the sequence to be amplified determined by the addition of primers complementary to regions of the DNA of interest. Through appropriate primer design, it can be tailored to be species specific, offering extremely high levels of specificity and sensitivity. For quantitative determinations, real-time PCR (RT-PCR)[29] is commonly used. This technique allows the measurement of the rate of formation of PCR product, which is dependent on the initial amount of target DNA. Allergenic foodstuff detection is most commonly performed by RT-PCR. Currently, there are commercial allergen test kits available for a variety of allergenic foods, such as soybean, walnut, sesame, mustard, fish, and celery. In addition, many laboratories utilize in-house methods, which are relatively easy to develop due to the ease of primer design and synthesis compared to antibody production.

PCR has several advantages over immunological detection. First, the use of PCR primers makes designing an assay that is selective for a particular foodstuff relatively simple and inexpensive. Much can be done *in silico* to ensure that PCR primers are specific to the target food, which often alleviates much of the work involved in eliminating cross-reactions with other foods. Second, amplification of the target DNA confers extremely good sensitivity on the technique. Theoretically, one copy of DNA is sufficient for detection, although practically detection limits will be higher depending on the reaction conditions used (e.g., 10 mg total plant material/kilogram in the case of peanut).[30] The DNA complement of a tissue is typically extremely stable and, unlike protein, is not prone to variations due to expression level. Thus, the amount of DNA detected will be consistently related to amount of allergen-containing tissue.

However, allergen detection based on species-specific DNA also has potentially serious drawbacks compared to protein-based detection techniques. Extraction of DNA is relatively involved, and laboratories performing DNA extraction and PCR amplification require special training. Quantitation requires RT-PCR machines, which can be expensive and require training to operate. There are also issues surrounding the use of DNA instead of protein as an analyte as allergens are themselves proteins. Processing techniques may affect the recovery of DNA and proteins differently, making under- or overestimation of allergen content possible. Similarly, allergens, as with other proteins, are differentially expressed in different tissues, at different times, and in response to different stimuli. Under these conditions, the recovery of DNA using RT-PCR will not change in response to decreasing or increasing allergen content. Because of inherent difficulties in equating recovery of DNA and protein allergens, it is advisable to use care when selecting PCR as a method for analysis, especially under conditions where recoveries may differ significantly (e.g., certain processing methods).

Immunoassay Methods

The original concept of raising antibodies to specific target molecules and then exploiting them in the development of an analytical method was described by Bersen and Yallow[31] in Nobel Prize-winning research, developing a radioimmunoassay (RIA) for the hormone insulin. Such an approach was applied early in the analysis of allergens in foods to determine the presence of allergenic peanut traces in foods using human allergic sera.[32] Soon after this work was published, the food analysis community began to apply a nonisotopic immunoassay, the enzyme-linked immunosorbent assay (ELISA), in a 96-well plate format, which has become one of the main analytical methods of choice for analysis of allergens in foods, both as published analytical methods and appearing in commercial kit form. They can employ either polyclonal antisera (polyclonal antibodies, Pabs), which are often raised to either purified allergens or extracted protein mixtures from allergenic foods. In general, such preparations have high affinity and can result in the development of sensitive immunoassays, although there can be problems of poor specificity since there may be prior sensitization of animals by allergenic proteins through the diet, as has been observed for gluten. To address such specificity issues, some researchers have developed monoclonal antibody (Mab) reagents, which have a more defined specificity and can supply (potentially) a homogeneous reagent. However, they often have poorer affinities than corresponding Pabs, resulting in less-sensitive assays. The ELISAs employed for allergen analysis have tended to adopt one of two common formats, one of which, the indirect ELISA, involves a competition for binding to the antibody reagent between allergen or protein extract adsorbed on the surface of the 96-well plate and either an allergenic standard or a food extract. In some cases, the specific antibody is labeled directly with an enzyme reporter, such as horseradish peroxidase, or a second, species-specific labeled antibody is used. Employing the last can avoid food extracts coming into direct contact with the enzyme reporter, which can be a source of matrix effects.

An alternative format employs a pair of antibodies to develop a sandwich or two-site assay in which the first antibody partner is adsorbed to the 96-well plate surface and to which either allergen standard or food extract is added; then, a second specific antibody (usually with an enzyme reporter) is added to complete the assay. In a 96-well plate format, ELISAs can give either quantitative or semiquantitative data on allergen levels in foods. It has been developed in a multianalyte format for detection of several tree nuts (peanut, hazelnut, almond, cashew, and Brazil nuts) in a single run.[33] They have also been adapted to dipstick formats, which give rapid semiquantitative analysis of allergens in foods and have found particular application in validation and monitoring of equipment cleaning.[34]

Mass Spectrometry

Advances in modern MS coupled with effective bioinformatic analysis are revolutionizing protein analysis. MS also offers the means of determining the presence of multiple allergens in a single analysis. This has been applied to the analysis of several foods, including the peanut, and involves digestion of food samples (either before or after extraction) by trypsin and quantification of resulting peptides using techniques such as liquid chromatography (LC) coupled with electrospray ionization tandem MS (ESI-MS-MS) and multiple-reaction monitoring (MRM). In general, at least two peptide markers need to be identified,[35] and limits of detection as low as 2 ppm have been achieved for the peanut allergen Ara h 1 in dark chocolate; employing a solid-phase extraction step LC-quadruple MS with full scan and MRM without an enzymatic digestion step allowed detection of cow's milk protein traces in protein-fortified mixed-fruit juices at around 1 µg/ml.[36] Others[37] have employed immuno-magnetic extraction to detect traces of the peanut allergen Ara h 3/4 in breakfast cereals at a level of around 3 µg peanuts/gram of matrix.

The ability to detect multiple allergens in a single chromatographic run combined with the excellent selectivity and rapid adaptability of MS methods make them an extremely promising method for allergen analysis. However, factors such as instrument cost and the expertise required in maintaining an MS platform are likely to slow uptake greatly. Initial uses of MS in allergen analysis are likely to focus on confirmation of immunological techniques, and as such they represent a valuable complementary technique.

METHOD APPLICATION, VALIDATION, AND STANDARDIZATION

Foodstuffs represent a complex and diverse range of matrices that food analysts have to tackle and can result in many different types of matrix effects that may affect analytical performance and may differentially affect different methods (Table 2.2). Thus, some foods are notoriously difficult to analyze for DNA-based methods of analysis, with egg a prime example since it frequently contains little if any DNA and does not allow egg to be discriminated from chicken. It is this lack of discriminating power coupled with the fact that DNA-based methods do not measure the protein components that present problems for allergy sufferers that makes them less well accepted than the other methods for allergen analysis.[38]

The major drawbacks of the immunological methods are the presence of allergenic contaminants from other foods, the complexity of the food matrix, and the

Table 2.2 General Characteristics of Allergen Detection Methods

Criteria	ELISA/Dipstick	PCR	Mass Spectrometry
Target	Protein (allergen)	DNA	Protein (allergen)
Basis of detection	Chemical (antibody)	Chemical (primer)	Physical
Cross reactions	Possible	Unlikely/avoidable	Unlikely/avoidable
Setup cost	Low	Moderate	High
Running cost	Moderate	Moderate	Moderate
Expertise needed	Low	Moderate	High
Multiplexing?	No	Yes	Yes

variable specificity of the antibody preparations used in commercial ELISA kits, making standardization difficult. In addition, cooking procedures have been shown to adversely affect the performance of ELISAs, in particular those for peanuts.[39] MS has much promise in overcoming many of the shortcomings of both PCR and ELISA, detecting low levels of allergenic proteins and, apparently, showing a more robust nature in terms of food-processing procedures. Thus, Chassaigne et al.[40,41] identified a set of highly stable peanut allergen peptides that can function as markers for either raw or roasted peanuts, including the identification of different isoforms of the peanut allergens Ara h 1 and Ara h 3/4. This confirms the suitability of MS for determining the allergen composition of natural or processed extracts.

The need for standardization in allergen analysis is emphasized by the fact that the European Committee for Standardization (CEN) set up an allergens working group (CEN/TC275/WG 12). The CEN WG 12 set up four ad hoc groups, one to address general considerations and validation of methods and the remaining three focused on molecular biological methods, protein-based methods for immunological detection of allergenic food and food ingredients, and chromatographical (including MS) methods. As a result of its activities, one standard has been published (British Standards Institution 2010 and associated European standards organizations[42]) with specific methods to be considered as a standard after collaborative or in-house validation. The activities of CEN are complemented by those of the Association of Analytical Communities (AOAC) Presidential Task Force to harmonize validation approaches for allergen ELISAs,[43] which have addressed the topic of the information to be provided by the method developer on various characteristics of the method (including the antibody reagents used in ELISAs) and the implementation of multilaboratory validation studies, illustrating them with two important food allergens, egg and milk. Last, harmonization of methods and of worldwide food quality and safety monitoring and control strategies in the food supply chain, including food allergens, is the major objective of the MoniQA project (www.moniqua.org), which through its working group on food allergens is specifically addressing the issues of standardization through the development of new reference materials incurred (RMIs) for allergen analysis focused on egg and milk in a baked cookie matrix and an infant formula mix, incorporating National Institute for Standards and Technology (NIST) reference materials for egg and milk. This will allow a collaborative trial to be undertaken using a range of commercial ELISA kits, enabling, for the first time, an adequate assessment to be made of matrix effects on analysis and the need for improved validation procedures.[39,44] When linked with other international efforts to develop effective reference materials, it will pave the way for providing the analytical community with much-needed materials in the future.

REFERENCES

1. Johansson SGO, Hourihane JO'B, Bousquet J, et al. 2001. A revised nomenclature for allergy. An EACCI position statement from the EACCI nomenclature task force. *Allergy,* 56, 813–824.

2. Steensma DP. 2003. The kiss of death: a severe allergic reaction to a shellfish induced by a good-night kiss. *Mayo Clinic Proceedings,* 78(2), 221–222.
3. Rona RJ, Keil T, Summers C, et al. 2007. The prevalence of food allergy: a meta-analysis. *Journal of Allergy and Clinical Immunology,* 120(3), 638–46.
4. Zuidmeer L, Goldhahn K, Rona RJ, et al. 2008 The prevalence of plant food allergies: a systematic review. *Journal of Allergy and Clinical Immunology,* 121(5), 1210–1218.
5. Schrander JJ, Oudsen S, Forget PP, et al. 1992. Follow up study of cow's milk protein intolerant infants. *European Journal of Pediatrics,* 151(10), 783–785.
6. Høst A and Halken S. 1990. A prospective study of cow milk allergy in Danish infants during the first 3 years of life. Clinical course in relation to clinical and immunological type of hypersensitivity reaction. *Allergy,* 45(8), 587–596.
7. Osterballe M, Hansen TK, Mortz CG, et al. 2005. The prevalence of food hypersensitivity in an unselected population of children and adults. *Pediatric Allergy and Immunology,* 16(7), 567–573.
8. Codex Alimentarius Commission. 1999. *Codex General Standard for the Labelling of Prepackaged Foods.* CODEX STAN 1-1985, Rev. 1-1991, 1–11. Joint FAO/WHO Food Standards Programme, FAO, Rome, Italy.
9. Codex Alimentarius Commission. 2008. *Codex General Standard for Foods for Special Dietary Use for Persons Intolerant to Gluten.* CODEX STAN 118-1979, Rev. 2008, 1–3. Joint FAO/WHO Food Standards Programme, FAO, Rome, Italy.
10. *Food Allergen Labeling and Consumer Protection Act.* 2004. Public Law 108-282, August 2. 18 STAT, 905. Office of the Federal Register, National Archives and Records Administration, College Park, MD.
11. European Parliament and Council. 2002. Directive 2002/178/EC. *Official Journal of the European Union,* L60, 70–80.
12. Food Standards Agency. 2006. Guidance on allergen management and consumer advice. http://www.food.gov.uk/multimedia/pdfs/maycontainguide.pdf.
13. Australian Food and Grocery Council. 2007. Food industry guide to allergen management and labelling. Consultation paper. http://www.allergenbureau.net/allergenguide/
14. British Retail Consortium. 2005. Guidance on directive 2005/26/EC. http://www.brc.org.uk/showDoc.asp?id=2513
15. Bush RK and Hefle SL. 1996. Food allergens. *Critical Reviews in Food Science and Nutrition,* 36(Suppl), S119–S163.
16. Imamura T, Kanagawa Y, and Ebisawa M. 2008. A survey of patients with self-reported severe food allergies in Japan. *Pediatric Allergy and Immunology,* 19(3), 270–274.
17. Park JW, Kang DB, Kim CW, et al. 2000. Identification and characterization of the major allergens of buckwheat. *Allergy,* 55(11), 1035–1041.
18. Dalal I, Binson I, Reifen R, et al. 2002. Food allergy is a matter of geography after all: sesame as a major cause of severe IgE-mediated food allergic reactions among infants and young children in Israel. *Allergy,* 57(4), 362–365.
19. Ballmer-Weber BK, Hoffmann A, Wüthrich B, et al. 2002. Influence of food processing on the allergenicity of celery: DBPCFC with celery spice and cooked celery in patients with celery allergy. *Allergy,* 57(3), 228–235.
20. Mills ENC, Mackie AR, Burney P, et al. 2007. The prevalence, cost and basis of food allergy across Europe. *Allergy,* 62(7), 717–722.
21. Breiteneder H and Mills ENC. 2005 Molecular properties of food allergens. *Journal of Allergy and Clinical Immunology,* 115, 14–23.
22. Aalberse R C. 1998. Clinical relevance of carbohydrate allergen epitopes. *Allergy,* 53, 54–57.

23. Crevel RW, Ballmer-Weber BK, Holzhauser T, et al. 2008. Thresholds for food allergens and their value to different stakeholders. *Allergy*, 63(5), 597–609.
24. Taylor SL, Hefle SL, Bindslev-Jensen C, et al. 2002. Factors affecting the determination of threshold doses for allergenic foods: how much is too much? *Journal of Allergy and Clinical Immunology*, 109, 24–30.
25. Madsen CB, Hattersley S, Buck J, et al. 2009. Approaches to risk assessment in food allergy: report from a workshop "developing a framework for assessing the risk from allergenic foods." *Food and Chemical Toxicology*, 47(2), 480–489.
26. Kruizinga AG, Briggs D, Crevel RW, Knulst AC, van den Bosch LM, and Houben GF. 2008. Probabilistic risk assessment model for allergens in food: sensitivity analysis of the minimum eliciting dose and food consumption. *Food and Chemical Toxicology*, 46(5), 1437–1443.
27. Brown HM. 2009. Validation of cleaning and cross-contact. In: *Management of food allergens* (Coutts J and Fielder R, eds.). Wiley-Blackwell, Oxford, UK, pp. 138–153.
28. Stephan O, Weisz N, Vieths S, et al. 2004. Protein quantification, sandwich ELISA, and real-time PCR used to monitor industrial cleaning procedures for contamination with peanut and celery allergens. *Journal of AOAC International*, 87(6), 1448–1457.
29. Higuchi R, Fockler C, Dollinger G, et al., 1993. Kinetic PCR analysis: real-time monitoring of DNA amplification reactions. *Biotechnology*, 11(9), 1026–1030.
30. Scaravelli E, Brohée M, Marchelli R, et al. 2007. Development of three real-time PCR assays to detect peanut allergen residue in processed food products. *European Food Research and Technology*, 227(3), 857–869.
31. Berson SA and Yallow RS. 1961. Immunochemical distinction between insulins with identical amino-acid sequences. *Nature*. 191, 1392–1393.
32. Keating MU, Jones RT, Worley NJ, et al. 1990. Immunoassay of peanut allergens in food-processing materials and finished foods. *Journal of Allergy and Clinical Immunology*, 86, 41–44.
33. Ben Rejeb S, Abbott M, Davies D, et al. 2005. Multi-allergen screening immunoassay for the detection of protein markers of peanut and four tree nuts in chocolate. *Food Additives and Contaminants*, 22(8), 709–715.
34. Röder M, Vieths S, and Holzhauser T. 2009. Commercial lateral flow devices for rapid detection of peanut (*Arachis hypogaea*) and hazelnut (*Corylus avellana*) cross-contamination in the industrial production of cookies. *Analytical Bioanalytical Chemistry*, 395(1), 103–109.
35. Shefcheck KJ, Callahan JH, and Musser SM. 2006. Confirmation of peanut protein using peptide markers in dark chocolate using liquid chromatography-tandem mass spectrometry (LC-MS/MS). *Journal of Agricultural and Food Chemistry*, 54(21), 7953–7959.
36. Monaci L and van Hengel AJ. 2008. Development of a method for the quantification of whey allergen traces in mixed-fruit juices based on liquid chromatography with mass spectrometric detection. *Journal of Chromatography Series A*, 1192, 113–120.
37. Careri M, Elviri L, Lagos JB, et al. 2008. Selective and rapid immunomagnetic bead-based sample treatment for the liquid chromatography–electrospray ion-trap mass spectrometry detection of Ara h3/4 peanut protein in foods. *Journal of Chromatography Series A*, 1206, 89–94.
38. van Hengel AJ. 2007. Food allergen detection methods and the challenge to protect food-allergic consumers. *Analytical and Bioanalytical Chemistry*, 389, 111–118.
39. Poms RE, Agazzi ME, Bau A, et al., 2005. Inter-laboratory validation study of five commercial ELISA test kits for the determination of peanut proteins in biscuits and dark chocolate. *Food Additives and Contaminants*, 22(2), 104–112.

40. Chassaigne H, Nørgaard JV, and Hengel A.J. 2007. Proteomics-based approach to detect and identify major allergens in processed peanuts by capillary LC-Q-TOF (MS/MS). *Journal of Agricultural and Food Chemistry,* 55, 4461–4473.
41. Chassaigne H, Trégoat V, Nørgaard JV, et al., 2009. Resolution and identification of major peanut allergens using a combination of fluorescence two-dimensional differential gel electrophoresis, Western blotting and Q-TOF mass spectrometry. *Journal of Proteomics,* 72, 511–526.
42. British Standards Institution. 2010. *Foodstuffs. Detection of food allergens. General considerations and validation of methods.* BS EN 15842:2010; EN 15842:2010 Identical. British Standards Institute, UK.
43. Abbott M, Benrejeb Godefroy S, Yeung JM, et al. In press. Guidance on a harmonized validation protocol for quantitative food allergen ELISA methods. *Journal of AOAC International.*
44. Kerbach S, Alldrick AJ, Crevel RWR, et al. 2009. Managing food allergens in the food supply chain—viewed from different stakeholders perspectives. *Quality Assurance and Safety of Crops and Foods,* 1(1), 50–60.

CHAPTER 3

Allergens in Peanut, Soybean, and Lupin

Christiane K. Fæste

CONTENTS

Introduction 30
Allergen Properties 31
    Allergen Databases 31
    Allergen Nomenclature 32
    Protein Families Containing Legume Allergens 33
    Peanut Allergens 36
    Soybean Allergens 40
    Lupin Allergens 45
Sample Extraction and Cleanup 48
    Preparation of Total Legume Extracts 49
        Peanut 50
        Soybean 50
        Lupin 50
    Isolation of Individual Allergens 50
        Peanut 51
        Soybean 51
        Lupin 51
Separation and Analysis Methods 52
    Peanut 54
    Soybean 54
    Lupin 54
Detection and Quantification Methods 55
    Peanut 55
    Soybean 58
    Lupin 58
References 63

INTRODUCTION

Peanut (*Arachis hypogea*), soybean (*Glycine max*), and lupin (*Lupinus* sp.) belong to the legume plant family (Leguminosae or Fabaceae), which includes 730 genera with about 19,400 species; among them are the much-used agricultural crops (www.ildis.org). Their main characteristics are the seed-containing pods (Latin *legumen*) (Figure 3.1). The Leguminosae contain most of the important groups of food and fodder plants and are also used as soil fertilizers due to their nitrogen-fixing ability. They are usually divided into three subfamilies (Papilionoideae [Faboideae], Caesalpinioideae, and Mimosoideae), which can be identified by their flowers. The Papilionoideae, known for their typical butterfly-like flowers, contain most of the important leguminous crop species, including peanut, soybean, and lupin, as well as common pea (*Pisum sativum*), chickpea (*Cicer arietinum*), French bean (*Phaseolus vulgaris*), lentil (*Lens culinaris*), and the curry spice fenugreek (*Trigonella foenum-graecum*).

Legume seeds (Figure 3.2) are valued as a protein source and food additive, and legume leaves and sprouts are consumed as vegetables. In addition, they are a source for a wide range of natural products, such as flavors, drugs, poisons, and dyes. The protein content of the seeds is high, ranging from 25% to 45% of the dry matter, and includes essential amino acids like threonine, leucine, and lysine. The seeds also contain considerable amounts of oil (5–48%) and fiber (9–17%). Their

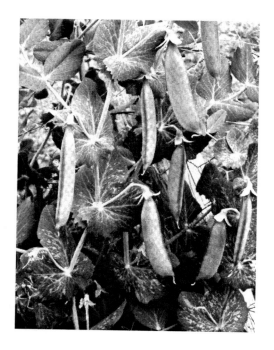

Figure 3.1 Legume plants with pods. (Modified from Wikimedia Commons.)

ALLERGENS IN PEANUT, SOYBEAN, AND LUPIN

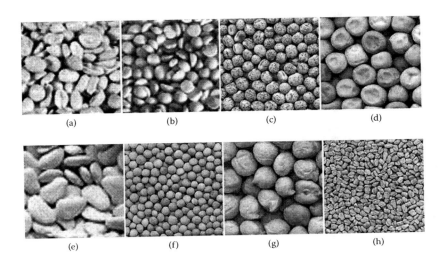

Figure 3.2 Legume seeds: (a) peanut, (b) soybean, (c) lupin, (d) pea, (e) bean, (f) lentil, (g) chickpea, (h) fenugreek.

high nutritional value combined with relatively low production costs make legumes an important part of the daily human diet. Being gluten free and with low starch content, they are also of interest for consumers with specific dietary needs; especially, soybean and lupin are commonly used in health foods and vegetarian products.

An increasing number of legume proteins have been identified as food allergens.[1] The prevalence of allergies to different legumes is geographically variant and apparently dependent on the dietary habits of the respective populations. Whereas allergies to lentils and chickpeas prevail in the Mediterranean area and India, peanut and soybean allergies are most important in Western Europe, Japan, and the United States.[2] The majority of patients experience allergic symptoms to more than one legume since the different species contain structurally homologous proteins, which give rise to cross-reactions with the serum immunoglobulin E (IgE).[3–5]

ALLERGEN PROPERTIES

Allergen Databases

Only relatively few protein families contain allergens, which have a limited number of biochemical functions connected to storage; hydrolysis of proteins, polysaccharides, and lipids; binding to metal ions and lipids; and cytoskeleton association.[6] There are several databases freely accessible on the Internet that provide comprehensive information about allergens (Table 3.1).

The allergen family database AllFam[6] has established a structural classification of allergens that are listed in the Allergome database[7] by using domain information from the larger protein family database Pfam[8] and amino acid sequence data from

Table 3.1 Allergen Information on the Internet

Database Name and Function	Web Address
Allergen Names	
IUIS Allergen Nomenclature Sub-Committee list.	www.allergen.org
Allergen Sequences	
The Allergen Database	www.allergen.csl.gov.uk
AllergenOnline (FARRP)	www.allergenonline.com
AllerMatch	www.allermatch.org
International Immunogenetics Information System	www.imgt.cines.fr
Allergen Database for Food Safety	www.allergen.nihs.go.jp/ADFS
Allergen Structures	
Structural Database of Allergen Proteins	www.fermi.utmb.edu/SDAP/sdap_ver.html
AllFam	www.meduniwien.ac.at/allergens/allfam
Pfam	www.pfam.sanger.ac.uk
General Information on Allergens	
Allergome	www.allergome.org
AllAllergy	www.allallergy.net
Informall	www.foodallergens.ifr.ac.uk
Protall	www.ifr.ac.uk/protall

the Uniprot database.[9] AllFam includes a total of 163 allergen families, containing 927 allergens (as of August 2010). The 377 known plant allergens are distributed in 42 plant allergen families. However, allergen databases should be updated on a regular basis, and data on sequence variants should be included.[10]

Sequence similarity has proven a useful tool for the comparison of allergenic proteins, although it has to be considered that the nature of allergenicity is local.[11] Distinct sequence motifs overlapping with IgE epitopes typically consisting of 6 to 15 amino acids have been identified and compiled in the Structural Database of Allergenic Proteins (SDAP).[12] This catalogue of characteristic allergenic motifs can be applied to determine fingerprints of allergenicity in candidate proteins by calculating the physicochemical property distance score providing the molecular basis for clinically observed cross-reactions.[13]

Allergen Nomenclature

Allergen nomenclature has been defined by the Allergen Nomenclature Subcommittee of the World Health Organization and International Union of Immunological Societies (WHO/IUIS).[14] The system uses the abbreviated Linnean genus and species names and an Arabic number to indicate the chronology of allergen purification (e.g., peanut Ara h 1, Ara h 2, etc.). This implies that allergens from different species belonging to the same plant family often do not have the same numbers. Isoallergens are multiple forms of the same allergen from one species that share extensive IgE cross-reactivity and have 67% or greater amino acid sequence identity. They are distinguished by additional numbers (e.g., Ara h 1.01, Ara h 1.02, etc.). *Isoforms* or *variants* refer to polymorphic variants of the same allergen, typically with greater than 90% sequence identity. Isoforms are distinguished in the nomenclature by two additional numbers (e.g., Ara h 1.0101, Ara h 1.0102, etc.). Even a few altered positions in a peptide sequence might affect T-cell responses or change allergenicity if polymorphism occurs in the antibody-binding sites.[12] Thus, a relationship of sequence homology in the IgE-binding epitopes of proteins to their allergenic cross-reactivity potential has been found. Regarding the observed cross-reactions between legume plants,[5,15] it was observed that the majority of peanut-sensitized patients were also sensitized to lupine and soybean. Clinically relevant sensitization to lupine and soybean occurred in about 35% of the study population.[16]

Protein Families Containing Legume Allergens

Four protein superfamilies comprise 65% of the known plant food allergens: prolamins, profilins, cupins, and pollinosis-associated proteins.[2,17,18] Furthermore, there are several other protein families (e.g., related to defense, lipid storage, or proteolysis) that contain considerable numbers of plant allergens.[19,20] The majority of allergens that have been identified in peanut, soybean, and lupin to date belong to the protein families shown in Table 3.2.

The prolamins (AllFam: AF050) constitute the largest plant allergen superfamily and include 73 known allergens (as of August 2010). All prolamins have a characteristic α-helical globular domain containing a conserved skeleton of six or eight cysteines that form three or four intramolecular disulfide bonds[21]; however, apart from the cysteine pattern, they share few sequence similarities. The superfamily comprises several minor and three major groups of plant food allergens, of which two have been identified in legume plants: 2S albumins and nonspecific lipid transfer proteins (nsLTPs). The 2S albumins are heterodimeric seed storage proteins consisting of two polypeptide chains of approximately 4 kDa and 9 kDa linked by four disulfide bridges.[19] Peanut and lupin conglutins as well as soybean albumin belong to this family. The nsLTPs are monomeric, ranging from 7 to 9 kDa, with a large internal hydrophobic tunnel-like cavity.[22] They show considerable resistance to proteolytic, acidic, and heat treatments and can refold after denaturation.[23] The nsLTPs have broad substrate-binding specificity and may have different functions, such as in phospholipid transfer or plant defense. Peanut and soybean nsLTPs belong to this family, and soybean hydrophobic protein from soy hulls[24] is related to this group.

The profilins (AF051) are calcium-binding ("EF-hand") cytosolic proteins of 12–15 kDa regulating the dynamics of actin polymerization and are found in all eukaryotic cells.[18] Profilins from higher plants (46 have been identified) occur in pollen and food. They constitute a family of highly cross-reactive allergens due to

Table 3.2 Database Entries for Peanut, Soybean, and Lupin Allergens

Allergen Family	Peanut (P), Soybean (S), Lupin (L)	Allergens in Peanut
AF050/PF00234 Prolamins	P S L	Ara h 2, Ara h 6, Ara h 7, Ara h 9 Gly m 1, Gly m 2S albumin, Gly m LTP Lup a δ-conglutin, Lup an δ-conglutin
AF051/PF00235 Profilins	P S	Ara h 5 Gly m 3
AF045/PF00190 Cupins	P S L	Ara h 1, Ara h 3/4 Gly m 5, Gly m 6, Gly m Bd28K, Gly m Bd 60K Lup a 1, Lup an 1, Lup a α-conglutin, Lup an α-conglutin
AF069/PF00407 Bet v 1-related proteins	P	Ara h 8 Gly m 4
AF090/PF01277 Oleosins	P S	Ara h 10, Ara h 11, Ara h oleosin 18kD Gly m oleosin
AF046/PF00197 Kunitz soybean trypsin inhibitors	S	Gly m TI, Gly m CPI
AF034 /PF00139 Legume lectins	P S	Ara h agglutinin Gly m agglutinin
AF030/Pfam PF00112 Papain-like endopeptidase	S	Gly m Bd30K
AF059/PF07333 Class A pollen coat protein	S	Gly m 2
AF004/PF00026 Eukaryotic aspartyl protease	L	Lup a γ-conglutin, Lup an γ-conglutin
AF-/PF03760 Late embryogenesis abundant group	S	Gly m EAP

sequence identities of at least 75% even between members from distantly related organisms. Several isoforms have been detected in the genome of plants, and differentiation between pollen-specific and constitutive profilins has been suggested.[25] Profilins are rather unstable and degenerate easily under digestion and heat treatment, so allergic reactions by profilins are usually limited to the oral allergy syndrome (OAS) occurring after the consumption of raw foods.[26] Peanut and soybean profilin belong to this family.

The cupins (AF045) are a large and functionally immensely diverse superfamily of proteins.[27] Common to all cupins is a β-barrel-formed core domain. Plant cupins are bicupins containing two such domains. They belong to the seed storage globulins constituting the major components of plant seeds and are generally stable. Cupins can be grouped into two families[28,29] vicilin-like proteins (7S globulins) and legumin-like proteins (11S globulins), which both have been recognized as major food allergens in legumes.[19,30] They share relatively low sequence identities of 35–45% but show high structural similarity.[31,32] The 7S globulins are heterotrimeric proteins of 150–190 kDa comprised of noncovalently assembled subunits that have molecular weights ranging from 40 to 80 kDa and can be glycosylated. The 11S globulins are hexameric proteins that are initially assembled as intermediate homologous trimers; these are proteolytically processed to yield an acidic 30- to 40-kDa polypeptide linked by a disulfide bond to a basic polypeptide of about 20 kDa.[19] Peanut conarachin and arachin, soybean glycinin and conglycinin, and lupin α-conglutin and β-conglutin belong to the cupin superfamily.

The Bet v 1-related proteins (pollinosis-associated proteins) (AF069) are divided into four subfamilies, of which the largest shows homology to family 10 pathogenesis-related proteins (PR10) of the plant defense system.[18] The PR10 have a molecular weight of about 17 kDa and are unstable to heat and digestion. They have been identified in 19 species, often expressed in several isoforms, and are primarily present in reproductive tissues of pollen (Fagales), fruits (Rosaceae and Apiaceae), and seeds (Fabaceae), including peanut and soybean. Homologous IgE epitopes in the different PR10 proteins cause considerable cross-reactivity, inducing the pollen-fruit-vegetable syndrome and OAS in allergic patients.[33]

Oleosins (AF090) are the proteinaceous components of the lipid storage bodies in the seeds of plants and may function as stabilizers of the lipid body.[34] Oleosin monomers have molecular weights ranging from 14 to 24 kDa; however, dimers and trimers have been detected by gel electrophoresis.[35] Seven plant oleosins are known. Peanut and soybean oleosins can elicit IgE-mediated reactions and may be involved in allergic cross-reactivity between the two species.

The Kunitz-type soybean trypsin inhibitors (STIs) (AF046) comprise a family of proteinase inhibitors that has four members. They have molecular weights of about 28 kDa and consist of a single polypeptide chain that is cross-linked by two disulfide bridges forming a β-trefoil structure.[36] The STI from soybean has been described as a minor allergen.[37]

Legume lectins (AF034) are one of the largest lectin families, with more than 70 members, of which 4 have been registered as allergens, including peanut and soybean agglutinin. Legume lectins consist of two or four subunits with molecular masses of 24–30 kDa, and each subunit has one carbohydrate-binding site.[38] The interaction with sugars requires tightly bound calcium and manganese ions. The exact function of legume lectins is not known yet; however, they may be involved in nitrogen fixation.

Papain-like proteins (AF030) are from a family of ubiquitous endopeptidases that are homologous in the catalytic site but share little similarities otherwise. Papain-like cysteine proteinases are synthesized as inactive proenzymes and posttranslationally processed into the mature enzyme.[21] A soybean papain-like protein has been identified as a major allergen.

Class A pollen coat proteins (AF059) are pollen-specific modular glycoproteins with a defensin-like and a hydroxyproline-rich domain.[39] A soybean hull protein provoking dust-induced asthma is related to this protein family.

Eukaryotic aspartyl proteases (AF004) contain two conserved aspartic domains in their catalytic centers.[40] The lupin γ-conglutins belong to this family.

Late embryogenesis abundant (LEA) proteins are involved in late embryogenesis in legume seeds. Family members are conserved along the entire coding region, especially within the hydrophobic internal 20-amino-acid motif. This motif may be repeated. Their allergenic potential is not clearly defined. One potential minor soybean allergen belongs to this protein family.

Peanut Allergens

Peanut, or groundnut (*Arachis hypogaea*), is native to South and Central America, but is now ranked globally 13th among food crops. It is an annual plant, developing legume fruits 3 to 7 cm long that contain one to four seeds (Figure 3.3). There are numerous peanut cultivars, although four major cultivar groups stand for most of the annual peanut production in the world, which amounts to about 34.5 million tons: Spanish, runner, Virginia, and valencia. In addition, the Tennessee red and Tennessee white groups are of some importance.

Peanut seeds are consumed raw, salted, roasted, boiled, and fried. Peanut butter is used on sandwiches or in confections, and peanut flour is popular as a flavor enhancer. Several types of peanut oil (cold pressed, refined, and roasted) are available. In addition, peanuts are utilized in cosmetics, nitroglycerine, plastics, dyes, and paints.

Peanut is considered a major food allergen with a high frequency of severe allergic incidents in Western countries.[41,42] The prevalence of peanut allergy is rather high, affecting almost 1% of the U.S. population.[43] In some cases, exposure to even small amounts of peanut protein, by eating, inhalation, or skin contact, can cause a fatal anaphylactic shock. Therefore, labeling of peanut ingredients in foods is mandatory in many countries, and much effort is made to protect peanut-allergic consumers.

Peanut allergens have been subject to extensive research. The main allergens have been sequenced and crystallized to determine their structure and functionality.[44,45] The currently available information on peanut allergens, including isoforms, has been compiled in Table 3.3, presenting the database accession numbers, protein family affiliations, sequence lengths, electrophoretical weights, and references. A detailed reference list of peanut allergens can also be found in the Allergome database for the entry "Ara h" (http://www.allergome.org) and for "Arachis" at AllergenOnline (http://www.allergenonline.org). In gel electrophoresis under denaturing conditions (sodium dodecyl sulfate, SDS), the peanut allergens are separated into their respective subunits (Figure 3.4).

Ara h 1 is a 7S vicilin-like protein from the cupin superfamily that is recognized by more than 90% of the peanut-allergic patients.[46,47] It has been shown to contain more than 20 IgE-binding epitopes, which are clustered in two regions of the molecule.[48] Information on the Ara h 1 domain structure is presented in the SDAP (http://fermi.utmb.edu/cgi-bin/SDAP/sdap_02?dB_Type=0&allid=324).

Ara h 2 is a 2S albumin from the prolamin superfamily. In some studies, it has been identified as the clinically most important allergen.[47,49] The heat- and protease-resistant core of the protein retains its IgE-binding capacity after rigorous

ALLERGENS IN PEANUT, SOYBEAN, AND LUPIN

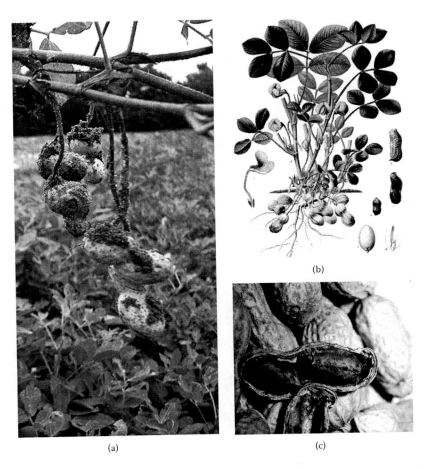

Figure 3.3 Peanut plants (a), pods (b), and seeds (c). (Peanut plants modified from Wikimedia Commons. Peanut graphic by Eugen Köhler, 1887, in *Köhlers Medizinal Pflanzen*.)

treatments.[50] Domain structure information also available in the SDAP (http://fermi.utmb.edu/cgi-bin/SDAP/sdap_02?dB_Type=0&allid=325).

Ara h 3 and Ara h 4 are no longer considered two different allergens but are regarded as isoforms of the more recently Ara h 3/4 assigned 11S legumin-like protein of the cupin superfamily, which produces multiple polypeptide bands in SDS gel electrophoresis.[51] The allergen is recognized by about 45% of peanut-allergic individuals.[47,52] The molecule contains sequential and conformational IgE-binding epitopes[53–55] in definite domains (http://fermi.utmb.edu/cgi-bin/SDAP/sdap_02?dB_Type=0&allid=326 and http://fermi.utmb.edu/cgi-bin/SDAP/sdap_02?dB_Type=0&allid=327).

Ara h 5 has been identified as profilin[44,56] that appears to be a minor peanut allergen, affecting about 15% of peanut-allergic-patients. (For domain information, see http://fermi.utmb.edu/cgi-bin/SDAP/sdap_02?dB_Type=0&allid=328.)

Table 3.3 Allergenic Peanut Proteins and Their Amino Acid Sequence Homologues

Allergen	Protein Family	MD (SDS-Page) (kDa)	UniProt Accession No.	NCBI Accession No.	Length (amino acids)
Ara h 1	Cupin (vicilin-like 7S globulin), conarachin	64			626
Ara h 1.0101			P43238	GI:602436	428
Ara h 1			Q6PSU4	GI:46560476	614
Unassigned			P43237	GI:620025	614
Unassigned			B3IXL2	GI:193850561	
Ara h 2	Prolamin (2 S albumin; conglutin), conglutin-7	17			
Ara h 2.0101			—	GI:52001226	179
Ara h 2.0102			C0LJJ1	GI:224747150	158
Ara h 2.0201			Q6PSU2	GI:26245447	172
Ara h 2.0202			—	—	151
Unassigned			—	GI:14347292	207
Unassigned			Q647G8	GI:52001231	158
Ara h 3/4	Cupin (legumin-like 11S globulin; glycinin, arachin)	37; 60			
Ara h 3.0101			O82580	GI:3703107	507
Ara h 3 iso.			B5TYU1	GI:199732457	530
iso-Ara h 3			Q0GM57	GI:112380623	512
Ara h 4.0101			Q9SQH7	GI:5712199	530
Ara h 3/4			Q8LKN1	GI:21314465	538
Ahy-1			Q647H4	GI:52001219	536
Ahy-2			Q647H3	GI:52001221	537
Ahy-3			Q647H2	GI:52001223	484
Ahy-4			Q5I6T2	GI:57669861	531
Arachin			Q6T2T4	GI:37789212	536
Arachin-6			A1DZF0	GI:118776570	529
Arachin-7			A1DZF1	GI:118776572	207
Gly1			Q9FZ11	GI:9864777	529
Glycinin			Q6IWG5	GI:47933675	510
Ara h 5	Profilin	15			
Ara h 5.0101			Q9SQI9	GI:5902968	131
Unassigned			Q5XXQ5	GI:52547772	128
Ara h 6	Prolamin (2 S albumin; conglutin 8)	15			
Ara h 6.0101			Q647G9	GI:52001229	145
conglutin 8			A1DZE9	GI:148613182	145
Unassigned			A5Z1R0	GI:148613179	145
Ara h 7	Prolamin (2 S albumin; conglutin)	15			
Ara h 7.0101			Q9SQH1	GI:5931948	160
Ara h 7.0201			B4XID4	GI:158121995	164
Ara h 8	Pathogenesis-related protein (PR-10), Bet v 1-like protein	17			
Ara h 8.0101			Q6VT83	GI:37499626	157
Ara h 8.0102			B0YIU5	GI:145904610	153
Ara h 8 iso 3			B1PYZ4	GI:169786740	157
Unassigned			Q5XXQ4	GI:52547774	150
Unassigned			B2ZGS2	GI:187940332	157
Ara h 9	Lipid-transfer protein (LPT)	9.8			
Ara h 9.0101			B6CEX8	GI:161087230	116
Ara h 9.0201			B6CG41	GI:161610580	92

ALLERGENS IN PEANUT, SOYBEAN, AND LUPIN

Table 3.3 (Continued) Allergenic Peanut Proteins and Their Amino Acid Sequence Homologues

Allergen	Protein Family	MD (SDS-Page) (kDa)	UniProt Accession No.	NCBI Accession No.	Length (amino acids)
Ara h 10	Oleosin-like protein 2	16			
Ara h 10.0101			Q647G5	GI:113200509	169
Ara h 10.0102			Q647G4	GI:52001239	150
Ara h 11	Oleosin-like protein 1	14	Q45W87	GI:71040655	137
Ara h 11.0101					
Ara h oleosin 18		18			
Unassigned			Q6J1J8	GI:86450991	176
Variant A			Q9AXI1	GI:13161005	176
Variant B			Q9AXI0	GI:13161008	176
Ara h agglutinin	D-Galactose-binding lectin	24–30	P02872	GI:253289	273
			Q38711	GI:951114	271
			Q43373	GI:951108	276
			Q8W0P8	GI:18072503	246
			Q43375	GI:951112	248

Source: Data compilation using the Allergome database, the AllergenOnline database, the UniProt database, and the National Center for Biotechnology Information (NCBI) database (November 2009).

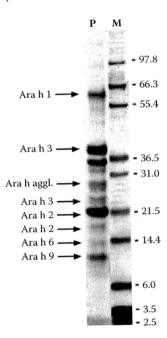

Figure 3.4 SDS gel of total peanut extract. M, molecular weight marker; P, peanut. Molecular weights (kDa) are indicated on the right side of the gel. (Image by C.K. Fæste.)

Ara h 6 and Ara h 7 are 2S albumins belonging to the prolamin superfamily. In contrast to Ara h 2, they appear to be minor allergens.[44,47] Domain information is available at http://fermi.utmb.edu/cgi-bin/SDAP/sdap_02?dB_Type=0&allid=329 and http://fermi.utmb.edu/cgi-bin/SDAP/sdap_02?dB_Type=0&allid=330.

Ara h 8 is a Bet v 1-related protein.[57] In geographical regions with high prevalence of birch pollen, considerable IgE binding to Ara h 8 has been measured, whereas the importance of Ara h 8 was low in the Mediterranean region. (For domain information, see http://fermi.utmb.edu/cgi-bin/SDAP/sdap_02?dB_Type=0&allid=780.)

Ara h 9 is a nsLTP from the prolamin superfamily that is relevant for the Mediterranean allergic population and is recognized by 60–90% of the peanut-allergic consumers.[58] In contrast, it is relatively unimportant in Northern countries.[59]

Ara h 10, Ara h 11, and Ara oleosin 18 kDa are peanut oleosins that have been identified as candidate allergens for IgE-mediated reactions.[60] In a French study, serum binding to monomeric or oligomeric oleosins was found for more than 20% of the peanut-allergic patients.[35]

Ara h agglutinin is a peanut lectin that has been identified as a minor allergen.[37,60,61] However, in one study IgE binding to the agglutinin was detected in many patients' sera even after heat processing.[62]

Soybean Allergens

Soybean (or soya, soy, soyabean) is an annual plant native to East Asia (Figure 3.5). Soybean varieties can be broadly classified as vegetable or oil types. The total world

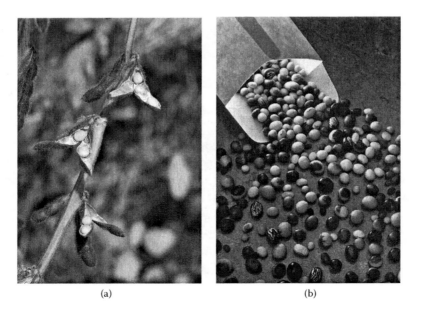

Figure 3.5 Soybean pods (a) and seeds (b). (Image b from Wikimedia Commons.)

soybean production in 2007 was 220.5 million tons. Soybeans provide about 35% of the global demand for human dietary protein. They are one of the "biotech food" crops that have been genetically modified.

Soybean is used in an increasing number of products.[63] For human consumption, soybeans must be cooked to destroy the protease inhibitors. Typical products are soy meal, soy flour, soy milk, soy paste, soy sauce, soy oil, soy lecithin, tofu, miso, tempeh, textured vegetable protein for vegetarian foods like meat and diary substitutes, and soy-based infant formula (SBIF). Soybeans are also used in industrial products, including oils, soap, cosmetics, resins, plastics, inks, crayons, solvents, and clothing.

Soybean has been counted among the eight major allergens and has to be labeled as a food ingredient in many countries; however, the prevalence of soybean allergy appears to be uncertain.[64] Although there are a number of reported cases of severe allergic incidents, especially in young people, a reliable estimate for the general population is difficult.[65] The prevalence of soy sensitization seems to be much higher than the occurrence of clinical symptoms.[66]

A considerable number of soybean proteins are allergenic and can be identified on immunoblot by IgE binding.[67] The main soybean allergens have been sequenced and intensively studied.[68,69] The currently available information on soybean allergens, including isoforms, has been compiled in Table 3.4, presenting the database accession numbers, protein family affiliations, sequence lengths, electrophoretical weights, and references. A detailed reference list of soybean allergens can also be found in the Allergome database for the entry "Gly m" (http://www.allergome.org) and for "Glycine" at AllergenOnline (http://www.allergenonline.org). In gel electrophoresis under denaturing conditions (SDS), the soybean allergens are separated into their respective subunits (Figure 3.6).

Gly m 1 is a hydrophobic seed protein belonging to the prolamin superfamily.[70] It has been identified as an aeroallergen, causing occupational asthma and respiratory allergies.[71] Information on the Gly m 1 domain structure is presented in the SDAP (http://fermi.utmb.edu/cgi-bin/SDAP/sdap_02?dB_Type=0&allid=321).

Gly m 2 is a hull protein from the defensin family. It has been found to be involved in soybean dust-connected epidemic asthma.[72] Domain information is available at http://fermi.utmb.edu/cgi-bin/SDAP/sdap_02?dB_Type=0&allid=322.

Gly m 3 is a profilin,[73] which might cause OAS in birch pollen-allergic patients.[74] (For domain information, see http://fermi.utmb.edu/cgi-bin/SDAP/sdap_02?dB_Type=0&allid=323.)

Gly m 4 is a Bet v 1-related soybean allergen[74] involved in severe OAS and anaphylactic reactions in pollen allergic consumers.[75] For domain information, see http://fermi.utmb.edu/cgi-bin/SDAP/sdap_02?dB_Type=0&allid=605.

Gly m 5, the soybean conglycinin, is a 7S vicilin-like cupin. Gly m Bd28K and Gly m Bd60K are isoforms. Up to 40% of the patients reacted to Gly m 5 in two clinical studies. All subunits of the protein were IgE reactive.[76] Domain information for Gly m 5 is available at http://fermi.utmb.edu/cgi-bin/SDAP/sdap_02?dB_Type=0&allid=681 and for Gly m Bd28K at http://fermi.utmb.edu/cgi-bin/SDAP/sdap_02?dB_Type=0&allid=684.

Table 3.4 Allergenic Soybean Proteins and Their Amino Acid Sequence Homologues

Allergen	Protein Family	MD (SDS-Page) (kDa)	UniProt Accession No.	NCBI Accession No.	Length (amino acids)
Gly m 1	Prolamin	7.5			
Gly m 1.0101	(hydrophobic		Q9S8F3	—	42
Gly m 1.0102	seed protein)		Q9S8F2	—	39
Gly m 1			P24337	—	80
Unassigned			Q9S7Z9	GI:5019730	119
HSP precursor			Q3HM29	GI:76782253	118
S5 peptide			Q9S904	—	34
HSP			Q3HM31	GI:76782247	134
Gly m 2	Defensin (hull	6			
Gly m 2.0101	allergen)		—	GI:1362049	20
Gly m 3	Profilin	14			
Gly m 3.0101			O65809	GI:3021375	131
Gly m 3.0102			O65810	GI:3021373	131
Unassigned			A7XZJ7	GI:156938901	131
Unassigned			C6SVT2	GI:255626021	131
Unassigned			Q0PPS3	GI:110729187	131
Unassigned			C6TLM1	GI:255646679	147
Gly m 4	Bet v 1-like	17			
Gly m 4.0101	protein		P26987	GI:18744	158
H4			Q43453	GI:18643	158
Unassigned			C6T1G1	GI:255630093	158
Unassigned			C6T3A2	GI:255631546	158
Unassigned			C6T588	GI:255633070	158
Unassigned			C6TFW4	GI:255640867	158
Unassigned			C6T206	GI:255630540	158
Unassigned			C6T3L5	GI:255631772	158
Gly m 5	Cupin (7S-vicilin;	60–80			
Gly m 5.0101	β-conglycinin,		O22120	GI:9967357	543
Gly m 5.0201	α-subunit)		Q9FZP9	GI:9967361	559
Gly m beta congl. a			Q4LER6	GI:68264913	621
Gly m beta congl. a			Q7XXT2	GI:32328882	621
Gly m beta congl. a			Q3V5S6	GI:74271743	605
Gly m beta congl. a			Q4LER5	GI:68264915	604
Gly m Bd60K			P13916	GI:18536	605
Gly m Bd60K			Q94LX2	GI:14245736	605
Gly m Bd28K			Q9AVK8	GI:12697782	473
Gly m beta congl. A			Q948Y0	GI:15425631	621
Gly m 5.0301	Cupin	36	P25974	GI:256427	439
Gly m 5.0302	(β-conglycinin, β-subunit)		P25974	GI:256427	439
Gly m 6	Glycinin	20; 40			
Gly m 6.0101/G1	(11S-legumin)		P04776	GI:169973	495
Gly m 6.0201/G2			P04405	GI:218265	485
Gly m 6.0301/G3			P11828	GI:18639	481
Gly m 6.0401/G4			P02858	GI:732706	562
Glycinin G4 subunit			Q9S9D0	-	560
Gy4 A5A4B3 subunit			Q39921	GI:806556	563
Gy4			Q43452	GI:18641	562
A5A4B3 subunit			A3KEY9	GI:126144648	563
A5A4B3 subunit			Q9SB11	GI:4249568	563

Table 3.4 (*Continued*) Allergenic Soybean Proteins and Their Amino Acid Sequence Homologues

Allergen	Protein Family	MD (SDS-Page) (kDa)	UniProt Accession No.	NCBI Accession No.	Length (amino acids)
Gly m 6.0501			Q7GC77	GI:10566449	517
A3B4 Glycinin			Q9SB12	GI:4249566	517
Gly 5 A3B4			Q39922	GI:736002	517
Gly A3B4			P93708	GI:1772308	517
Gly A3B4			P93707	GI:1772306	517
Gly A3B4			A3KEY8	GI:126144646	513
Glycinin A3B4			P04347	GI:169969	516
mGly A3B4			C0KG62	GI:223649560	534
Proglycinin A2B1			Q549Z4	GI:32328880	485
Glycinin A1bB2–455			Q852U5	GI:27922971	481
Glycinin A1bB2–784			Q852U4	GI:27922973	482
mGlycinin A1aB1b			C7EA91	GI:254029113	386
mGlycinin A1aB1b			C7EA92	GI:254029115	386
Gly m 2S albumin	Prolamin (2S albumin)	17			
Unassigned			P19594	GI:2305020	158
Napin-type 2S alb.3			Q53WV6	GI:4097896	158
Napin-type 2S alb.1			Q9ZNZ4	GI:4097894	155
Unassigned			C6T1Q7	GI:255630323	155
Gly m Bd30k	Maturing seed protein (peptidase C1-like; papain-like)	30	O64458	GI:84371705	379
			P22895	GI:1199563	379
Gly m LTP	Lipid transfer protein	9			
Unassigned			C6TFP9	GI:255640734	122
Unassigned			C6TFC1	GI:255640474	122
Gly m oleosin	Oleosin	24			
Oleosin			C3VHQ8	GI:226897921	165
Oleosin isoform A			P29530	GI:476214	226
Oleosin isoform B			P29531	GI:944830	223
Unassigned			C6SZ13	GI:255628283	147
Gly m agglutinin	Lectin	22–35	P05046	GI:170006	285
Gly m TI	Kunitz-type trypsin inhibitor	28	P01070	GI:256428	216
Trypsin inhibitor A			Q9LLX2	GI:9367042	168
Trypsin inhibitor			B1ACD3	GI:168259032	214
Gly m CPI	Cysteine protease inhibitor	25	C6SWI5	GI:255626526	198
			C4XVM5	GI:239992735	208
			C6TLR5	GI:255646769	209
			C6T1F1	GI:255630073	217
			C6SY93	GI:255627743	203
			Q9ATY1	GI:13375349	216
			C6T5E	GI:255633198	199

Continued

Table 3.4 (*Continued*) Allergenic Soybean Proteins and Their Amino Acid Sequence Homologues

Allergen	Protein Family	MD (SDS-Page) (kDa)	UniProt Accession No.	NCBI Accession No.	Length (amino acids)
Gly m EAP	Late embryonic abundant protein	15	Q9ZTZ2	GI:4102692	133
			Q2XSK1	GI:82394554	133

Note: congl = conglutin.
Source: Data compilation using the Allergome database, the AllergenOnline database, the UniProt database, and the National Center for Biotechnology Information (NCBI) database (November 2009).

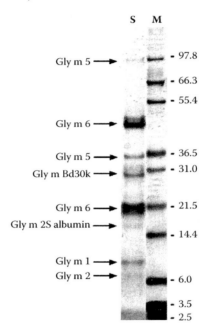

Figure 3.6 SDS gel of total soybean extract. M, molecular weight marker; S, soybean. Molecular weights (kDa) are indicated on the right side of the gel. (Image by C.K. Fæste.)

Gly m 6, the soybean glycinin, is an 11S legumin-like cupin.[54] It has been described as a major soybean allergen, showing IgE reactivity in up to 40% of the patients in a number of clinical studies. (For domain information for Gly m glycinin G1 see http://fermi.utmb.edu/cgi-bin/SDAP/sdap_02?dB_Type=0&allid=680 and for Gly m glycinin G2 see http://fermi.utmb.edu/cgi-bin/SDAP/sdap_02?dB_Type=0&allid=795.)

Gly m 2S albumin has to be considered as a minor soybean allergen. In a relatively small cohort, IgE binding was not detected in any of the patients' sera.[77]

Gly m Bd30K (P34) is an immunodominant soybean allergen occurring in the seed storage vacuoles.[68] It shows sequence similarity to papain-like proteases but lacks their enzymatic activity.[78] In a clinical study, about 65% of the patients reacted to Gly m 30K. Thermal processing can decrease the allergenicity, and there are soybean cultivars with low levels of this allergen.

Gly m LTP (lipid transfer protein) is a hydrophobic protein from the prolamin family,[24] like Gly m 1. The heat-labile soybean LTP might be involved in cross-reactions causing OAS. However, it has to be considered a minor allergen.

Gly m oleosin occurs in the soybean oil bodies,[79] and residual oleosin in soybean oils is a potential danger for allergic consumers. However, the oleosin fraction was shown to be a minor IgE-binding constituent of total soybean protein.[80]

Gly m agglutinin is a legume lectin considered a minor soybean allergen.[37] About 16% of the patients' sera showed IgE reactivity to soybean agglutinin in a clinical study. (For domain information, see http://fermi.utmb.edu/cgi-bin/SDAP/sdap_02?dB_Type=0&allid=682.)

Gly TI belongs to the Kunitz soybean trypsin inhibitor family.[81] It has been described as a minor allergen.[37] Fewer than 10% of the patients in a clinical study had IgE-mediated reactions to Gly TI. Domain information is available at http://fermi.utmb.edu/cgi-bin/SDAP/sdap_02?dB_Type=0&allid=683.

Gly m CPI is a cysteine protease inhibitor[82] that is related to the same protein family as Gly TI. Homologous allergens, for example, are the major potato allergens. The allergic potential of the soybean Gly m CPI is unclear.

Gly m EAP (embryonic abundant protein) has been identified as a late EAP belonging to the seed maturation proteins.[82] However, its relevance in soybean allergy is unclear.

Lupin Allergens

Lupin belongs to the genus *Lupinus*, which includes 450 species. It is widely grown as ornamental flowers; however, garden species contain high alkaloid levels and are unsuited for human consumption. Selective breeding has led to lupine varieties with reduced alkaloid content, the "sweet lupines." Four edible species are cultivated in different geographical regions: white lupine (*Lupinus albus*) in the Mediterranean countries, blue or narrow-leaved lupin (*Lupinus angustifolius*) in Australia, yellow lupine (*Lupinus luteus*) in Central Europe, and the Andean lupine (*Lupinus mutabilis*) in South America (Figure 3.7).

The total global yearly production of lupin is about 2 million tonnes, of which 4% are used for human consumption and the rest for animal feed. Sweet lupin products include lupin flour, lupin bran, lupin-tofu, and lupin-derived "milk." Typical foods containing lupin are breads, biscuits, pasta, sauces, milk substitutes, soy substitutes, chocolate spread, sausages, and pastes.[83,84] Lupin is also used to clarify wine and for Asian fermented foods such as tempeh and miso. In addition, seeds from bitter lupin cultivars are traditionally eaten as "lupini" snacks in southern Europe.

Lupin allergy occurs by primary sensitization to ingested lupin protein,[85–87] by sensitization through inhalation,[88,89] and by occupational exposures.[90] More often, lupin

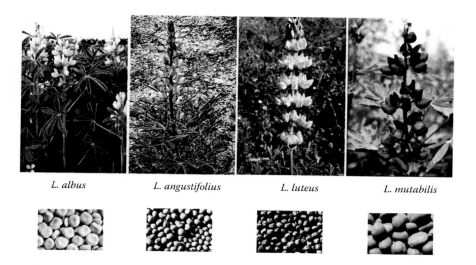

Figure 3.7 Sweet lupin plants and seeds.

allergy seems to arise by cross-reactivity in patients with existing peanut allergy.[91–94] Due to the increasing number of incidents of lupin allergy, lupin-derived ingredients in processed foods have had to be mandatorily labeled in Europe since 2006.

A number of lupin allergens have been identified. They are homologous to known legume allergens from peanut and soybean. The currently available information on lupin allergens, including isoforms, has been compiled in Table 3.5, enumerating allergenic proteins from *Lupinus albus* (Lup a), *Lupinus angustifolius* (Lup an), and *Lupinus luteus* (Lup l). A detailed reference list of lupin allergens can also be found in the Allergome database for the entry "lup" (http://www.allergome.org) and for "Lupinus" at AllergenOnline (http://www.allergenonline.org). In gel electrophoresis under denaturing conditions (SDS), the lupin allergens are separated into their respective subunits (Figure 3.8).

Lupin α-conglutins are 11S legumin-like globulins belonging to the cupin superfamily.[95] In contrast to most other 11S globulins, the acidic subunits, which are larger than the basic ones, are glycosylated in the mature protein.[96] Lupin α-conglutins are considered major lupin allergens.[97] In a clinical study, about 40% of the patients showed IgE-mediated reactions to Lup a α-conglutin.[98] Lup an α-conglutin demonstrated, in a study with sera from lupin-allergic patients, considerable cross-reactivity to the homologous peanut allergen Ara h 3.[49]

Lupin β-conglutins are 7S vicilin-like globulins.[95] The endogenous cleavage of these proteins is in lupin greatly enhanced in comparison to other legumes.[99] Lupin β-conglutins are major lupin allergens. Almost 60% of the patients in a recent study reacted to Lup a 1, the Lup a β-conglutin.[98] The Lup an β-conglutin, Lup an 1,100 was shown to cross-react with the homologous Ara h 1 from peanut.[49]

Table 3.5 Allergenic Lupin Proteins and Their Amino Acid Sequence Homologues

Allergen	Protein Family	MD (SDS-Page) (kDa)	UniProt Accession No.	NCBI Accession No.	Length
Lup α congl.	11 S legumin-like protein; α conglutin)	69–89			
Lup a α congl.			Q53I54	GI:85361412	512
Lup a α congl.			Q53I53	GI:62816188	365
Lup a α congl.			Q53I55	GI:62816184	254
Lup an α congl.			Q96475	GI:2313076	131
Lup an seed storage			C9WC98	GI:224184735	493
Lup β congl.	Cupin (7S vicilin-like protein; β conglycinin)	19–60			
Lup a 1			Q53HY0	GI:89994190	531
Lup a β congl.			Q6EBC1	GI:46451223	533
Lup an 1.0101			B8Q5G0	GI:169950562	611
Lup an β congl.			B0YJF7	GI:169950562	611
Lup an β congl.			B0YJF8	GI:149208403	455
Lup γ congl.	Cupin (basic 7S globulin)	17; 29			
Lup a γ congl.			Q7M1N2	—	40
Lup a γ congl.			Q9FEX1	GI:67966634	448
Lup a γ congl.			Q9FSH9	GI:11191819	452
Lup a γ congl.			Q9S8M6	—	31
Lup an γ congl.			Q42369	GI:666056	449
Lup δ congl.	2S albumin	4.6; 9.4			
Lup a δ congl.			Q333K7	GI:80221495	148
Lup an δ congl.			P09931	—	80
Lup an δ congl.			P09930	—	37
Lup an δ congl.			Q99235	GI:19141	153
Lup PR-10 protein	Bet v 1-like protein	17			
Lup a			O24010	GI:2398666	158
Lup a			Q93XI0	GI:15341238	158
Lup l LIR 18A			P52778	GI:1039334	156
Lup l LIR 18B			P52779	GI:1039336	156
Lup l PR-10 2A			Q9LLQ3	GI:8574575	158
Lup l PR-10 2B			Q9LLQ2	GI:8574577	158
Lup l PR-10 2C			Q9AXK2	GI:12958727	158
Lup l PR-10 2D			Q9AXK1	GI:12958729	158
Lup l PR-10 2E			Q7Y1W5	GI:30962008	157
Lup l PR-10 2F			Q7XZT8	GI:31790202	157

Note: congl. = conglutin.
Source: Data compilation using the Allergome database, the AllergenOnline database, the UniProt database, and the National Center for Biotechnology Information (NCBI) database (November 2009).

Lupin γ-conglutins are basic proteins with homogeneous tetramers consisting of two different disulfide-linked monomers.[101–103] They belong to the protein family of eukaryotic aspartyl proteases, which also includes the major cockroach allergen Bla g 2. The allergenic potential of the lupin γ-conglutin, however, is under discussion. Cross-reactivity to peanut allergens has not been detected so far,[49] although about 30% of the patients in a clinical study had IgE to lupin γ-conglutin.[98]

Lupin delta-conglutins are 2S albumins.103 About 25% of the patients in a clinical study showed IgE-mediated reactions to Lup a delta-conglutin.[98] Lup an delta-conglutin cross-reacted considerably with the homologous peanut Ara h 2.[49]

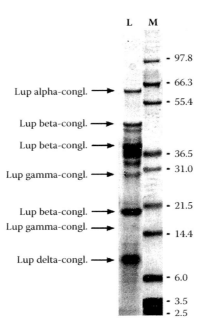

Figure 3.8 SDS gel of total lupin (*L. albus*) extract. L, lupin; M, molecular weight marker. Molecular weights (kDa) are indicated on the right side of the gel. (Image by C.K. Fæste.)

Lupin pathogenesis-related proteins (PR10 proteins) from the Bet v 1-like family are encoded by multigenes. In yellow lupin, the different homologous allergens have been divided into two subclasses sharing 60% sequence identity.[104] By cross-reaction to the homologous peanut PR10 Ara h 8 and the major birch pollen allergen Bet v1, Lup a PR10[105] and Lup l PR10 might be involved in OAS reactions to lupin.

There are no entries for lupin in the SDAP so far.

SAMPLE EXTRACTION AND CLEANUP

The analysis of food matrices for the presence of food allergens requires several steps, which all have influence on the analytical results. The procedure can be considered a two-step process consisting of sample preparation and sample analysis. The sample preparation includes sample taking, extraction, and cleanup. If the test material is inhomogeneous, it might be difficult to take representative samples. Low protein contents and adsorbent materials like flours and powders are additional challenges. The retrieved samples have to be homogenized and extracted for the analyte (i.e., the allergenic proteins or the DNA marker molecules). Optimally, the extraction will be almost compete or at least proportional to the analyte content of the test material. In many cases, the extracted analytes are further purified by specific cleanup procedures before they are finally submitted to analyses by a dedicated method.

The influence of sampling, subsampling, and analytical variances on the determination of the allergen content in foods has been shown for peanut in bars and in milk chocolate.[106] The variability of the analytical results was greater than 95% and greater than 60% chocolate, respectively. By increasing the sample size, subsample size, and number of analyses, variabilities were considerably reduced.

The extractability of the analyte from the food matrix depends on a number of factors, like matrix constituents, analyte structure changes by food-processing techniques, and the extraction buffer used. Detection might be impaired by food matrix interaction (e.g., by binding to other proteins, carbohydrates like in a Maillard reaction,[107] or tannins in chocolate), and heat denaturing of proteins can lead to reduced solubility and antibody-binding differences.[108–113] Furthermore, optimum allergen extractability is buffer dependent, and no single buffer is appropriate for use as a universal extraction solution for all allergenic foods.[114,115] Therefore, a thorough evaluation of sample preparation buffers (e.g., with regard to ionic strength and pH) needs to be performed for every individual allergenic food.

Analytes with different molecular properties, like proteins and DNA, need different extraction methods,[116] although the general issues with regard to sampling, homogeneity, and modifications by food processing apply to both groups. In the following description of specific separation techniques, however, the focus is proteinaceous analytes.

Preparation of Total Legume Extracts

Sample homogenization and solubilization are of great importance for sample preparation. With regard to the breaking up and releasing of the allergenic protein from the food matrix for analysis, peanut and soybean are considered among the most difficult analytes.[117]

Legume seed extraction is generally performed following a common strategy: The milled samples are defatted by shaking at 4°C, room temperature, or 37°C with lipophilic solvents such as n-hexane, acetone, or n-pentane, optionally by using a Soxhlet apparatus.[118]

In the following discussion, the proteins are extracted from the air-dried legume flours by buffer addition in ratios ranging from 1:5 to 1:20 (w/v). A commonly used extraction buffer is Tris-HCl at pH 7.5.[119]

The extraction of legume proteins from complex food matrices may require additional purification steps. The raw extract can be filtered through glass wool, sieves (0.2 mm), or, for example, a 1.2-μm cellulose acetate filter. The proteins of interest can be separated by immunoaffinity purification using specific antibodies that are coupled to columns or magnetic beads.[120,121] Furthermore, gel filtration columns (e.g., Superose 12HR10/30 column in 0.1M Tris-HCl buffer at pH 7.5 or Superdex S200 equilibrated with 25 mM Tris-HCl at pH 7.4/200 mM NaCl/3 mM NaN$_3$) or reversed-phased solid phase extraction cartridges might be applied. Buffer changes can be achieved by dialysis through low cutoff membranes (1- to 3.5-kDa pore sizes). In general, all extracts have to be further diluted before they are submitted to analysis.

Peanut

As a major food allergen, peanut has been well studied, and numerous analytical methods for the detection of allergen in foods have been developed. Each method includes specific sample preparation steps. As a consequence, many different cleanup techniques for peanut have been described involving various different buffers and procedures.[122] As an alternative to Tris-HCl from the consensus method discussed in the preceding section, phosphate-buffered saline (PBS) buffer (e.g., 20 mM Na$_2$PO$_4$/1M NaCl at pH 7.0) is often used to extract peanut proteins from homogenized peanuts.[123] Commercially available kits for peanut allergen detection always include dedicated extraction buffers and procedures.[122]

Soybean

Soybean analytical methods include specific buffers as described for peanut. Besides PBS (pH 7.4) and Tris-HCl, buffers containing 25 mM N-[tris(hydroxymethyl) methyl]glycine (Tricine) and 2 mM calcium lactate at pH 8.6 have been used.[124] A comparison of different extraction procedures showed that recoveries for soybean protein from matrices were considerably improved if the pH of the extraction buffer was raised to above pH 12.0.[125]

Lupin

Lupin proteins can be extracted from seeds and food matrices using Tris-HCl at pH 8.0 for 4 h at 4°C.[95] More recent procedures demonstrated good extraction results by increasing the pH, the extraction time, and the temperature, applying 1M Tris/0.5M glycine buffer at pH 8.7 at 45°C overnight.[93,100,126]

Isolation of Individual Allergens

The three groups of major legume seed proteins are different in hydrophilicity: Whereas albumins are soluble in aqueous buffers, globulins are better extracted by saline solutions, and prolamins afford a mixture of alcohol and water.

A single improved methodology for the extraction, fractionation, and purification of the legume seed storage 11S and 7S globulins and 2S albumins has been proposed[119]: The seeds are milled and defatted with n-hexane (34 ml/g flour) for 4 h with agitation. The n-hexane is decanted, and the seed flour is air-dried. The albumin fraction is extracted by stirring with water (pH 8.0) containing 10 mM CaCl$_2$, 10 mM MgCl$_2$, and 1 mM phenylmethylsulfonyl fluoride (PMSF) (34 mg/g flour) for 4 h and collected from the supernatant after centrifugation at 30,000g for 1 h. The total globulin fraction is extracted from the precipitate by stirring with 0.1M Tris-HCl buffer at pH 7.5 containing 10% w/v NaCl, 0.05% NaN$_3$, 1 mM PMSF, 10 mM ethylenediaminetetraacetic acid (EDTA), and 10 mM ethylene glycol bis(β-aminoethyl ether)-N,N,N,N-tetraacetic acid (EGTA) for 4 h. After centrifugation at 30,000g for 1 h, the prolamins are in the pellet, and the globulins can be collected from the supernatant by precipitation with 80% ammonium sulfate (561 g/L). The globulins are separated at 30,000g for 20 min, resuspended in 50 mM Tris-HCl at pH 7.5, and desalted on PD-10 columns. All steps are performed at 4°C.

The globulin fraction can be further separated by anion exchange chromatography (e.g., on a Mono Q HR5/5 or Resource Q column) applying fast liquid protein chromatography (FPLC) and optical detection (A_{280} peaks) of the globulins.[95,119,127] Finally, the different globulins can be separated by isopycnic sucrose density gradient centrifugation.[128] Sucrose layers consisting of 10–30% sucrose in 35 mM phosphate buffer at pH 7.6 containing 10 mM mercaptoethanol and 0.4M NaCl are assembled in ultracentrifuge tubes to generate a stepwise gradient. This is converted to a continuous gradient by thawing and incubation at 4°C for 24 h. After ultracentrifugation at 100,000g for 24 h at 4°C, the globulins are separated according to their sedimentation coefficients and can be collected from the respective layers in the tubes. Alternatively to using sucrose, the density gradient can be prepared with glycerol consisting of layers of 5–45% glycerol in 50 mM Tris-HCl buffer at pH 7.5.

Peanut

Many protocols intended for the purification of the major peanut allergens[45] are variations of the universally applicable legume protein isolation method. However, alternative procedures have been described, such as the separation by reversed-phase high-performance liquid chromatography (RP-HPLC). The proteins were dissolved from the defatted peanut kernels by 0.05% trifluoroacetic acid (TFA) and analyzed by RP-HPLC with a 0–100% gradient of methanol containing 0.05% TFA. The protein peaks were recovered and tested in SDS-PAGE (polyacrylamide gel electrophoresis).[129]

Soybean

The major soybean allergens can be fractionated by the general legume protein isolation method. A fast and simple fractionation technique using 10 mM Ca^{2+} was developed by which about 87% of the soybean seed storage globulins glycinin and β-conglycinin are removed from the raw extract by precipitation, allowing the detection of 541 previously inconspicuous proteins present in soybean seed by proteomic methods.[130]

Lupin

The lupin conglutins can be separated without chromatographic methods or density gradient centrifugation by fractionated extraction and precipitation steps.

The 2S albumin delta-conglutin is extracted from the defatted seeds with cold deionized water at pH 8.0–8.5 and precipitated by lowering the pH to 4.5. The albumin is resuspended from the pellet, which still contains contaminating α-, β-, and γ-conglutins, with 0.1M calcium carbonate buffer at pH 4.0 containing 0.4M

NaCl and 40% ethanol, separated by centrifugation, and finally collected by cold precipitation.[118]

The globulin fraction, consisting of α-conglutin, β-conglutin, and to a lesser degree γ-conglutin, is extracted from the lupin seeds with 10% (w/v) NaCl. Cold-insoluble γ-conglutin can be removed by dialysis from the cold-soluble α- and β-conglutin. These were separated by differential ammonium sulfate precipitation, with a 64–66% cut for α-conglutin and a 70–90% cut for β-conglutin.[95,131] Purified conglutins are dissolved in 0.15M phosphate buffer. For the isolation of γ-conglutin, lupin seeds were soaked in deionized water for 16 h and heated at 60°C for 4 h.[127] Precipitated γ-conglutin is obtained by centrifugation and dissolved in 50 mM Tris-HCl buffer and pH 7.5.

In a more compact procedure,[118] defatted lupin flour is suspended in water (1:20 w/v), brought to pH 8.0–8.5 with diluted NaOH solution, stirred for 3 h at room temperature, and centrifuged for 30 min at 10,000g, removing insoluble fractions like, for example, prolamins. The supernatant is diluted with HCl to pH 4.5 and centrifuged again to precipitate α-, β-, and δ-conglutin. γ-Conglutin can be obtained from the supernatant at pH 7.0 (adjusted with NaOH) by adding $ZnCl_2$ to a final concentration of 20 mM. The pellet containing α-, β-, and δ-conglutin is resuspended in 0.1M Na-acetate pH 4.0/0.4M NaCl/40% ethanol for 1 h at room temperature under stirring, resulting in the resolubilization of δ-conglutin. The δ-conglutin can be recovered from the supernatant by cold precipitation at −20°C overnight, whereas α- and β-conglutin can be redissolved from the pellet and separated by differential ammonium sulfate precipitation or FPLC.

SEPARATION AND ANALYSIS METHODS

Many different analytical techniques have been applied for the detection, identification, and characterization of allergens. They target either all or specific proteins or DNA fragments encoding for species-specific proteins. Therefore, the analysis methods can be divided into protein-based and DNA-based techniques.

Most protein-based assays are immunoassays making use of the specific antibody-antigen binding. Therefore, selective antibodies are a prerequisite for successful allergen detection. IgE from allergic patients can be applied; however, this is a limited resource and difficult to standardize. The majority of immunological detection assays employ polyclonal antibodies from rabbit, sheep, or goat or monoclonal antibodies from mice.[122]

Mass spectrometric (MS) methods have been developed for the detection of allergenic proteins in foods. MS techniques have the advantage of directly detecting allergen-specific peptides by their characteristic mass/charge ratios and are therefore less influenced by potential protein structure changes due to food processing. However, MS requires advanced instruments and has not been used in routine analysis so far.[132]

In DNA-based methods, a specific DNA segment is amplified by polymerase chain reaction (PCR). The generated DNA is either detected afterward on agarose gel or measured in parallel while the PCR is performed (real-time PCR).[133] (Table 3.6).

Table 3.6 Methods for Allergen Analysis

Method	Principle	Characteristics LOD [mg/kg]	Reference
Immundiffusion "Ouchterlony"	Agarose gel (1%): six peripheral wells containing test proteins surround central well with antibody: formation of antibody-protein precipitates	Qualitative	134
Rocket immunoelectrophoresis	Antibody-containing agarose gel: electrophoresis of proteins results in rocket-shaped precipitations	Quantitative; > 20	134
Polyacrylamide gel electrophoresis (on-gel proteomics)	SDS-PAGE: separation of proteins by electrophoresis (1-DE, 2-DE); protein staining; comparison to molecular weight standards	Semiquantitative; stain intensities comparable to standards	135
Dot blot	Nitrocellulose membrane: protein dots applied, signal development with antibodies	Semiquantitative; stain intensities comparable to standards, > 0.1	136
Immunoblot (Western blot)	Transfer of protein from 1-DE or 2-DE on nitrocellulose membrane: protein dots applied, signal development with antibodies	Semiquantitative, > 5; stain intensities comparable to standards	137
Enzyme immunoassays (EIAs)	Formats: competitive, inhibition, sandwich, dipstick (lateral flow); using monoclonal or polyclonal antibody; second antibody for signal development	Quantitative; > 0.1	138
Radioallergosorbent test (RAST)/enzyme-allergosorbent test (EAST)	Surface-bound allergen, competitive binding of human IgE, isotope-labeled or enzyme-coupled second antibody	Quantitative; > 1	139
Fluorescence polarization-based immunoassay	Completive binding assay in cuvette, fluorescence detection of tagged molecule	Quantitative	140
Biosensor	Antibodies or gene sequences on chip; optical detection or plasmon resonance	Quantitative; 1 – 12.5	141 142
Basophile histamine release assay	Allergen-induced IgE-mediated histamine release from blood basophiles; fluorescence or radioactive immunoassay for detection	Semi-quantitative; > 1	143

Continued

Table 3.6 (*Continued*) Methods for Allergen Analysis

Method	Principle	Characteristics LOD [mg/kg]	Reference
PCR	Formats: PCR, real-time PCR, PCR-ELISA; DNA of allergen or marker protein is detected	(Semi-)quantitative; > 1	122
Chromatography, mass spectrometry (gel-free proteomics)	High-performance liquid chromatography (reversed phase or perfusion): separation of proteins/tryptic peptides; detection by mass spectrometry: single MS, MS-MS; different ionization and detector types.	Quantitative; > 1 ng	144 132

Note: DE = dimensional electrophoresis.

Peanut

Peanut residues in foods have been analyzed by numerous techniques varying in sensibility, specificity, and performance.[145] For the investigation of the peanut seed proteome (i.e., all proteins expressed in the seed), proteomic analyses are applied. Results of gel-assisted proteomics obtained by one- and two-dimensional gel electrophoresis and immunoblot[55,135] are available at http://www.oilseedproteomics.missouri.edu. Peanut protein profiling by MS[60,146,147] using alkylated and trypsinated peptides, capillary or nano-HPLC, electrospray ionization, and quadruple time-of-flight (Q-TOF) or linear ion trap mass analyzers resulted in the identification of specific peptide markers of the major allergens Ara h 1, Ara h 2, and Ara h 3, which are suitable analytes for quantitation experiments. The relative quantities of the peanut allergens Ara h 1, Ara h 2, Ara h 3/4, Ara h 6, Ara h 7, Ara h 8, and Ara h 10 became determinable.

Soybean

Soybean protein in foods can be detected by various methods. In addition, many PCR assays have been developed for the identification of genetically modified soybeans. However, there are also several PCR methods that target soybean allergen genes. Differences in performance and applicability have been examined in comparative studies.[124] The soybean seed proteome has been studied,[148,149] revealing the glycinin subunit G4 as a suitable marker peptide for the detection of soybean residues in foods.

Lupin

Lupin can be analyzed by a number of different techniques, including immunochemical, genomic, and chromatographic assays. Lupin proteins have been studied by differential sedimentation,[119,128] isoelectrofocusing, 150 crystallization,[151] and proteomic analysis by one- and two-dimensional gel electrophoresis[99,100,152] or liquid chromatography/electrospray ionization tandem mass spectrometry.[103,153,154]

DETECTION AND QUANTIFICATION METHODS

Traces of peanut, soybean, or lupin in processed foods supposedly free of these allergens might be introduced by contamination under production. In addition, mislabeling might occur. Therefore, reliable detection methods are necessary to ensure consumer protection. The analyses target either the proteins themselves or typical biomarkers for their presence (e.g., DNA).

Method validation is an important issue to guarantee the reliability and applicability of the allergen detection methods. Standard validation protocols have been developed that give numbers to the essential method characteristics specificity, sensitivity, linearity, precision, recovery, and robustness.[155,156]

The detection of allergens in food can be impaired by matrix effects. Furthermore, reference standards are only available for a few allergens. For peanut, a standard prepared containing roasted and raw material has been produced by the European Joint Research Centre (JRC). Alternatively, the peanut butter standard from the National Institute of Standards and Technology (NIST) has been used in a number of validation studies. If well-characterized reference material is lacking, such as for soybean allergen and lupin allergen, the protein fraction used in an assay has to be sufficiently described.

The homogeneity and contents of the test material are of great importance for the determination of assay recoveries. There is consensus that incurred standards are preferable to spiked standards.[157] Whereas incurred samples are produced by incorporating allergenic food residues incorporated into various representative food matrices and processing them in a manner similar to "real-world" food processing, spiking is performed by addition of standard protein to blank food matrix and subsequent homogenization.

Assays for the detection of food allergens have to be sensitive enough to ensure consumer protection. Considering that patients had eliciting doses for objective symptoms in food provocation studies as low as 1 mg for peanut,[158] 2 mg for soybean,[159,160] and 265 mg for lupin,[15,86,92] and that subject OASs were observed at even lower allergen contents (e.g., 1 mg for lupin[86]), allergen detection methods have to have limits of detection (LODs) between 1 and 100 mg/kg, depending on the respective food.[122]

A great number of methods for the detection of peanut, soybean, and lupin in foods have been developed, delivering qualitative or quantitative results. They include single-laboratory assays, either thoroughly validated or of more experimental character, and commercially available kits, which sometimes have been validated in multilaboratory tests. The assays show considerable differences in their extraction procedures and buffers, method protocols, standards, incubation times and temperatures, and performance.[161]

Peanut

Published experimental methods and commercial kits for the detection of peanut in foods are enumerated in Table 3.7. With respect to the seriousness of peanut allergy, great efforts are being made regarding assay validation and applicability. Thus, several test kit performance studies for enzyme-linked immunosorbent assay (ELISA), dipstick, and PCR methods have been performed.[113,136,162–170]

Table 3.7 Methods for Peanut Analysis

Method	LOD (mg/kg)	Characteristics	Matrix	References
Immundiffusion	>1,000.0	Antipeanut polyclonal sheep antibody	Cake	134
Rocket immuno-electrophoresis	2	Antipeanut polyclonal sheep antibody	Cake	134
	25	Antipeanut polyclonal rabbit antibody	Candy, chocolate, Cereals, ice cream	171
Dot blot	>2.5	Dot blot cloth-based EIA system; cloth precoated with anti-peanut IgY	Cookies, bars, ice Cream, chocolate	172
	0.1	Multiplex immunoassay	Cookie, chocolate	173
	>2.5	Dot blot	Cookies, ice creams, chocolate	174
Enzyme immunoassays	>2.5	Peanut sandwich ELISA (Veratox)	Cereals, chocolate, cookies, ice cream	Neogen
	>5	Peanut sandwich ELISA (Alert)		Neogen
	1.6	Peanut sandwich ELISA (Prolisa)		Pro-Lab Diagnostics
	0.5	Peanut sandwich ELISA (Via)		Tecra
	>5	Competitive peanut ELISA (Diagnokit)		Abkem Iberia
	2.5	Peanut sandwich ELISA (Ridascreen)		R-Biopharm
	1.5	Ara h 1 sandwich ELISA (Ridas. Fast)		R-Biopharm
	0.1	Ara h 1 sandwich ELISA (BioKits)		Tepnel BioSystems
	>2.5	Ara h 1 - ELISA (Peanut ELISA)		Eurofins Scientific
	1	Ara h 2 sandwich ELISA		Elisa Systems
	1	Ara h 2 sandwich ELISA		Morinaga
	>5	Peanut dipstick (Reveal)		Neogen
	>1	Peanut dipstick		Tepnel Biosystems
	>10	Ara h 1 dipstick (Biokits rapid 3D)		Tepnel Biosystems
	>5	Ara h 1 dipstick (RidaQuick)		R-Biopharm

Table 3.7 (*Continued*) Methods for Peanut Analysis

Method	LOD (mg/kg)	Characteristics	Matrix	References
	87.5	Radioimmuno inhibition assay (IgE)	Var. foods	175
	40	Peanut sandwich ELISA	Cookies, bars, ice cream, chocolate	123
	>0.1	Peanut/sandwich Ara h 1 ELISA	Cookies, bars, Sauce, chocolate	176
	0.4	Peanut competitive ELISA	Cookies, bars, sauce, chocolate	177
	2	Peanut sandwich ELISA	Nuts, cookie, bars, chocolate, Raisins	178
	2	Peanut indirect competitive ELISA	Var. foods	179
	0.1	Immunoaffinity chromatography & ELISA	Chocolate	180
	1	Competitive indirect multiassay	Var. foods	181
	1	Ara h 1 sandwich ELISA	Var. foods	182
	>0.5/12	Competitive ELISA, Ara h1 & Ara h 2	Peanut foods	183
	>10	Peanut sandwich ELISA (sheep/rabbit)	Var. foods	184
	0.2	Monoclonal antibody-polyclonal antibody sandwich ELISA	Var. foods	185
	>100	Ara h 1 peanut dipstick immunoassay	Chocolate, marzipan	186
	1	Dipstick sandwich immunoassay	Var. foods	187
	158	Ara h 1 antibody-based lateral flow	Chocolate	188
RAST/EAST	>3	Patient serum	Peanut products	189
		Patient serum	Sunflower butter	190
		Patient serum	Peanut oil	191
Biosensor	7	Antibody as recognition molecule, SPR	Chocolate	192
	1	Polyclonal antibody, sandwich, plasmon resonance	Chocolate	142

Continued

Table 3.7 (*Continued*) Methods for Peanut Analysis

Method	LOD (mg/kg)	Characteristics	Matrix	References
PCR	>10	PCR agarose gel (Biokits DNA)		Tepnel Biosystems
	>10	RT-PCR (SureFood)		R-Biopharm
	10	PCR-ELISA		R-Biopharm
	12	RT-PCR (Single-AllerGene)		Eurofins Scientific
	6	RT-PCR (Multi-AllerGene)		Eurofins Scientific
	2	RT-PCR, Ara h 2 gene	Cookies, others	193
	>10	RT-PCR, Ara h 2 gene	Var. foods	184
	10	PCR-agarose gel, agglutinin precursor gene	Var. foods	194
	>10	Multiplex PCR, agarose-gel, agglutination precursor gene	Var. Foods	195
	10	RT-PCR, Ara h 3 gene	Var. foods	196
	>1	Qualitative PCR, ITS region		197
Chromatography, mass spectrometry	10	Ara h 1, μLC-ESI-Q-TOF MS	Ice cream	198
	2	Ara h 1, μLC-ESI-Q-TOF MS	Dark chocolate	199
	>1/5	Ara h3/4 and Ara h 2 LC-ESI-MS-MS	Chocolate	200
	3	Ara h 3/4, LC-ESI-IP MS-MS	Breakfast cereals	201
	>7	EU-tagged coupled MS immunoassay	Chocolate	202

Note: ITS = internal transcribed spacer; MS-MS = tandem mass spectrometry; RT = real time; SPR = surface plasmon resonance; Var. = various.

Soybean

Published experimental methods and commercial kits for the detection of soybean in foods are enumerated in Table 3.8. Several of the methods have been evaluated in a comparison study.[124]

Lupin

Lupin has only recently been counted among the major allergens. Consequently, fewer analytical methods for the detection of lupin in foods have been developed. These are enumerated in Table 3.9. Comparative studies have not been published.

Table 3.8 Methods for Soybean Analysis

Method	LOD (mg/kg)	Characteristics	Matrix	References
SDS-gel electrophoresis	600	Improved sample treatment	Melted cheese	203
	100	SDS gel capillary electrophoresis	Milk powder	204
Dot blot	200	Antisoybean rabbit serum	Meat	205
	500	Polyclonal antisoybean rabbit antibody	Crab sticks, kebob, hamburger	134
Immunoblot	>1,000	Kunitz soybean trypsin inhibitor antibody	Meat	206
	200	Antisoybean rabbit serum	Meat	205
	—	Antisoybean rabbit serum	Milk substitutes	207
Enzyme immunoassays	3,000	Competitive assay, polyclonal rabbit antibody	Crab sticks, kebob	Cortecs Diagnostics
	1,400	Soybean competitive ELISA		Tepnel BioSystems
	>100	Soy ELISA		Eurofins Scientific
	0.3	Soy noncompetitive ELISA (BioKits)		Tepnel BioSystems
	1	Soy trypsin inhibitor sandwich ELISA		Elisa Systems
	2.5	Soy flour sandwich ELISA (Veratox)		Neogen
	10	Soy protein sandwich ELISA (Veratox)		Neogen
	>5	Soy flour sandwich ELISA (Alert)		Neogen
	>10	Soy protein sandwich ELISA (Alert)		Neogen
	>5	Dipstick soy protein (rapid 3D)		Tepnel Biosystems
	>1,000	Antisoybean ELISA	Meat	208
	>1,000	Antisoybean ELISA	Meat	209
	100	Antisoybean ELISA	Margarine, soy oil	210
	>1,000	Antisoybean ELISA	Meat	211
	>1,000	Antiglycinin ELISA	Meat	212
	500	Gly m Bd30k sandwich ELISA	Milk, tofu, meat	213

Continued

Table 3.8 (*Continued*) Methods for Soybean Analysis

Method	LOD (mg/kg)	Characteristics	Matrix	References
	140	Gly m Bd28k sandwich ELISA	Milk, tofu	214
	>50	Kunitz soybean trypsin inhibitor monoclonal antibody	Processed foods	215
	2.5	Antiactive soybean lectin ELISA	Hamburger, milk, sprouts	216
	10	Soybean sandwich ELISA	Various foods	125
	0.4	Soybean competitive ELISA	Various foods	125
	1	Soybean direct ELISA	Soy sauce	217
	2	Anticonglycinin competitive ELISA	Paste, meal	218
	0.2	Anti-Gly m 1 sandwich ELISA	Dust samples	219
	0.04	Anti-Gly m 1 sandwich ELISA	Air samples	71
	0.2	Anti-Gly m Bd30k sandwich ELISA	Processed foods	220
	0.05	Direct total soy flake sandwich ELISA	Processed foods	124
	20	Competitive total soy flake ELISA	Processed foods	124
RAST/EAST	—	RAST	Soybean products	221
	1.5	RAST	Soy sauce	217
	—	RAST (2 ng IgE/mg protein)	Soybean ingredients	222
	0.8	EAST (serum 1)	Processed foods	124
	12	EAST (serum 2)	Processed foods	124
Biosensor		Biotinylated soybean lectin gene sequences on chip	Var. foods	223
		Ara h 1-impedance biosensor		224
Cell-based release assay	—	Release of β-N-acetylhexosaminase from rat mucosal mast cells by Gly m Bd 30K; mouse antiserum	Var. food products	225
	0.2	Basophil histamine release assay	Processed foods	124

ALLERGENS IN PEANUT, SOYBEAN, AND LUPIN

Table 3.8 (Continued) Methods for Soybean Analysis

Method	LOD (mg/kg)	Characteristics	Matrix	References
PCR	>10	Soy lectin, PCR-gel (Biokits DNA)	Meat	Tepnel BioSystems
	>10	Soy DNA RT-PCR	Soy sauce	GeneScan USA
	5	Soy DNA RT-PCR (SureFood)	Var. foods	r-Biopharm
	>10	RT-PCR (Single-AllerGene)		Eurofins Scientific
	>10	RT-PCR (Multi-AllerGene)		Eurofins Scientific
	100	Soy lecithin gene PCR	Processed meat	159
	>1	RT-PCR	Var. foods	226
	1	Soy DNA PCR	Milk, diary products	227
	>1	RT-PCR	Var. foods	228
	>1	Qualitative PCR, ITS region		197
Chromatography, mass spectrometry	>1,000	HPLC (polyphenols)	Meat	229
	>100	Retention time by RP-perfusion	Var. foods	230
	138	HPLC-ESI-MS, $\varepsilon(\gamma$-glutamyl)lysine	Plant proteins	231

Note: ESI = electrospray ionization; ITS = internal transcribed spacer; Var. = various.

Table 3.9 Methods for Lupin Analysis

Method	LOD (mg/kg)	Characteristics	Matrix	References
Enzyme immunoassays	1	Polyclonal antibody sandwich ELISA	Var. foods	Hallmark Analytical Ventures
	0.6	Polyclonal antibody sandwich ELISA (Ridascr. Fast)	Var. foods	R-Biopharm
	1	Polyclonal antibody sandwich ELISA	Var. foods	126
	1	Monoclonal antibody-polyclonal antibody lupin sandwich ELISA	Bread, cake, Pasta, chocolate	232
	1	Polyclonal antibody sandwich ELISA	Beef, muffins	233
PCR	10,000	PCR – agarose gel		Coring System Diagnostix
	>100	RT-PCR		Institute for Product Quality
	>5	RT-PCR (SureFood)		R-Biopharm
	0.1	RT-PCR	Var. foods	234
RAST/EAST	>50	Serum IgE	Pasta	123
Chromatography, mass spectrometry	>1,000	HPLC (polyphenols)	Meat	229
	138	HPLC-ESI-MS, $\varepsilon(\gamma$-glutamyl) lysine	Plant proteins	231
	>50	Tryptic peptides, RP-µHPLC-Electrospray MS-MS; *L. albus*	Lupin flakes, lupin beverage	235

Note: Var. = various.

REFERENCES

1. J. P. Lallès and G. Peltre. Biochemical features of grain legume allergens in humans and animals. *Nutr Rev*, 54, 101–107, 1996.
2. M.J. Pereira, M.T. Belver, C.Y. Pascual, and M. Martín Esteban. [The allergenic significance of legumes]. *Allergol Immunopathol (Madr)*, 30, 346–353, 2002.
3. M.D. Ibáñez, M. Martinez, J.J. Sánchez, and E. Fernández-Caldas. [Legume cross-reactivity]. *Allergol Immunopathol (Madr)*, 31, 151–161, 2003.
4. L.B. Jensen, M.H. Pedersen, P.S. Skov, L.K. Poulsen, C. Bindslev-Jensen, S.B. Andersen, and A.M. Torp. Peanut cross-reacting allergens in seeds and sprouts of a range of legumes. *Clin Exp Allergy*, 38, 1969–1977, 2008.
5. C.K. Fæste and E. Namork. Differentiated patterns of legume sensitisation in peanut-allergic patients. *Food Anal Methods*, DOI: 10.1007/s12161–009–9096-x, 2010.
6. C. Radauer, M. Bublin, S. Wagner, A. Mari, and H. Breiteneder. Allergens are distributed into few protein families and possess a restricted number of biochemical functions. *J Allergy Clin Immunol*, 121, 847–852, 2008.
7. A. Mari, C. Rasi, P. Palazzo, and E. Scala. Allergen databases: current status and perspectives. *Curr Allergy Asthma Rep*, 9, 376–383, 2009.
8. R.D. Finn, J. Tate, J. Mistry, P.C. Coggill, S.J. Sammut, H.R. Hotz, G. Ceric, K. Forslund, S.R. Eddy, E.L. Sonnhammer, and A. Bateman. The Pfam protein families database. *Nucleic Acids Res*, 36, D281–D288, 2008.
9. UniProt Consortium. The Universal Protein Resource (UniProt) 2009. *Nucleic Acids Res*, 37, D169–D174, 2009.
10. M.B. Stadler and B.M. Stadler. Allergenicity prediction by protein sequence. *FASEB J*, 17, 1141–1143, 2003.
11. O. Ivanciuc, T. Garcia, M. Torres, C.H. Schein, and W. Braun. Characteristic motifs for families of allergenic proteins. *Mol Immunol*, 46, 559–568, 2009.
12. O. Ivanciuc, C.H. Schein, T. Garcia, N. Oezguen, S.S. Negi, and W. Braun. Structural analysis of linear and conformational epitopes of allergens. *Regul Toxicol Pharmacol*, 54, S11–S19, 2009.
13. M.D. Chapman, A. Pomés, H. Breiteneder, and F. Ferreira. Nomenclature and structural biology of allergens. *J Allergy Clin Immunol*, 119, 414–20, 2007.
14. T.P. King, D. Hoffman, H. Løwenstein, D.G. Marsh, T.A. Platts-Mills, and W. Thomas. Allergen nomenclature. *Allergy*, 50, 765–774, 1995.
15. H. Lindvik, L. Holden, M. Løvik, M. Cvancarova, and R. Halvorsen. Lupin sensitization and clinical allergy in food allergic children in Norway. *Acta Paediatr*, 97, 91–95, 2008.
16. K.A. Peeters, S.J. Koppelman, A.H. Penninks, A. Lebens, C.A. Bruijnzeel-Koomen, S.L. Hefle, S.L. Taylor, E. van Hoffen, and A.C. Knulst. Clinical relevance of sensitization to lupine in peanut-sensitized adults. *Allergy*, 64, 549–55, 2009.
17. H. Breiteneder and E.N.C. Mills. Plant food allergens—structural and functional aspects of allergenicity. *Biotechnol Adv*, 23, 395–399, 2005.
18. C. Radauer and H. Breiteneder. Evolutionary biology of plant food allergens. *J Allergy Clin Immunol*, 120, 518–525, 2007.
19. H. Breiteneder and C. Radauer. A classification of plant food allergens. *J Allergy Clin Immunol*, 113, 821–830, 2004.
20. H. Breiteneder and E.N. Mills. Molecular properties of food allergens. *J Allergy Clin Immunol*, 115, 14–23, 2005.

21. E.N. Mills, J.A. Jenkins, M.J. Alcocer, and P.R. Shewry. Structural, biological, and evolutionary relationships of plant food allergens sensitizing via the gastrointestinal tract. *Crit Rev Food Sci Nutr*, 44, 379–407, 2004.
22. G. Salcedo, R. Sánchez-Monge, D. Barber, and A. Díaz-Perales. Plant non-specific lipid transfer proteins: an interface between plant defence and human allergy. *Biochim Biophys Acta*, 771, 781–791, 2007.
23. R. van Ree. Clinical importance of non-specific lipid transfer proteins as food allergens. *Biochem Soc Trans*, 30, 910–913, 2002.
24. F. Baud, E. Pebay-Peyroula, C. Cohen-Addad, S. Odani, and M.S. Lehmann. Crystal structure of hydrophobic protein soybean; a member of a new cysteine-rich family. *J Mol Biol*, 231, 877, 1993.
25. S. Huang, J.M. McDowell, M.J. Weise, and R.B. Meagher. The *Arabidopsis* profilin gene family. Evidence for an ancient split between constitutive and pollen-specific profilin genes. *Plant Physiol*, 111, 115–126, 1996.
26. C. Radauer and H. Breiteneder. Pollen allergens are restricted to few protein families and show distinct patterns of species distribution. *J Allergy Clin Immunol*, 117, 141–147, 2006.
27. J.M. Dunwell, A. Purvis, and S. Khuri. Cupins: the most functionally diverse protein superfamily? *Phytochemistry*, 65, 7–17, 2004.
28. E. Derbyshire, D.J. Wright, and D. Boulter. Legumin and vicilin, storage proteins of legume seeds. *Phytochemistry*, 15, 3–24, 1976.
29. P. Argos, S.V. Narayana, and N.C. Nielsen. Structural similarity between legumin and vicilin storage proteins from legumes. *EMBO J*, 4, 1111–7, 1985.
30. E.N.C. Mills, C. Madsen, P.R. Shewry, and H.J. Wichers. Food allergens of plant origin—their molecular and evolutionary relationships. *Trends Food Sci Technol*, 14, 145–156, 2003.
31. N. Maruyama, M. Adachi, K. Takahashi, K. Yagasaki, M. Kohno, Y. Takenaka, E. Okuda, S. Nakagawa, B. Mikami, and S. Utsumi. Crystal structures of recombinant and native soybean beta-conglycinin beta homotrimers. *Eur J Biochem*, 268, 3595–3604, 2001.
32. M. Adachi, J. Kanamori, T. Masuda, K. Yagasaki, K. Kitamura, B. Mikami, and S. Utsumi. Crystal structure of soybean 11S globulin: glycinin A3B4 homohexamer. *Proc Natl Acad Sci USA*, 100, 7395–7400, 2003.
33. J. Jenkins, S. Griffiths-Jones, P. Shewry, H. Breiteneder, and E. Mills. Structural relatedness of plant food allergens with specific reference to cross-reactive allergens: an in silico analysis. *J Allergy Clin Immunol*, 115, 163–170, 2005.
34. F. Capuano, F. Beaudoin, J.A. Napier, and P.R. Shewry. Properties and exploitation of oleosins. *Biotechnol Adv*, 25, 203–206, 2007.
35. L. Pons, C. Chery, A. Romano, F. Namour, M.C. Artesani, and J.L. Guéant. The 18 kDa peanut oleosin is a candidate allergen for IgE-mediated reactions to peanuts. *Allergy*, 57, 88–93, 2002.
36. R.F. Steiner. Accessibility and structural function of particular amino acid residues of soy bean trypsin inhibition. *Arch Biochem Biophys*, 115, 257–270, 1966.
37. A.W. Burks, G. Cockrell, C. Connaughton, J. Guin, W. Allen, and R.M. Helm. Identification of peanut agglutinin and soybean trypsin inhibitor as minor legume allergens. *Int Arch Allergy Immunol*, 105, 143–149, 1994.
38. N. Sharon and H. Lis. Legume lectins-a large family of homologous proteins. *FASEB J*, 4, 3198–3208, 1990.

39. M. Himly, B. Jahn-Schmid, A. Dedic, P. Kelemen, N. Wopfner, F. Altmann, R. van Ree, P. Briza, K. Richter, C. Ebner, and F. Ferreira. Art v 1, the major allergen of mugwort pollen, is a modular glycoprotein with a defensin-like and a hydroxyproline-rich domain. *FASEB J*, 17, 106–108, 2003.
40. P.B. Szecsi. The aspartic proteases. *Scand J Clin Lab Invest Suppl*, 210, 5–22, 1992.
41. J.O. Hourihane. Recent advances in peanut allergy. *Curr Opin Allergy Clin Immunol*, 2, 227–231, 2002.
42. S.A. Bock, A. Muñoz-Furlong, and H.A. Sampson. Fatalities due to anaphylactic reactions to foods. *J Allergy Clin Immunol*, 107, 191–193, 2001.
43. J. Grundy, S. Matthews, B. Bateman, T. Dean, and S.H. Arshad. Rising prevalence of allergy to peanut in children: data from two sequential cohorts. *J Allergy Clin Immunol*, 110, 784–789, 2002.
44. T. Kleber-Janke, R. Crameri, U. Appenzeller, M. Schlaak, and W.M. Becker. Selective cloning of peanut allergens, including profilin and 2S albumins, by phage display technology. *Int Arch Allergy Immunol*, 119, 265–274, 1999.
45. J. Marsh, N. Rigby, K. Wellner, G. Reese, A. Knulst, J. Akkerdaas, R. van Ree, C. Radauer, A. Lovegrove, A. Sancho, C. Mills, S. Vieths, K. Hoffmann-Sommergruber, and P.R. Shewry. Purification and characterisation of a panel of peanut allergens suitable for use in allergy diagnosis. *Mol Nutr Food Res*, 52, S272–S285, 2008.
46. D.S. Shin, C.M. Compadre, S.J. Maleki, R.A. Kopper, H. Sampson, S.K. Huang, A.W. Burks, and G.A. Bannon. Biochemical and structural analysis of the IgE binding sites on Ara h 1, an abundant and highly allergenic peanut protein. *J Biol Chem*, 273, 13753–13759, 1998.
47. S.J. Koppelman, M. Wensing, M. Ertmann, A.C. Knulst, and E.F. Knol. Relevance of Ara h 1, Ara h 2 and Ara h 3 in peanut-allergic patients, as determined by immunoglobulin E Western blotting, basophil-histamine release and intracutaneous testing: Ara h 2 is the most important peanut allergen. *Clin Exp Allergy*, 34, 583–590, 2004.
48. A.W. Burks, D. Shin, G. Cockrell, J.S. Stanley, R.M. Helm, and G.A. Bannon. Mapping and mutational analysis of the IgE-binding epitopes on Ara h 1, a legume vicilin protein and a major allergen in peanut hypersensitivity. *Eur J Biochem*, 245, 334–339, 1997.
49. M.M. Dooper, C. Plassen, L. Holden, H. Lindvik, and C.K. Faeste. Immunoglobulin E cross-reactivity between lupine conglutins and peanut allergens in serum of lupine-allergic individuals. *J Investig Allergol Clin Immunol*, 19, 283–291, 2009.
50. K. Lehmann, K. Schweimer, G. Reese, S. Randow, M. Suhr, W.M. Becker, S. Vieths, and P. Rösch. Structure and stability of 2S albumin-type peanut allergens: implications for the severity of peanut allergic reactions. *Biochem J*, 395, 463–472, 2006.
51. S.R. Piersma, M. Gaspari, S.L. Hefle, and S.J. Koppelman. Proteolytic processing of the peanut allergen Ara h 3. *Mol Nutr Food Res*, 49, 744–755, 2005.
52. P. Rabjohn, E.M. Helm, J.S. Stanley, C.M. West, H.A. Sampson, A.W. Burks, and G.A. Bannon. Molecular cloning and epitope analysis of the peanut allergen Ara h 3. *J Clin Invest*, 103, 535–542, 1999.
53. A. Barre, G. Jacquet, C. Sordet, R. Culerrier, and P. Rougé. Homology modelling and conformational analysis of IgE-binding epitopes of Ara h 3 and other legumin allergens with a cupin fold from tree nuts. *Mol Immunol*, 44, 3243–3255, 2007.
54. E.L. van Boxtel, L.A. van den Broek, S.J. Koppelman, and H. Gruppen. Legumin allergens from peanuts and soybeans: effects of denaturation and aggregation on allergenicity. *Mol Nutr Food Res*, 52, 674–682, 2008.

55. B. Guo, X. Liang, S.Y. Chung, and S.J. Maleki. Proteomic screening points to the potential importance of Ara h 3 basic subunit in allergenicity of peanut. *Inflamm Allergy Drug Targets*, 7, 163–166, 2008.
56. T. Kleber-Janke, R. Crameri, S. Scheurer, S. Vieths, and W.M. Becker. Patient-tailored cloning of allergens by phage display: peanut (*Arachis hypogaea*) profilin, a food allergen derived from a rare mRNA. *J Chromatogr B Biomed Sci Appl*, 756, 295–305, 2001.
57. S. Riecken, B. Lindner, A. Petersen, U. Jappe, and W.M. Becker. Purification and characterization of natural Ara h 8, the Bet v 1 homologous allergen from peanut, provides a novel isoform. *Biol Chem*, 389, 415–423, 2008.
58. S. Krause, G. Reese, S. Randow, D. Zennaro, D. Quaratino, P. Palazzo, M.A. Ciardiello, A. Petersen, W.M. Becker, and A. Mari. Lipid transfer protein (Ara h 9) as a new peanut allergen relevant for a Mediterranean allergic population. *J Allergy Clin Immunol*, 124, 771–778, 2009.
59. I. Lauer, N. Dueringer, S. Pokoj, S. Rehm, G. Zoccatelli, G. Reese, M.S. Miguel-Moncin, A. Cistero-Bahima, E. Enrique, J. Lidholm, S. Vieths, and S. Scheurer. The non-specific lipid transfer protein, Ara h 9, is an important allergen in peanut. *Clin Exp Allergy*, 39, 1427–1437, 2009.
60. S.E. Stevenson, Y. Chu, P. Ozias-Akins, and J.J. Thelen. Validation of gel-free, label-free quantitative proteomics approaches: applications for seed allergen profiling. *J Proteomics*, 72, 555–566, 2009.
61. E. Rodriguez-Arango, R. Arango, R. Adar, G. Galili, and N. Sharon. Cloning, sequence analysis and expression in *Escherichia coli* of the cDNA encoding a precursor of peanut agglutinin. *FEBS Lett*, 307, 185–189, 1992. Erratum in: *FEBS Lett*, 310, 204, 1992.
62. P. Gruber, W.M. Becker, and T. Hofmann. Influence of the Maillard reaction on the allergenicity of rAra h 2, a recombinant major allergen from peanut (*Arachis hypogaea*), its major epitopes, and peanut agglutinin. *J Agric Food Chem*, 53, 2289–2296, 2005.
63. E.W. Lusas and M.N. Rias. Soy protein products: processing and use. *J Nutr*, 125, 573S–580S, 1995.
64. B.K. Ballmer-Weber and S. Vieths. Soy allergy in perspective. *Curr Opin Allergy Clin Immunol*, 8, 270–275, 2008.
65. M. Osterballe, C.G. Mortz, T.K. Hansen, K.E. Andersen, and C. Bindslev-Jensen. The prevalence of food hypersensitivity in young adults. *Pediatr Allergy Immunol*, 20, 686–692, 2009.
66. L. Zuidmeer, K. Goldhahn, R.J. Rona, D. Gislason, C. Madsen, C. Summers, E. Sodergren, J. Dahlstrom, T. Lindner, S.T. Sigurdardottir, D. McBride, and T. Keil. The prevalence of plant food allergies: a systematic review. *J Allergy Clin Immunol*, 121, 1210–1218, 2008.
67. C. Gagnon, V. Poysa, E.R. Cober, and S. Gleddie. Soybean allergens affecting North American patients identified by 2D Gels and mass spectrometry. *Food Anal Meth*, DOI 10.1007/s12161-009-9090-3, 2009.
68. T. Ogawa, M. Samoto, and K. Takahashi. Soybean allergens and hypoallergenic soybean products. *J Nutr Sci Vitaminol*, 46, 271–279, 2000.
69. M. Hajduch, A. Ganapathy, J.W. Stein, and J.J. Thelen. A systematic proteomic study of seed filling in soybean. Establishment of high-resolution two-dimensional reference maps, expression profiles, and an interactive proteome database. *Plant Physiol*, 137, 1397–1419, 2005.
70. R. González, J. Varela, J. Carreira, and F. Polo. Soybean hydrophobic protein and soybean hull allergy. *Lancet*, 346, 48–49, 1995.

71. S. Gómez-Ollés, M.J. Cruz, A. Renström, G. Doekes, F. Morell, and M.J. Rodrigo. An amplified sandwich EIA for the measurement of soy aeroallergens. *Clin Exp Allergy*, 36, 1176–1183, 2006.
72. R. Codina, L. Ardusso, R.F. Lockey, C.D. Crisci, C. Jaén, and N.H. Bertoya. Identification of the soybean hull allergens involved in sensitization to soybean dust in a rural population from Argentina and N-terminal sequence of a major 50 KD allergen. *Clin Exp Allergy*, 32, 1059–1063, 2002.
73. H.P. Rihs, Z. Chen, F. Ruëff, A. Petersen, P. Rozynek, H. Heimann, and X. Baur. IgE binding of the recombinant allergen soybean profilin (rGly m 3) is mediated by conformational epitopes. *J Allergy Clin Immunol*, 104, 1293–1301, 1999.
74. D. Mittag, S. Vieths, L. Vogel, W.M. Becker, H.P. Rihs, A. Helbling, B. Wüthrich, and B.K. Ballmer-Weber. Soybean allergy in patients allergic to birch pollen: clinical investigation and molecular characterization of allergens. *J Allergy Clin Immunol*, 113, 148–154, 2004.
75. J. Kleine-Tebbe, L. Vogel, D.N. Crowell, U.F. Haustein, and S. Vieths. Severe oral allergy syndrome and anaphylactic reactions caused by a Bet v 1-related PR-10 protein in soybean, SAM22. *J Allergy Clin Immunol*, 110, 797–804, 2002.
76. T. Holzhauser, O. Wackermann, B.K. Ballmer-Weber, C. Bindslev-Jensen, J. Scibilia, L. Perono-Garoffo, S. Utsumi, L.K. Poulsen, and S. Vieths. Soybean (*Glycine max*) allergy in Europe: Gly m 5 ([beta]-conglycinin) and Gly m 6 (glycinin) are potential diagnostic markers for severe allergic reactions to soy. *J Allergy Clin Immunol*, 123, 452–458, 2009.
77. J. Lin, P.R. Shewry, D.B. Archer, K. Beyer, B. Niggemann, H. Haas, P. Wilson, and M.J.C. Alcocer. The potential allergenicity of two 2S albumins from soybean (*Glycine max*): a protein microarray approach. *Int Arch Allergy Immunol*, 141, 91–102, 2006.
78. S. Wilson, C. Martinez-Villaluenga, and E.G. de Mejia. Purification, thermal stability, and antigenicity of the immunodominant soybean allergen P34 in soy cultivars, ingredients, and products. *J Food Sci*, 73, T106–T114, 2008.
79. C. Sarmiento, J.H. Ross, E. Herman, and D.J. Murphy. Expression and subcellular targeting of a soybean oleosin in transgenic rapeseed. Implications for the mechanism of oil-body formation in seeds. *Plant J*, 11, 783–796, 1997.
80. A. Yagami, Y. Inaba, Y. Kuno, K. Suzuki, A. Tanaka, S. Sjolander, H. Saito, and K. Matsunaga. 2009. Two cases of pollen-food allergy syndrome to soy milk diagnosed by skin prick test, specific serum immunoglobulin E and microarray analysis. *J Dermatol*, 36, 50–55, 2009.
81. C. Gotor, J.A. Pintor-Toro, and L.C. Romero. Isolation of a new member of the soybean Kunitz-type proteinase inhibitors. *Plant Physiol*, 107, 1015–1016, 1995.
82. R. Batista, I. Martins, P. Jeno, C.P. Ricardo, and M.M. Oliveira. A proteomic study to identify soya allergens—the human response to transgenic versus non-transgenic soya samples. *J Int Arch Allerg Immunol*, 144, 29–38, 2007.
83. R. Uauy, V. Gattas, and E. Yañez. Sweet lupins in human nutrition. *World Rev Nutr Diet*, 77, 75–88, 1995.
84. Y.P. Lee, T.A. Mori, S. Sipsas, A. Barden, I.B. Puddey, V. Burke, R.S. Hall, and J.M. Hodgson. Lupin-enriched bread increases satiety and reduces energy intake acutely. *Am J Clin Nutr*, 84, 975–980, 2006.
85. S. Brennecke, W.M. Becker, U. Lepp, and U. Jappe. Anaphylactic reaction to lupine flour. *J Dtsch Dermatol Ges*, 5, 774–776, 2007.
86. K.A. Peeters, J.A. Nordlee, A.H. Penninks, L. Chen, R.E. Goodman, C.A. Bruijnzeel-Koomen, S.L. Hefle, S.L. Taylor, and A.C. Knulst. Lupine allergy: not simply cross-reactivity with peanut or soy. *J Allergy Clin Immunol*, 120, 647–653, 2007.

87. B. Wüthrich. Anaphylactic reaction to lupine flour because of a primary sensitization. *Allergy*, 63, 476–477, 2008.
88. E. Novembre, M. Moriondo, R. Bernadini, C. Azzari, M.E. Rossi, and A. Vierucci. Lupin allergy in a child. *J Allergy Clin Immunol*, 103, 1214–1216, 1999.
89. A.M. Reis, N.P. Fernandes, S.L. Marques, M.J. Paes, S. Sousa, F. Carvalho, T. Conde, and M. Trindade. Lupine sensitisation in a population of 1,160 subjects. *Allergol Immunopathol (Madr)*, 35, 162–163, 2007.
90. C.P. Campbell, A.S. Jackson, A.R. Johnson, P.S. Thomas, and D.H. Yates. Occupational sensitization to lupin in the workplace: occupational asthma, rhinitis, and work-aggravated asthma. *J Allergy Clin Immunol*, 119, 1133–1139, 2007.
91. S.L. Hefle, R.F. Lemanske Jr, and R.K. Bush. Adverse-reaction to lupine-fortified pasta. *J Allergy Clin Immunol*, 94, 167–172, 1994.
92. D.A. Moneret-Vautrin, L. Guérin, G. Kanny, J. Flabbé, S. Frémont, and M. Morisset. Cross-allergenicity of peanut and lupine: the risk of lupine allergy in patients allergic to peanuts. *J Allergy Clin Immunol*, 104, 883–888, 1999.
93. C.K. Fæste, M. Løvik, H.G. Wiker, and E. Egaas. A case of peanut cross-allergy to lupine flour in a hot dog bread. *Int Arch Allergy Immunol*, 135, 36–39, 2004.
94. J. Shaw, G. Roberts, K. Grimshaw, S. White, and J. Hourihane. Lupin allergy in peanut-allergic children and teenagers. *Allergy*, 63, 370–373, 2008.
95. T.S. Melo, R.B. Ferreira, and A.N. Teixeira. The seed storage proteins from *Lupinus albus*. *Phytochemistry*, 37, 641–648, 1994.
96. M. Duranti, C. Gius, F. Sessa, and G. Vecchio. The saccharide chain of lupin seed conglutin gamma is not responsible for the protection of the native protein from degradation by trypsin, but facilitates the refolding of the acid-treated protein to the resistant conformation. *Eur J Biochem*, 230, 886–891, 1995.
97. L. Holden, G.B.G. Sletten, H. Lindvik, C.K. Fæste, and M.M.B.W. Dooper. Characterization of IgE binding to lupin, peanut and almond with sera from lupin-allergic patients. *Int Arch Allergy Immunol*, 146, 267–276, 2008.
98. A. Fiocchi, P. Sarratud, L. Terracciano, E. Vacca, R. Bernardini, D. Fuggetta, C. Ballabio, M. Duranti, C. Magni, and P. Restani. Assessment of the tolerance to lupine-enriched pasta in peanut-allergic children. *Clin Exp Allergy*, 39, 1045–1051, 2009.
99. M. Duranti, F. Sessa, and A. Carpen. Identification, purification and properties of the precursor of conglutin β, the 7S storage globulin in *Lupinus albus* L. seeds. *J Exp Bot*, 43, 1373–1378, 1992.
100. D.E. Goggin, G. Mir, W.B. Smith, M. Stuckey, and P.M. Smith. Proteomic analysis of lupin seed proteins to identify conglutin beta as an allergen, Lup an 1. *J Agric Food Chem*, 56, 6370–6377, 2008.
101. S.C. Ilgoutz, N. Knittel, J.M. Lin, S. Sterle, and K.R. Gayler. Transcription of genes for conglutin gamma and a leginsulin-like protein in narrow-leafed lupin. *Plant Mol Biol*, 34, 613–627, 1997.
102. A. Scarafoni, A. di Cataldo, T.D. Vassilevskaia, E.P. Bekman, C. Rodrigues-Pousada, F. Ceciliani, and M. Duranti. Cloning, sequencing and expression in the seeds and radicles of two *Lupinus albus* conglutin γ genes. *Biochim Biophys Acta*, 1519, 147–151, 2001.
103. C. Magni, A. Scarafoni, A. Herndl, F. Sessa, B. Prinsi, L. Espen, and M. Duranti. Combined 2D electrophoretic approaches for the study of white lupin mature seed storage proteome. *Phytochemistry*, 68, 997–1007, 2007.

104. O. Pasternak, J. Biesiadka, R. Dolot, L. Handschuh, G. Bujacz, M.M. Sikorski, and M. Jaskolski. Structure of a yellow lupin pathogenesis-related PR-10 protein belonging to a novel subclass. *Acta Crystallogr D Biol Crystallogr*, 61, 99–107, 2005.
105. B. Bantignies, J. Séguin, I. Muzac, F. Dédaldéchamp, P. Gulick, and R. Ibrahim. Direct evidence for ribonucleolytic activity of a PR-10-like protein from white lupin roots. *Plant Mol Biol*, 42, 871–881, 2000.
106. M.W. Trucksess, T.B. Whitaker, A.B. Slate, K.M. Williams, V.A. Brewer, P. Whittaker, and J.T. Heeres. Variation of analytical results for peanuts in energy bars and milk chocolate. *J AOAC Int*, 87, 943–949, 2004.
107. S.J. Maleki and B.K. Hurlburt. Structural and functional alterations in major peanut allergens caused by thermal processing. *J AOAC Int*, 87,1475–1479, 2004.
108. D.A. Moneret-Vautrin. Modifications of allergenicity linked to food technologies. *Allerg Immunol (Paris)*, 30, 9–13, 1998.
109. P. Franck, D.A. Moneret Vautrin, B. Dousset, G. Kanny, P. Nabet, L. Guénard-Bilbaut, and L. Parisot. The allergenicity of soybean-based products is modified by food technologies. *Int Arch Allergy Immunol*, 128, 212–219, 2002.
110. R.E. Poms, C. Capelletti, and E. Anklam. Effect of roasting history and buffer composition on peanut protein extraction efficiency. *Mol Nutr Food Res*, 48, 459–464, 2004.
111. F. van Wijk, S. Nierkens, I. Hassing, M. Feijen, S.J. Koppelman, G.A. de Jong, R. Pieters, and L.M. Knippels. The effect of the food matrix on in vivo immune responses to purified peanut allergens. *Toxicol Sci*, 86, 333–341, 2005.
112. J. Alvarez-Alvarez, E. Guillamon, J.F. Crespo, C. Cuadrado, C. Burbano, J. Rodriguez, C. Fernandez, and M. Muzquiz. Effects of extrusion, boiling, autoclaving, and microwave heating on lupine allergenicity. *J Agric Food Chem,* 53, 1294–1298, 2005.
113. E. Scaravelli, M. Brohée, R. Marchelli, and A.J. van Hengel. The effect of heat treatment on the detection of peanut allergens as determined by ELISA and real-time PCR. *Anal Bioanal Chem*, 395, 127–137, 2009.
114. C.D. Westphal, M.R. Pereira, R.B. Raybourne, and K.M. Williams. Evaluation of extraction buffers using the current approach of detecting multiple allergenic and nonallergenic proteins in food. *J AOAC Int*, 871458–871465, 2004.
115. C.K. Fæste, K.E. Løvberg, H. Lindvik, and E. Egaas. Extractability, stability, and allergenicity of egg white proteins in differently heat-processed foods. *J AOAC Int*, 90, 427–436, 2007.
116. K. Supli, N. Gryson, K. Messens, M. De Loose, and K. Dewettinck. Extraction and PCR analysis of soy DNA in chocolate. *Meded Rijksuniv Gent Fak Landbouwkd Toegep Biol Wet*, 66, 631–634, 2001.
117. P.R. Goodwin. Food allergen detection methods: a coordinated approach. *J AOAC Int*, 87, 1383–1890, 2004.
118. E. Sironi, F. Sessa, and D. Marcello. A simple procedure of lupin seed protein fractionation for selective food applications. *Eur Food Res Technol*, 221, 145–150, 2005.
119. R.L. Freitas, R.B. Ferreira, and A.R. Teixeira. Use of a single method in the extraction of the seed storage globulins from several legume species. Application to analyse structural comparisons within the major classes of globulins. *Int J Food Sci Nutr*, 51, 341–352, 2000.
120. A.W. Burks, G. Cockrell, C. Connaughton, and R.M. Helm. Epitope specificity and immunoaffinity purification of the major peanut allergen, Ara h I. *J Allergy Clin Immunol*, 93, 743–750, 1994.

121. H. Tsuji, N. Bando, M. Hiemori, R. Yamanishi, M. Kimoto, K. Nishikawa, and T. Ogawa. Purification of characterization of soybean allergen Gly m Bd 28K. *Biosci Biotechnol Biochem*, 61, 942–947, 1997.
122. R.E. Poms, C.L. Klein, and E. Anklam. Methods for allergen analysis in food: a review. *Food Addit Contam*, 21, 1–31, 2004.
123. S.L. Hefle, R.K. Bush, J.W. Yunginger, and F.S. Chu. A sandwich enzyme-linked immunosorbent assay (ELISA) for the quantitation of selected peanut proteins in foods. *J Food Protec*, 57, 419–423, 1994.
124. M.H. Pedersen, T. Holzhauser, C. Bisson, A. Conti, L.B. Jensen, P.S. Skov, C. Bindslev-Jensen, D.S. Brinch, and L.K. Poulsen. Soybean allergen detection methods--a comparison study. *Mol Nutr Food Res*, 52, 1486–1496, 2008.
125. S.J. Koppelman, C.M. Lakemond, R. Vlooswijk, and S.L. Hefle. Detection of soy proteins in processed foods: literature overview and new experimental work. *J AOAC Int*, 87, 1398–1407, 2004.
126. L. Holden, C.K. Faeste, and E. Egaas. Quantitative sandwich ELISA for the determination of lupine (*Lupinus* spp.) in foods. *J Agric Food Chem*, 53, 5866–5871, 2005.
127. M.M. Dooper, L. Holden, C.K. Fæste, K.M. Thompson, and E. Egaas. Monoclonal antibodies against the candidate lupin allergens alpha-conglutin and beta-conglutin. *Int Arch Allergy Immunol*, 143, 49–58, 2007.
128. E. Franco, R.B. Ferreira, and A.N. Teixeira. Utilization of an improved methodology to isolate *Lupinus albus* conglutins in the study of their sedimentation coefficients. *J Agric Food Chem*, 45, 3908–3913, 1997.
129. H.F. Moutete, A. Olszewski, I. Gastin, F. Namour, D.A. Moneret-Vautrin, and J.L. Guéant. Purification of allergenic proteins from peanut for preparative of the reactive solid phase of a specific IgE radioimmunoassay. *J Chromatogr B Biomed Appl*, 64, 211–217, 1995.
130. H.B. Krishnan, N.W. Oehrle, and S.S. Natarajan. A rapid and simple procedure for the depletion of abundant storage proteins from legume seeds to advance proteome analysis: a case study using *Glycine max*. *Proteomics*, 9, 3174–3188, 2009.
131. R.J. Blagrove and J.M. Gillespie. Isolation, purification and characterization of the seed globulins of *Lupinus angustifolius*. *Austr J Plant Physiol*, 2, 13–27, 1975.
132. S. Kirsch, S. Fourdrilis, R. Dobson, M.-L. Scippo, G. Maghuin-Rogister, and E. De Pauw. Quantitative methods for food allergens: a review. *Anal Bioanal Chem*, 395, 57–67, 2009.
133. R.E. Poms, E. Anklam, and M. Kuhn. Polymerase chain reaction techniques for food allergen detection. *J AOAC Int*, 87, 1391–1397, 2004.
134. I. Malmheden Yman, A. Eriksson, T. Karlsson, and L. Yman. Adverse reactions to food. Analysis of food proteins for verification of contamination or mislabelling. *Food Agric Immunol*, 6, 167–172, 1994.
135. J.J. Thelen. Proteomics tools and resources for investigating protein allergens in oilseeds. *Regul Toxicol Pharmacol*, 54, S41–S45, 2009.
136. P. Koch, G.F. Schäppi, R.E. Poms, B. Wüthrich, E. Anklam, and R. Battaglia. Comparison of commercially available ELISA kits with human sera-based detection methods for peanut allergens in foods. *Food Addit Contam*, 20, 797–803, 2003.
137. B. Scheibe, W. Weiss, F. Ruëff, B. Przybilla, and A. Görg. Detection of trace amounts of hidden allergens: hazelnut and almond proteins in chocolate. *J Chromatogr B Biomed Sci Appl*, 756, 229–237, 2001.
138. S.L. Taylor and J.A. Nordlee. Immunological analysis of food allergens and other food proteins. *Food Technol*, 50, 231, 1996.

139. S.J. Koppelman, A.C. Knulst, W.J. Koers, A.H. Penninks, H. Peppelman, R. Vlooswijk, I. Pigmans, G. van Duijn, and M. Hessing. Comparison of different immunochemical methods for the detection and quantification of hazelnut proteins in food products. *J Immunol Methods*, 229, 107–120, 1999.
140. R.E. Poms and E. Anklam. Tracking and tracing for allergen-free food production chains. *Wageningen UR Frontis Series*, 10, 77–83, 2006.
141. L.C. Shriver-Lake, C.R. Taitt, and F.S. Ligler. Applications of array biosensor for detection of food allergens. *J AOAC Int*, 87, 1498–1502, 2004.
142. I. Malmheden Yman, A. Eriksson, M.A. Johansson, and K.E. Hellenäs. Food allergen detection with biosensor immunoassays. *J AOAC Int*, 89, 856–861, 2006.
143. S.T. Holgate, M.K. Church, and L.M. Lichtenstein. Effector cells of allergy. In: S.T. Holgate, M.K. Church, L.M. Lichtenstein, eds., *Allergy*, 2nd ed. London: Mosby, pp. 303–310, 2001.
144. M. Careri and A. Mangia. Analysis of food proteins and peptides by chromatography and mass spectrometry. *J Chromatogr A*, 1000, 609–635, 2003.
145. H.-W. Wen, W. Borejsza-Wysocki, T.R. DeCory, and R.A. Durst. Peanut allergy, peanut allergens, and methods for the detection of peanut contamination in food products. *Compr Rev Food Sci Food Safety*, 6, 47–58, 2007.
146. H. Chassaigne, J.V. Nørgaard, and A.J. Hengel. Proteomics-based approach to detect and identify major allergens in processed peanuts by capillary LC-Q-TOF (MS/MS). *J Agric Food Chem*, 55, 4461–4473, 2007.
147. H. Chassaigne, V. Trégoat, J.V. Nørgaard, S.J. Maleki, and A.J. van Hengel. Resolution and identification of major peanut allergens using a combination of fluorescence two-dimensional differential gel electrophoresis, Western blotting and Q-TOF mass spectrometry. *J Proteomics*, 72, 511–526, 2009.
148. A. Leitner, F. Castro-Rubio, M.L. Marina, and W. Lindner. Identification of marker proteins for the adulteration of meat products with soybean proteins by multidimensional liquid chromatography-tandem mass spectrometry. *J Proteome Res*, 5, 2424–2430, 2006.
149. S.S. Natarajan, H.B. Krishnan, S. Lakshman, and W.M. Garrett. An efficient extraction method to enhance analysis of low abundant proteins from soybean seed. *Anal Biochem*, 394, 259–268, 2009.
150. R.R. Quaresma, R. Viseu, L.M. Martins, E. Tomaz, and F. Inácio. Allergic primary sensitization to lupine seed. *Allergy*, 62, 1473–1474, 2007.
151. J. Biesiadka, M.M. Sikorski, G. Bujacz, and M. Jaskólski. Crystallization and preliminary x-ray structure determination of *Lupinus luteus* PR10 protein. *Acta Crystallogr D Biol Crystallogr*, 55, 1925–1927, 1999.
152. C. Magni, A. Herndl, E. Sironi, A. Scarafoni, C. Ballabio, P. Restani, R. Bernardini, E. Novembre, A. Vierucci, and M. Duranti. One- and two-dimensional electrophoretic identification of IgE-binding polypeptides of *Lupinus albus* and other legume seeds. *J Agric Food Chem*, 53, 4567–4571, 2005.
153. T. Schwend, I. Redwanz, T. Ruppert, A. Szenthe, and M. Wink. Analysis of proteins in the spent culture medium of *Lupinus albus* by electrospray ionisation tandem mass spectrometry. *J Chromatogr A*, 1009, 105–110, 2003.
154. R. Wait, E. Gianazza, D. Brambilla, I. Eberini, S. Morandi, A. Arnoldi, and C.R. Sirtori. Analysis of *Lupinus albus* storage proteins by two-dimensional electrophoresis and mass spectrometry. *J Agric Food Chem*, 53, 4599–4606, 2005.
155. M. Thompson, S.L.R. Ellison, and R. Wood. Harmonized guidelines for single-laboratory validation of methods of analysis. *Pure Appl Chem*, 74, 835–855, 2002.

156. M.J. Walker, P. Colwell, S. Elahi, K. Gray, and I. Lumley. Food allergen detection: a literature review 2004–2007. *J Assoc Publ Analysts*, 36, 1–18, 2008.
157. S.L. Taylor, J.A. Nordlee, L.M. Niemann, and D.M. Lambrecht. Allergen immunoassays--considerations for use of naturally incurred standards. *Anal Bioanal Chem*, 395, 83–92, 2009.
158. S.L. Taylor, S.L. Hefle, C. Bindslev-Jensen, S.A. Bock, A.W. Burks Jr, L. Christie, D.J. Hill, A. Host, J.O. Hourihane, G. Lack, D.D. Metcalfe, D.A. Moneret-Vautrin, P.A. Vadas, F. Rance, D.J. Skrypec, T.A. Trautman, I.M. Yman, and R.S. Zeiger. Factors affecting the determination of threshold doses for allergenic foods: how much is too much? *J Allergy Clin Immunol*, 109, 24–30, 2002.
159. R. Meyer, U. Candrian, and J. Lüthy. Polymerase chain reaction (PCR) in the quality and safety assurance of food: detection of soya in processed meat products. *Z Lebensm Untersuch Forsch*, 203, 339–344, 1996.
160. B.K. Ballmer-Weber, T. Holzhauser, J. Scibilia, D. Mittag, G. Zisa, C. Ortolani, M. Oesterballe, L.K. Poulsen, S. Vieths, and C. Bindslev-Jensen. Clinical characteristics of soybean allergy in Europe: a double-blind, placebo-controlled food challenge study. *J Allergy Clin Immunol*, 119, 1489–1496, 2007.
161. P. Schubert-Ullrich, J. Rudolf, P. Ansari, B. Galler, M. Führer, A. Molinelli, and S. Baumgartner. Commercialized rapid immunoanalytical tests for determination of allergenic food proteins: an overview. *Anal Bioanal Chem*, 395, 69–81, 2009.
162. W.J. Hurst, E.R. Krout, and W.R. Burks. A comparison of commercially available peanut ELISA test kits on the analysis of samples of dark and milk chocolate. *J Immunoassay Immunochem*, 23, 451–459, 2002.
163. R.E. Poms, C. Lisi, C. Summa, J. Stroka, and E. Anklam. In-house validation of commercially available ELISA test kits for peanut allergens in food. Report from the Institute for Reference Materials and Measurements, Joint Research Centre, European Commission, EUR 20767EN, 2003.
164. H. Akiyama, K. Nakamura, N. Harikai, H. Watanabe, K. Iijima, H. Yamakawa, Y. Mizuguchi, R. Yoshikawa, M. Yamamoto, H. Sato, M. Watai, F. Arakawa, T. Ogasawara, R. Nishihara, H. Kato, A. Yamauchi, Y. Takahata, F. Morimatsu, S. Mamegoshi, S. Muraoka, T. Honjoh, T. Watanabe, K. Sakata, T. Imamura, M. Toyoda, R. Matsuda, and T. Maitani. [Inter-laboratory evaluation studies for establishment of notified ELISA methods for allergic substances (peanuts)]. *Shokuhin Eiseigaku Zasshi*, 45, 325–331, 2004.
165. R.E. Poms, M.E. Agazzi, A. Bau, M. Brohee, C. Capelletti, J.V. Nørgaard, and E. Anklam. Inter-laboratory validation study of five commercial ELISA test kits for the determination of peanut proteins in biscuits and dark chocolate. *Food Addit Contam*, 22, 104–112, 2005.
166. D.L. Park, S. Coates, V.A. Brewer, E.A. Garber, M. Abouzied, K. Johnson, B. Ritter, and D. McKenzie. Performance Tested Method multiple laboratory validation study of ELISA-based assays for the detection of peanuts in food. *J AOAC Int*, 88, 156–160, 2005.
167. T.B. Whitaker, K.M. Williams, M.W. Trucksess, and A.B. Slate. Immunochemical analytical methods for the determination of peanut proteins in foods. *J AOAC Int*, 88, 161–174, 2005.
168. A.J. van Hengel, C. Capelletti, M. Brohee, and E. Anklam. Validation of two commercial lateral flow devices for the detection of peanut proteins in cookies: interlaboratory study. *J AOAC Int*, 89, 462–468, 2006.
169. L. L'Hocine, J.I. Boye, and C. Munyana. Detection and quantification of soy allergens in food: study of two commercial enzyme-linked immunosorbent assays. *J Food Sci*, 72, C145–C153, 2007.

170. M. Röder, S. Vieths, and T. Holzhauser. Commercial lateral flow devices for rapid detection of peanut (*Arachis hypogaea*) and hazelnut (*Corylus avellana*) cross-contamination in the industrial production of cookies. *Anal Bioanal Chem*, 395, 103–109, 2009.
171. T. Holzhauser, L.I. Dehne, A. Hoffmann, D. Haustein, and S. Vieths. Rocket immunoelectrophoresis (RIE) for determination of potentially allergenic peanut proteins in processed foods as a simple means for quality assurance and food safety. *Z Lebensm Unters Forsch*, 206, 1–8, 1998.
172. B.W. Blais and L.M. Philippe. A cloth-based enzyme immunoassay for detection of peanut proteins in foods. *Food Agric Immunol*, 12, 243–248, 2000.
173. B.W. Blais, M. Gaudreault, and L.M. Philippe. Multiplex enzyme immunoassay system for the simultaneous detection of multiple allergens in foods. *Food Control*, 14, 43–47, 2003.
174. G.F. Schäppi, V. Konrad, D. Imhof, R. Etter, and B. Wüthrich. Hidden peanut allergens detected in various foods: findings and legal measures. *Allergy*, 56, 1216–1220, 2001.
175. M.U. Keating, R.T. Jones, N.J. Worley, C.A. Shively, and J.W. Yunginger. Immunoassay of peanut allergens in food processing materials and finished foods. *J Allergy Clin Immunol*, 86, 41–44, 1990.
176. S.J. Koppelmann, H. Bleeker-Marcelis, G. Duijn, and M. Hessing. Detecting peanut allergens. The development of an immunochemical assay for peanut proteins. *Word Ingred*, 12, 35–38, 1996.
177. J.M. Yeung and P.G. Collins. Enzyme immunoassay for determination of peanut proteins in food products. *J AOAC Int*, 79, 1411–1416 1996.
178. B. Keck-Gassenmeier, S. Benet, C. Rosa, and C. Hirschenhuber. Determination of peanut traces in food by a commercially-available ELISA test. *Food Agric Immunol*, 11, 243–50, 1999.
179. T. Holzhauser, S. Vieths. Indirect competitive ELISA for determination of traces of peanut (*Arachis hypogaea* L.) protein in complex food matrices. *J Agric Food Chem*, 47, 603–611, 1999.
180. W.H. Newsome and M. Abbott. An immunoaffinity column for the determination of peanut protein in chocolate. *J AOAC Int*, 82, 666–668, 1999.
181. S. Ben Rejeb, M. Abbott, D. Davies, C. Cléroux, and P. Delahaut. Multi-allergen screening immunoassay for the detection of protein markers of peanut and four tree nuts in chocolate. *Food Addit Contam*, 22, 709–715, 2005.
182. A. Pomés, R.M. Helm, G.A. Bannon, A.W. Burks, A. Tsay, and M.D. Chapman. Monitoring peanut allergen in food products by measuring Ara h 1. *J Allergy Clin Immunol*, 111, 640–645, 2003.
183. D.A. Schmitt, H. Cheng, S.J. Maleki, and A.W. Burks. Competitive inhibition ELISA for quantification of Ara h 1 and Ara h 2, the major allergens of peanuts. *J AOAC Int*, 87, 1492–1497, 2004.
184. O. Stephan and S. Vieths. Development of a real-time PCR and a sandwich ELISA for detection of potentially allergenic trace amounts of peanut (*Arachis hypogaea*) in processed foods. *J Agric Food Chem*, 52, 3754–360, 2004.
185. M. Kiening, R. Niessner, E. Drs, S. Baumgartner, R. Krska, M. Bremer, V. Tomkies, P. Reece, C. Danks, U. Immer, and M.G. Weller. Sandwich immunoassays for the determination of peanut and hazelnut traces in foods. *J Agric Food Chem*, 53, 3321–3327, 2005.
186. E.N.C. Mills, A. Potts, G.W. Plumb, and N. Lambert. Development of a rapid dipstick immunoassay for the detection of peanut contamination of food. *Food Agricul Immunol*, 9, 37–50, 1997.

187. O. Stephan, N. Möller, S. Lehmann, T. Holzhauser, and S. Vieths. Development and validation of two dipstick type immunoassays for determination of trace amounts of peanut and hazelnut in processed foods. *Eur Food Res Technol*, 215, 431–436, 2002.
188. H.-W. Wen, W. Borejsza-Wysocki, T.R. DeCory, and R.A. Durst. Development of a competitive liposome-based lateral flow assay for the rapid detection of the allergenic peanut protein Ara h1. *Anal Bioanal Chem*, 382, 1217–1226, 2005.
189. J.A. Nordlee, S.L. Taylor, R.T. Jones, and J.W. Yunginger. Allergenicity of various peanut products as determined by RAST inhibition. *J Allergy Clin Immunol*, 68, 376–382, 1981.
190. J.W. Yunginger, M.B. Gauerke, R.T. Jones, M.J.E. Dahlberg, and S.J. Ackerman. Use of radioimmunoassay to determine the nature, quantity, and source of allergenic contamination of sunflower butter. *J Food Prot*, 46, 625–628, 1983.
191. A. Olszewski, L. Pons, F. Moutete, I. Aimone-Gastin, G. Kanny, and D.A. Moneret-Vautrin. Isolation and characterization of proteic allergens in refined peanut oil. *Clin Exp Allergy*, 28, 850–859, 1998.
192. I. Mohammed, W.M. Mullett, E.P.C. Lai, and J.M. Yeung. Is biosensor a viable method for food allergen detection? *Analyt Chim Acta*, 444, 97–102, 2001.
193. H. Hird, J. Lloyd, R. Goodier, J. Brown, and P. Reece. Detection of peanut using real-time polymerase chain reaction. *Eur Food Res Technol*, 217, 265–268, 2003.
194. T. Watanabe, H. Akiyama, S. Maleki, H. Yamakawa, K. IIjima, F. Yamazaki, T. Matsumoto, S. Futo, F. Arakawa, M. Watai, and T. Maitani. A specific qualitative detection method for peanut (*Arachis hypogaea*) in foods using polymerase chain reaction. *J Food Biochem*, 30, 215–233, 2006.
195. H. Hashimoto, Y. Makabe, Y. Hasegawa, J. Sajiki, and F. Miyamoto. [Detection of allergenic substances in foods by a multiplex PCR method]. *Shokuhin Eiseigaku Zasshi*, 48, 132–138, 2007.
196. E. Scaravelli, M. Brohée, R. Marchelli, and A.J. van Hengel. Development of three real-time PCR assays to detect peanut allergen residue in processed foods. *Eur Food Res Technol*, 227, 857–869, 2008.
197. T. Hirao, S. Watanabe, Y. Temmei, M. Hiramoto, and H. Kato. Qualitative polymerase chain reaction methods for detecting major food allergens (peanut, soybean, and wheat) by using internal transcribed spacer region. *J AOAC Int*, 92, 1464–1471, 2009.
198. K.J. Shefcheck and S.M. Musser. Confirmation of the allergenic peanut protein, Ara h 1, in a model food matrix using liquid chromatography/tandem mass spectrometry (LC/MS/MS). *J Agric Food Chem*, 52, 2785–2790, 2004.
199. K.J. Shefcheck, J.H. Callahan, and S.M. Musser. Confirmation of peanut protein using peptide markers in dark chocolate using liquid chromatography-tandem mass spectrometry (LC-MS/MS). *J Agric Food Chem*, 54, 7953–7959, 2006.
200. M. Careri, A. Costa, L. Elviri, J.B. Lagos, A. Mangia, M. Terenghi, A. Cereti, and L.P. Garoffo. Use of specific peptide biomarkers for quantitative confirmation of hidden allergenic peanut proteins Ara h 2 and Ara h 3/4 for food control by liquid chromatography-tandem mass spectrometry. *Anal Bioanal Chem*, 389, 1901–1907, 2007.
201. M. Careri, L. Elviri, M. Maffini, A. Mangia, C. Mucchino, and M. Terenghi. Determination of peanut allergens in cereal-chocolate-based snacks: metal-tag inductively coupled plasma mass spectrometry immunoassay versus liquid chromatography/electrospray ionization tandem mass spectrometry. *Rapid Commun Mass Spectrom*, 22, 807–811, 2008.
202. M. Careri, L. Elviri, J.B. Lagos, A. Mangia, F. Speroni, and M. Terenghi. Selective and rapid immunomagnetic bead-based sample treatment for the liquid chromatography-electrospray ion-trap mass spectrometry detection of Ara h3/4 peanut protein in foods. *J Chromatogr A*, 1206, 89–94, 2008.

203. T.M.P. Cattaneo, A. Feroldi, P.M. Toppino, and C. Olieman. Sample preparation for selective and sensitive detection of soya proteins in dairy products wich chromatographic and electrophoretic techniques. *Nederlands melk en Zuiveltijdschrift*, 48, 225–234, 1994.
204. J. Lopez-Tapia, M.R. Garcia-Risco, M.A. Manso, and R. Lopz-Fandiño. Detection of the presence of soya protein in milk powder by sodium dodecyl sulphate capillary electrophoresis. *J Chromatogr A*, 836, 153–160, 1999.
205. F.W. Janssen, G. Voortman, and J.A. de Baaij. Detection of soya proteins in heated meat products by "blotting" and "dot blot." *Z Lebensm Unters Forsch*, 182, 479–483, 1986.
206. N. Catsimpoolas and E. Leuthner. Immunochemical methods for detection and quantitation of Kunitz soybean trypsin inhibitor. *Anal Biochem*, 31, 437–447, 1969.
207. B.L. Ventling and W.L. Hurley. Soy proteins in milk replacers identified by immunoblotting. *J Food Sci*, 54, 766–767, 1988.
208. C.H.S. Hitchcock, F.J. Bailey, A.A. Crimes, D.A.G. Dean, and P.J. Davis. Determination of soya proteins in food using an enzyme-linked immunosorbent assay procedure. *J Sci Food Agric*, 32, 157–165, 1981.
209. N.M. Griffith, M.J. Billington, A.A. Crimes, and C.H.S. Hitchcock. An assessment of commercially available reagents for an enzyme-linked immunosorbent assay (ELISA) of soya protein in meat products. *J Sci Food Agric*, 35, 1255–1260, 1984.
210. O. Porras, B. Carlsson, S.P. Fällström, and L.A. Hanson. Detection of soy protein in soy lecithin, margarine and, occasionally, soy oil. *Int Arch Allergy Appl Immunol*, 78, 30–32, 1985.
211. J.H. Rittenburg, A. Adams, J. Palmer, and J.C. Allen. Improved enzyme-linked immunosorbent assay for determination of soy protein in meat products. *J Assoc Off Anal Chem*, 70, 582–587, 1987.
212. K. Yasumoto, M. Sudo, and T. Suzuki. Quantitation of soya protein by enzyme linked immunosorbent assay of its characteristic peptide. *J Sci Food Agric*, 50, 377–389, 1990.
213. H. Tsuji, N. Okada, R. Yamanishi, N. Bando, M. Kimoto, and T. Ogawa. Measurement of Gly m Bd 30K, a major soybean allergen, in soybean products by a sandwich enzyme-linked immunosorbent assay. *Biosci Biotechnol Biochem*, 59, 150–151, 1995.
214. N. Bando, H. Tsuji, M. Hiemori, K. Yoshizumi, R. Yamanishi, M. Kimoto, and T. Ogawa. Quantitative analysis of Gly m Bd 28K in soybean products by a sandwich enzyme-linked immunosorbent assay. *J Nutr Sci Vitaminol (Tokyo)*, 44, 655–664, 1998.
215. D.L. Brandon and M. Friedman. Immunoassays of soy proteins. *J Agric Food Chem*, 50, 6635–6642, 2002.
216. C. Rizzi, L. Galeoto, G. Zoccatelli, S. Vincenzi, R. Chignola, and A.D.B. Peruffo. Active soybean lectin in foods: quantitative determination by ELISA using immobilised asialofetuin. *Food Res Int*, 36, 815–821, 2003.
217. S.L. Hefle, D.M. Lambrecht, and J.A. Nordlee. Soy sauce retains allergenicity through the fermentation/production process. *J Allergy Clin Immunol*, 115, S32, 2005.
218. J. You, D. Li, S. Qiao, Z. Wang, P. He, D. Ou, and B. Dong. Development of a monoclonal antibody-based competitive ELISA for detection of β-conglycinin, an allergen from soybean. *Food Chem*, 106, 352–360, 2008.
219. R. González, O. Duffort, B. Calabozo, D. Barber, J. Carreira, and F. Polo. Monoclonal antibody-based method to quantify Gly m 1. Its application to assess environmental exposure to soybean dust. *Allergy*, 55, 59–64, 2000.
220. N. Morishita, K. Kamiya, T. Matsumoto, S. Sakai, R. Teshima, A. Urisu, T. Moriyama, T. Ogawa, H. Akiyama, and F. Morimatsu. Reliable enzyme-linked immunosorbent assay for the determination of soybean proteins in processed foods. *J Agric Food Chem*, 56, 6818–6824, 2008.

221. A.M. Herian, S.L. Tayor, and R.K. Bush. Allergenic reactivity of various soybean products as determined by RAST inhibition. *J Food Sci*, 58, 385–388, 1993.
222. Y.S. Song, C. Martinez-Villaluenga and E.G. de Meijia. Quantification of human IgE immunoreactive soybean proteins in commercial soy ingredients and products. *J Food Sci*, 73, T90–T99, 2008.
223. G. Feriotto, M. Borgatti, C. Mischiati, N. Bianchi, and R. Gambari. Biosensor technology and surface plasmon resonance for real-time detection of genetically modified Roundup Ready soybean gene sequences. *J Agric Food Chem*, 50, 955–962, 2002.
224. Y. Huang, M.C. Bell, and I.I. Suni. Impedance biosensor for peanut protein Ara h 1. *Anal Chem*, 80, 9157–9161, 2008.
225. R. Yamanishi. H. Tsuji, N. Bando, I. Yoshimoto, and T. Ogawa. Micro-assay method for evaluating the allergenicity of the major soybean allergen, Gly m Bd 30K, with mouse antiserum and RBL-2H3 cells. *Biosci Biotechnol Biochem*, 61, 19–23, 1997.
226. H. Hörtner. Nachweismöglichkeiten gentechnisch hergestellter Lebensmittel. *Ernährung (Nutrition)*, 21, 443–446, 1997.
227. R.E. Poms, J. Glössl, and H. Foissy. Increased sensitivity for detection of specific target DNA in milk by concentration in milk fat. *Eur Food Res Technol*, 213, 361–365, 2001.
228. C.F. Terry, D.J. Shanahan, L.D. Ballam, N. Harris, D.G. McDowell, and H.C. Parkes. Real-time detection of genetically modified soya using Lightcycler and ABI 7700 platforms with TaqMan, Scorpion, and SYBR Green I chemistries. *J AOAC Int*, 85, 938–944, 2002.
229. O. Mellenthin and R. Galensa. Analysis of polyphenols using capillary zone electrophoresis and HPLC: detection of soy, lupin, and pea protein in meat products. *J Agric Food Chem*, 47, 594–602, 1999.
230. M.C. Garcia, M. Torre, and M.L. Marina. Characterization of commercial soybean products by conventional and perfusion reversed-phase high-performance liquid chromatography and multivariate analysis. *J Chromatogr A*, 881, 47–57, 2000.
231. C. Schäfer, M. Schott, F. Brandl, S. Neidhart, and R. Carle. Identification and quantification of epsilon-(gamma-glutamyl)lysine in digests of enzymatically cross-linked leguminous proteins by high-performance liquid chromatography-electrospray ionization mass spectrometry (HPLC-ESI-MS). *J Agric Food Chem*, 20, 2830–2837, 2005.
232. L. Holden, L.H. Moen, G.B. Sletten, and M.M. Dooper. Novel polyclonal-monoclonal-based ELISA utilized to examine lupine (*Lupinus* species) content in food products. *J Agric Food Chem*, 55, 2536–2542, 2007.
233. C.H. Kaw, S.L. Hefle, and S.L. Taylor. Sandwich enzyme-linked immunosorbent assay (ELISA) for the detection of lupine residues in foods. *J Food Sci*, 73, T135–T140, 2008.
234. A. Demmel, C. Hupfer, E. Ilg Hampe, U. Busch, and K.H. Engel. Development of a real-time PCR for the detection of lupine DNA (*Lupinus* species) in foods. *J Agric Food Chem*, 56, 4328–4332, 2008.
235. D. Locati, S. Morandi, M. Zanotti, and A. Arnoldi. Preliminary approaches for the development of a high-performance liquid chromatography/electrospray ionization tandem mass spectrometry method for the detection and label-free semi-quantitation of the main storage proteins of *Lupinus albus* in foods. *Rapid Commun Mass Spectrom*, 20, 1305–1316, 2006.

CHAPTER 4

Allergens in Tree Nuts, Sesame Seeds, Mustard, and Celery

Thomas Holzhauser and Martin Röder

CONTENTS

Introduction 78
Prevalence Data 78
Eliciting Thresholds and Symptoms of Allergic Reactions 78
    Allergen Labeling 80
Allergenic Properties 81
General Aspects on Methodology 83
Sample Preparation 99
    For Protein Detection 99
    For Nucleic Acid Detection 99
Detection and Quantification 100
    Protein Detection 100
    Nucleic Acid Detection 101
Potential and Limitations of Published Methods 102
    Almond 102
    Brazil Nut 103
    Cashew 104
    Hazelnut 106
    Pecan 109
    Pistachio 110
    Macadamia 111
    Walnut 111
    Tree Nuts Multiplex Assays 113
    Sesame Seeds 114
    Mustard 115
    Celery 116

Commercial Test Kits for Allergen Detection 118
Summary and Conclusion 119
References 121

INTRODUCTION

This chapter deals with important allergenic foods of plant origin for human consumption. The term *tree nuts* includes a variety of seeds that originate from different botanical families, which is true for sesame, mustard, and celery (Table 4.1). Tree nuts are common ingredients in salty snacks, bakery products, breakfast cereals and muesli, and sweets like chocolate and ice cream. Sesame seeds are usually ingredients of bakery products and seasonings. Mustard seeds and celery seeds are both used as spices. In addition, celery and celeriac are consumed as vegetables.

PREVALENCE DATA

The prevalence of allergy to tree nuts, sesame seeds, and mustard may vary between different countries. The true prevalence of allergy to the listed foods is yet unknown. Peanut and tree nuts were estimated to affect approximately 1% of the general population in the United Kingdom and the United States,[1,2] with between 0.4% and 0.6% specifically affected by tree nuts.[2] A meta-analysis of published data based on surveys or challenge studies ranged the prevalence of tree nut allergy between 0.1% and 4.3%, with a similar range for hazelnut.[3] In Europe, hazelnut allergy is common and often associated with birch pollinosis,[4] whereas in the United States allergy to walnut, cashew, almond, pecan, and Brazil nut appears to be more common than to hazelnut.[2] However, data from Europe, the United States, and Australia identified hazelnut as the food with the highest sensitization rate.[5] Sesame was identified as one of the most frequent causes of food allergy in a study cohort of infants and children in Israel,[6] and prevalence estimates ranged between 0.05% and 0.6%.[3] Mustard allergy appears to be common in France,[7] whereas allergy to celery is common in Europe, especially in Switzerland.[8,9]

ELICITING THRESHOLDS AND SYMPTOMS OF ALLERGIC REACTIONS

Life-threatening anaphylaxis and even fatal episodes have been reported for several of the allergenic foods listed.[10-14] Data about the most harmful tree nut species are limited. However, in the United Kingdom, 12% of 784 investigated tree nut- and peanut-allergic children had their worst ever reaction to Brazil nut.[15] Clinically relevant lowest observed adverse effect levels (LOAELs) within this group of foods were determined by titrated double-blind, placebo-controlled food challenge (DBPCFC) and ranged from 6.4 mg hazelnut[16] to 30 mg sesame seed.[17] Other studies based on comparable challenge protocols are unfortunately lacking. However, the observed

ALLERGENS IN TREE NUTS, SESAME SEEDS, MUSTARD, AND CELERY

Table 4.1 Tree Nuts, Sesame Seed, Mustard, and Celery Species as Listed for Allergen Labeling in Various Countries

Food	Botanical Systematics (Order/Family/Genus)	Labeling Required in
Coconut (*Cocos nucifera*)	Arecales/Arecaceae/Cocos	US/AU
Brazil nut (*Bertholletia excelsa*)	Ericales/Lecythidaceae/Bertholletia	EU/US/AU/CA/HK
Sapucaia nut (*Lecythis* spp.)	Ericales/Lecythidaceae/Lecythis	AU
Sheanut (*Butyrospermum parkii* = *Vitellaria paradoxa*)	Ericales/Sapotaceae/Butyrospermum	US
Hazelnut (*Corylus avellana*)	Fagales/Betulaceae/Corylus	EU/US/AU/CA/HK
Filbert/Hazelnut (*Corylus* spp.)	Fagales/Betulaceae/Corylus	US/AU/CA
Chestnut (Chinese, American, European, Seguin) (*Castanea* spp.)	Fagales/Fagaceae/Castanea	US/AU
Chinquapin (*Castanea pumila*)	Fagales/Fagaceae/Castanea	US
Beechnut (*Fagus* spp.)	Fagales/Fagaceae/Fagus	US/AU
Hickory nut (*Carya* spp.)	Fagales/Juglandaceae/Carya	US/AU
Pecan nut (*Carya illinoiesis* (*Wangenh.*) K. Koch)	Fagales/Juglandaceae/Carya	EU/US/AU/CA/HK
Butternut (*Juglans cinera*)	Fagales/Juglandaceae/Juglans	US/CA
Walnut (*Juglans regia*)	Fagales/Juglandaceae/Juglans	EU/US/AU/CA/HK
Walnut/heartnut/butternut (*Juglans* spp.)	Fagales/Juglandaceae/Juglans	US/AU/CA
Ginko nut (*Ginkgo biloba*)	Ginkgoales Ginkgoaceae/Ginkgo	US
Pine nut/pinon nut (*Pinus* spp.)	Pinales/Pinaceae/Pinus	US/AU/CA
Macadamia nut and Queensland nut (*Macadamia ternifolia*)	Proteales/Proteaceae/Macadamia	EU/US/AU/CA/HK
Bush nut Macadamia spp. (*Macadamia* spp.)	Proteales/Proteaceae/Macadamia	US/AUS/CA
Almond (*Amygdalus communis* L.; *Prunis dulcis*)	Rosales/Rosaceae/Prunus	EU/US/AU/CA/HK
Japanese horse-chestnut (*Aesculus turbinata*)	Sapindales/Sapindaceae/Aesculus	AU
Cashew (*Anacardium occidentale*)	Sapindales/Anacardiaceae/Anacardium	EU/US/AU/CA/HK
Pistachio nut (*Pistacia vera*)	Sapindales/Anacardiaceae/Pistacia	EU/US/AU/CA/HK
Pili nut (*Canarium ovatum*)	Sapindales/Burseraceae/Canarium	US/AU
Lichee nut (*Litchi chinensis*)	Sapindales/Sapindaceae/Litchi	US

Continued

Table 4.1 (*Continued*) Tree Nuts, Sesame Seed, Mustard, and Celery Species as Listed for Allergen Labeling in Various Countries

Food	Botanical Systematics (Order/Family/Genus)	Labeling Required in
Celery (*Apium graveolens*)	Araliales/Apiaceae/Apium	EU/US/HK
Mustard (*Brassica* spp.)	Brassicales/Brassicaceae/Brassica	EU/US/CH/CA
Sesame (*Sesamum indicum*)	Lamiales/Pedaliaceae/Sesamum	EU/US/AU/CA/HK

Note: AU = Australia; CA = Canada; HK = Hong Kong; UK = United Kingdom; US = United States.

LOAELs reflect those levels found for other allergenic foods, for example, 10 mg soybean[18] or 5 mg peanut.[17] Even though not part of this chapter, data on eliciting doses of allergenic peanut are highly interesting because peanut (1) appears to be one of the most allergenic, and it is one of the (2) most intensively studied foods with (3) a fairly low LOAEL. Based on a probability distribution model of a challenge series of 286 peanut-allergic individuals, Taylor and colleagues determined with 95% confidence that 5.2 mg whole peanut was the lower limit of ED_{05}, the eliciting dose to provoke a reaction in only 5% of the peanut-allergic population.[19] Avoidance of hidden allergens at this level would thus help to avoid severe allergic reactions in the majority of food-allergic individuals. Taking into account such a low level of eliciting dose, analytical methods should be able to detect the allergenic food in the low milligram/kilogram range to allow verifying compliance with allergen labeling regulations and avoiding relevant levels of hidden allergens due to cross-contact.

Allergen Labeling

Within the European Union, mandatory labeling of tree nuts used as ingredients was specified with Directives 2003/89/EC and 2007/68/EC, amending Directive 2000/13/EC. Although tree nuts are defined in Annex IIIa of Directive 2007/68/EC with common names, the botanical name of only certain varieties is given in parenthesis.[20–22] The tree nut list comprises eight different "nuts." Switzerland adopted the E.U. list in its own legislation.[23] In the United States, the *Food Allergen Labeling and Consumer Protection Act of 2004* (FALCPA)[24] established labeling requirements for packaged foods that contain certain food allergens. FALCPA does not provide a clear definition of tree nuts since only three examples are given. In 2006, the U.S. Food and Drug Administration (FDA) published an open list with currently 18 hits that "reflect FDA's current best judgement as to those nuts that are tree nuts within the meaning of section 201 (qq) of FALCPA."[25]

Health Canada has published on its homepage proposed regulatory amendments to clarify requirements for food allergen labeling. Therein, the mandatory labeling of nine different tree nuts is required.[26] Within Australia and New Zealand, in December 2002 the *Australia New Zealand Food Standards Code* came into force. Standard 1.2.3, Clause 4 of the code requires the declaration of tree nuts among other certain allergenic substances. The general term *tree nut* is not specified in detail in this regulation.[27] Hence, for Australia a listing of 14 commodities is given for tree nuts.[28] In Japan, the Ministry of Health, Labor, and Welfare (MHLW), responsible for food safety regulations, enumerated five items as foods containing allergens for which obligatory labeling is necessary, and there are 19 food items that are recommended for labeling, including the general term *tree nuts*.[29]

In Hong Kong, pursuant to paragraph 2(4E) of Schedule 3 to the Food and Drugs (Composition and Labelling) Regulations, Cap 132W, the name of any tree nut and nut product shall be specified in the list of ingredients if present in the final food products (Food and Drugs (Composition and Labelling) Regulations). A definition for tree nuts is not given; however, the Center for Food Safety of Hong Kong has published a list of eight nuts.[30]

ALLERGENIC PROPERTIES

Proteins are the allergenic fraction to which susceptible atopic individuals may develop an allergy with clinical symptoms on repeated uptake. Many single allergens have so far been identified and characterized. Table 4.2 summarizes those single allergens from allergenic foods within this chapter that were officially assigned by the International Union of Immunological Societies (IUIS) Allergen Nomenclature Subcommittee. Other immunoglobulin E (IgE)-binding proteins, thus potential allergens, have been described but not yet accepted as allergens. According to protein residue identities, their function, and their structures, proteins are grouped into protein families. Evolutionary-related proteins are grouped into superfamilies. Until February 23, 2009, the Structural Classification of Proteins (SCOP) database (http://scop.mrc-lmb.cam.ac.uk/scop/index.html) counted 3,902 families and 1,962 superfamilies. By contrast, most plant food allergens are found in a limited number of families and superfamilies. Only four families include approximately 60% of all plant food allergens: the prolamin superfamily, which includes 2S albumin seed storage proteins and nonspecific lipid transfer proteins (nsLTP); the cupin superfamily, which includes vicilin (7S) and legumin-type (11S) seed storage proteins; the profilins, which constitute regulatory proteins; and allergens related to birch pollen Bet v 1 within the family 10 pathogenesis-related protein (PR10) family.[31] Moreover, lipophilic allergenic oil bodies have been identified in fatty or oily plant food seeds, such as sesame[32] and hazelnut.[33] In food-allergic subjects, serological and clinical cross-reactivity between different allergenic foods may be caused by homologous allergens within the described protein families.[34,35] Also, animal antibodies that are specifically generated by immunization against single allergens or extracts from allergenic plant foods may thus show cross-sensitivity to homologous proteins or allergens of other plant food species. When developing specific antibodies to allergenic foods, such potential cross-sensitivity should be taken into account.

Tree nuts and seeds are usually consumed as both raw and heat-treated food. Storage proteins and nsLTPs, of which several have been described as allergens (Table 4.2), have been shown to retain stability to heat (summarized in Mills and

Table 4.2 Known Single Allergens of Allergenic Tree Nuts, Sesame, Mustard, and Celery, as Assigned by the International Union of Immunological Societies (IUIS) Allergen Nomenclature Subcommittee, Grouped into Protein Families

Plant food	PR10 Protein	Profilin	nsLTP	2S Albumin	11S Globulin	7S Globulin	Oleosin	Others
Brazil nut (*Bertholletia excelsa*)				Ber e 1	Ber e 2			
Hazelnut (*Corylus avellana*)	Cor a 1	Cor a 2	Cor a 8	Cor a 14	Cor a 9	Cor a 11	Cor a 12 Cor a 13	
Chestnut (Chinese, American, European, Seguin) (*Castanea* spp.)			Cas s 8					Cas s 5 Cas s 9
Pecan nut (*Carya illinoiesis* (Wangenh.) K. Koch)				Car i 1	Car i 4			
Walnut (*Juglans* spp.)			Jug r 3	Jug r 1 Jug n 1	Jug r 4	Jug r 2 Jug n 2		
Almond (*Amygdalus communis* L.; *Prunus dulcis*)		Pru du 4	Pru du 3		Pru du 6			Pru du 5
Cashew (*Anacardium occidentale*)				Ana o 3	Ana o 2	Ana o 1		
Pistachio nut (*Pistacia vera*)				Pis v 1	Pis v 2 Pis v 5	Pis v 3		Pis v 4
Lichee nut (*Litchi chinensis*)		Lit c 1						
Celery (*Apium graveolens*)	Api g 1	Api g 4	Api g 2					Api g 3 Api g 5
Oriental/yellow mustard (*Brassica* spp./*Sinapis alba*)		Sin a 4	Sin a 3	Bra j 1 Sin a 1	Sin a 2			
Sesame (*Sesamum indicum*)				Ses i 1 Ses i 2	Ses i 6 Ses i 7	Ses i 3	Ses i 4 Ses i 5	

Mackie[36]) and digestion[37] to a certain extent. By contrast, allergens of the PR10 family and profilins that are associated with birch and mugwort allergy appear to be more susceptible to heat (summarized in Mills and Mackie[36]) and digestion.[38] Nonetheless, systemic and severe allergic reactions may also be elicited in pollen-associated food allergy, such as is the case for celery.[39] Moreover, celery-allergic subjects still reacted to cooked celery, which is thought to refer only to partially inactivated allergens,[9] and a sensitizing potential may be retained even after digestion.[38]

The following paragraphs highlight details of the qualification of methods to detect tree nuts, sesame seeds, mustard, and celery with special regard to general aspects of the potential of methodologies, sample preparation, and detection and quantification. Finally, published methods are reviewed with special emphasis on potential and limitations to detect or quantify allergenic foods discussed in this chapter. For better comparison of the characteristics of the published methods, Table 4.3 and Table 4.4 summarize protein-based and DNA-based detection methods, respectively. The tables summarize the published methods as comprehensively as possible but without claiming completeness because of the fast evolution in method development since the introduction of legal labeling requirements.

GENERAL ASPECTS ON METHODOLOGY

The first methods for the detection of tree nuts and seeds are based on protein detection because of the protein nature of allergens. The technique most often applied and accepted is the enzyme-linked immunosorbent assay (ELISA) for its easy handling and readout. ELISA tests make use of specific animal antibodies, in most cases polyclonal antisera of limited availability or occasionally monoclonal antibodies with, in theory, unrestricted availability. In most cases of tests based on polyclonal antisera, the entire selectivity in terms of single-allergen detection is not fully known. Moreover, not all relevant single allergens or allergen isoforms are known at the molecular level. Whereas food allergens that elicit an immediate-type allergic reaction are proteins or glycoproteins, not each protein of the detectable protein fraction is an allergen. Hence, the protein fraction that is detected by animal antisera still has to be considered as a marker fraction for the presence of the allergenic food rather than a proof of detected allergens. This should be taken into account when interpreting ELISA test results. Further, antibody specificity may be limited due to its natural binding to structures, especially if similar structures are present in conserved protein families described in this chapter. Hence, detecting a molecular sequence would be the most specific approach to detect a species such as an allergenic food. Mass spectrometric (MS) methods have the capability to detect specific sequences of marker peptides. Ideally, based on specific multiple-reaction monitoring (MRM) transitions, specific sequences of all allergenic proteins of the allergenic food would be detected. However, this task appears to be a mission impossible from the point of complexity.

Table 4.3 Published Protein-Based Methods for the Detection of Tree Nuts, Sesame, Mustard, and Celery (as of April 2010)

Allergenic Food	Year	Ref.	Technique	Antibody (Source and Type)	Immunogen/Standard	Standard	Detection	Cross-Reactivity/Tested Foods	Sensitivity in Matrix	Recovery Studies in Spiked/Incurred Matrices
Almond	1999	78	Competitive ELISA	Rabbit Ab, polyclonal	purified AMP	Purified AMP	AP	4/8: Cashew globulin (0.27%) Tepary bean phaseolin (0.12%) Walnut albumin (0.021%) Rice globulin (0.017%)	No data	No data
Almond	2000	81	Sandwich ELISA	Sheep Ab, rabbit Ab, both polyclonal	Roasted almond of different varieties	Roasted almond of different varieties	AP	7/38: Black walnut, Brazil nut, cashew, hazelnut, macadamia, pistachio, sesame seed	1 mg/kg almond	Incurred samples: Milk chocolate Spiked samples: Corn, wheat, breakfast cereal mixture
Almond	2001	79	Competitive ELISA	Rabbit Ab, polyclonal from Reference 78	Purified AMP	Purified AMP	AP	Same as Reference 78	5–37 mg/kg almond	Spiked samples: Raisin bran cereal, rolled oats, cookie, candy, rice cereal
Almond	2001	96	Immunoblot	Commercially available rabbit Ab, polyclonal	No data		AP	1/3: Hazelnut	5 mg/kg almond protein	Spiked chocolates from 5 to 50,000 mg/kg
Almond	2002	80	Sandwich ELISA	Rabbit Ab, goat Ab, both polyclonal	Raw almond protein extract	Raw almond protein extract	AP	No data	No data	No data

Allergen	Year	Method	Antibody	Calibrator	Extract	Detection	Cross-reactivity	LOD	Spiked samples
Almond	2005	95	Competitive ELISA (multi-allergen)	Rabbit IgG polyclonal	Roasted almond extract	Roasted almond extract	HRP	5/24: Cashew (very strong) Beef, lamb, pork poultry	<1 mg/kg almond protein	spiked sample: dark and milk chocolate
Brazil nut	2002	54	Sandwich ELISA	Hen's egg yolk IgY, polyclonal	Brazil nut	Brazil nut	HRP	0/5	1 mg/kg Brazil nut protein	Spiked samples: Chocolate, granola bars, cereals, tofu burger, cake, ice cream
Brazil nut	2003	94	Sandwich dot blot (multiallergen)	Hen's egg IgY, polyclonal	Brazil nut extract	Not applicable (qualitative)	HRP	0/2	0.1–0.5 mg/kg Brazil nut	Spiked samples: Cookies, chocolate, ice cream
Brazil nut	2004	82	Competitive ELISA	Rabbit Ab, polyclonal	Purified 2S albumin	Raw or roasted protein extracts	HRP	0/7	No data	No data
Brazil nut	2005	95	Competitive ELISA (multiallergen)	Rabbit IgG, polyclonal	Roasted Brazil nut extract	Roasted Brazil nut extract	HRP	0/24	<1 mg/kg Brazil nut protein	Spiked sample: Dark and milk chocolate
Brazil nut	2009	83	Competitive ELISA	Rabbit Ab, polyclonal	Brazil nut protein extract	Brazil nut protein extract	AP	1/66: Cinnamon (1.36%)	No data	Spiked samples: Lowest matrix spike level: 100 mg/kg: Wheat flour, dark chocolate, oat cereal, shortbread cookies

Continued

Table 4.3 (*Continued*) Published Protein-Based Methods for the Detection of Tree Nuts, Sesame, Mustard, and Celery (as of April 2010)

Allergenic Food	Year	Ref.	Technique	Antibody (Source and Type)	Immunogen/ Standard	Standard	Detection	Cross-Reactivity/ Tested Foods	Sensitivity in Matrix	Recovery Studies in Spiked/incurred Matrices
Cashew	2003	85	Sandwich ELISA	Goat Ab, rabbit Ab, both polyclonal	Purified anacardein and cashew protein	Purified anacardein	AP	4/15: Pecan (0.004%) Sunflower seeds (0.0023%) Pistachio (0.002%) Walnut (0.0018%)	1 mg/kg cashew major protein	Spiked samples: Whole wheat flour, rolled oats, chocolate, raisin bran cereal, cookies, rice cereal
Cashew	2005	95	Competitive ELISA (multiallergen)	Rabbit IgG, polyclonal	Roasted cashew extract	Roasted cashew extract	HRP	0/24	<1 mg/kg cashew protein	Spiked sample: Dark and milk chocolate
Hazelnut	1994	49	RIE	Rabbit Ab, polyclonal	Corylin	Corylin	Coomassie staining	No data	No data	Chocolate
Hazelnut	1999	42	Sandwich ELISA	Rabbit Ab, sheep Ab, both polyclonal	Native and heated corylin	Roasted hazelnut protein extract	HRP	3/39: Walnut (0.0004%) Pumpkin seed (0.0006%) Cashew (0.0002%)	0.03–0.43 mg/kg hazelnut protein	Spiked samples: Cookie, cereal bar, chocolate; Incurred sample: Chocolate
Hazelnut	1999	43	Sandwich ELISA	Rabbit IgG, polyclonal	Crude hazelnut protein extract	Native hazelnut protein extract	HRP	6/27: Walnut (0.0787%) Cashew (0.0034%) Brazil nut (0.0028%) Pinenut (0.0010%) Peanut (0.0011%) Almond (0.0028%)	1 mg/kg hazelnut	No data

ALLERGENS IN TREE NUTS, SESAME SEEDS, MUSTARD, AND CELERY

Allergen	Year	Ref	Method	Antibody	Calibrator	Reference	Label	Cross-reactivity	Detection limit	Samples
Hazelnut	2001	47	Sandwich ELISA	Hen's egg yolk IgY, polyclonal	Hazelnut globulin fraction	Raw hazelnut protein extract	HRP	0/4	1 mg/kg hazelnut protein	Spiked samples: Cake, cookies, fruit bar, muesli, chocolate, ice cream
Hazelnut	2001	97	Biosensor	Polyclonal	Corylin	No data	Surface plasmon resonance	No data	10 mg/kg corylin	No data
Hazelnut	2001	96	Immunoblot	Rabbit Ab, polyclonal	No data	No data	AP	1/4: Almond	5 mg/kg hazelnut protein	Spiked samples: Chocolates
Hazelnut	2002	52	Sandwich ELISA (dipstick)	Rabbit Ab, sheep Ab, both polyclonal	Native and heated corylin	Not applicable (qualitative)	HRP	5/23: Kidney bean (weak) Walnut (clear) Pine seed (weak) Coconut (weak) Cereals (weak)	0.2 mg/kg hazelnut protein	Recovery verified versus ELISA: Chocolate, cereal bar, cookies,
Hazelnut	2003	44	Competitive ELISA	Rabbit IgG, polyclonal	Roasted hazelnut extract	Roasted hazelnut extract	HRP	0/39: At < 1mg/ml	0.25 mg/kg hazelnut protein	Spiked samples: Milk chocolate, cookies, breakfast cereals, ice cream
Hazelnut	2003	94	Sandwich dot blot (multiallergen)	Hen's egg IgY, polyclonal	Raw hazelnut extract	Not applicable (qualitative)	HRP	0/2	0.1–1 mg/kg hazelnut	Spiked samples: Cookies, chocolate, ice cream
Hazelnut	2004	93	Competitive ELISA	Hen's egg IgY, polyclonal	Roasted hazelnut extract	Hazelnut extract	HRP	13/29: At %-level	Unclear data	Spiked sample: Cookie

Continued

Table 4.3 (Continued) Published Protein-Based Methods for the Detection of Tree Nuts, Sesame, Mustard, and Celery (as of April 2010)

Allergenic Food	Year	Ref.	Technique	Antibody (Source and Type)	Immunogen/	Standard	Detection	Cross-Reactivity/ Tested Foods	Sensitivity in Matrix	Recovery Studies in Spiked/incurred Matrices
Hazelnut	2005	95	Competitive ELISA (multiallergen)	Rabbit IgG, polyclonal	Roasted hazelnut extract	Roasted hazelnut extract	HRP	4/24: Almond Cashew Egg Lobster	<1 mg/kg hazelnut protein	Spiked sample: dark and milk chocolate
Hazelnut	2005	45	Sandwich ELISA	Mouse, monoclonal; rabbit Ab, polyclonal	Roasted hazelnut extract	Hazelnut extract	HRP	5/20: Walnut (0.0012%) Almond (0.0001%) Cashew (0.0001%) Macadamia (0.0001%) Soybean (0.0001%)	0.2–1.2 mg/kg hazelnut	Spiked samples: Cookie, cereals, ice cream, milk chocolate, dark chocolate
Hazelnut	2006	68	Sandwich ELISA	Rabbit Ab, polyclonal	Native hazelnut corylin	Raw hazelnut extract	Europium chelate	1/26: Walnut (0.0001%)	0.1 mg/kg hazelnut protein	Spiked samples: Cereals, cookies, milk chocolate, dark chocolate
Hazelnut	2006	46	Biosensor	Rabbit IgG, hen's egg IgY, both polyclonal	Hazelnut protein fraction	No data	Surface plasmon resonance	No data	5 mg/kg hazelnut	No data
Hazelnut	2009	51	Biosensor	Mouse, monoclonal	Raw and roasted hazelnut extract	Hazelnut protein in olive oil	Surface plasmon resonance	0/40	0.1 mg/kg hazelnut protein	Spiked samples: olive oil

ALLERGENS IN TREE NUTS, SESAME SEEDS, MUSTARD, AND CELERY

Allergen	Year	Ref	Method	Antibody	Standard	Target	Detection	Specificity	LOD/LOQ	Samples
Hazelnut	2009	56	Mass spectrometry	Not applicable	Not applicable	No data	ESI LC-MS/MS and MALDI TOF MS(/MS)	No data	No data	No data
Pecan	2006	102	Competitive ELISA	Rabbit Ab, polyclonal	Pecan protein extract	Pecan protein extract	AP	No data	No specific data available	No data
Pecan	2009	103	Competitive ELISA	Rabbit Ab, polyclonal	Pecan protein extract	Pecan protein extract	HRP	1/65: Walnut (7.8%)	No specific data available	Spiked sample: Chocolate
Walnut	2008	55	Sandwich ELISA	Rabbit Ab, polyclonal	Purified 2S albumin from the roasted walnut variety *Chandler*	Walnut variety *Chandler*	HRP	2/153: Pecan (0.01%), Hazelnut (0.0001%)	LOQ 0.31 mg/kg walnut protein (LOD 0.156)	Incurred samples: Rice porridge, chicken meat balls, bread, sponge cake, biscuits, jelly, orange juice
Walnut	2009	53	Sandwich ELISA	Rabbit Ab, sheep Ab, both polyclonal	Roasted mixture of several brands of English walnuts	English walnut or black walnut	AP	5/100: Pecan (2.5%), minimal with hazelnut, mustard, mace, poppy seed	English walnut: LOQ 1 mg/kg	Incurred samples: Chocolate Spiked samples: Cookies, ice cream, muffins chocolate
Sesame	2006	46	Biosensor	Rabbit IgG, hen's egg IgY, both polyclonal	Sesame protein	Not specified	Surface plasmon resonance	No data	12.5 mg/kg sesame seed protein	No data

Continued

Table 4.3 (*Continued*) Published Protein-Based Methods for the Detection of Tree Nuts, Sesame, Mustard, and Celery (as of April 2010)

Allergenic Food	Year	Ref.	Technique	Antibody (Source and Type)	Immunogen/ Standard	Standard	Detection	Cross-Reactivity/ Tested Foods	Sensitivity in Matrix	Recovery Studies in Spiked/Incurred Matrices
Sesame	2010	50	Competitive ELISA	Hen's egg IgY, polyclonal	Sesame protein extract	Sesame protein extract	HRP	1/13: Chocolate (0.7%)	5–10 mg sesame seed protein	Protein spikes: Crisp toasts, snacks, rolls Sesame seed spikes: Cookies, muesli
Mustard	2007	110	Competitive ELISA	Rabbit Ab, polyclonal	Mustard protein extract	Mustard protein extract	HRP	3/16: Soy (0.016%) Milk (0.28%) Egg yolk (0.2 %)	1.5 mg/kg mustard protein	Spiked sample: Mustard seed oil
Mustard	2008	48	Sandwich ELISA	Rabbit Ab, sheep Ab, both polyclonal	Mustard protein extract	Mustard protein extract	AP	1/>90: Rapeseed (1.2–1.7%)	1–3 mg/kg mustard flour	Incurred samples: Sausages

Food	Year	Ref	Method	Antibody	Capture	Detection	Label	Cross-reactivity	LOD/LOQ	Matrix
Mustard	2008	111	Sandwich ELISA	Rabbit IgG, polyclonal	Sin a 1	Sin a 1	HRP	No data	No data	No data
Celery	2010	57	Sandwich ELISA	Rabbit Ab, polyclonal	Celeriac powder extract	Celeriac powder extract	HRP	18/36: Especially: Potato (>100%) Carrot (>100%) Parsnip (41%) Parsley (18%) Cabbage (19%) Cherry (12%) Dill (12%)	0.5–1.7 mg/kg celeriac protein	Spikes: Taco mix, Swedish sausage, dressing, pasta sauce
Celery	2010	57	Mass spectrometry	Not applicable	No data	No data	NanoLC-ion trap MS/MS QQQ MS/MS	No data	No data	No data

Note: Ab = antibody: antiserum or purified fraction thereof; AP = alkaline phosphatase; ESI = electrospray ionization; HRP = horseradish peroxidase; LC = liquid chromatography; MALDI TOF = matrix-assisted laser desorption/ionization time of flight; QQQ = triple quadrupole.

Table 4.4 Published DNA-Based Methods for the Detection of Tree Nuts, Sesame, Mustard, and Celery (as of April 2010)

Allergenic Food	Year	Ref.	Target Gene Coding for	Method	Amplicon Size (bp)	Cross-Reactivity/Tested Foods	Sensitivity	Recovery Studies in Spiked/Incurred Matrices
Almond	2009	74	Pru 1 (11S globulin), sequence not specified	Real-time PCR; SYBR Green; melting curve	76	0/8	1 template copy	No data
Almond	2009	74	1,5-Bisphosphate carboxylase	Real-time PCR; SYBR Green; melting curve	69	6/8	1 template copy	No data
Almond	2009	72	extensin gene	Ligation-dependent probe amplification	116	4/48: Apricot Nectarine Peach Plum	No data	No data
Almond	2010	101	Pru av 1	Tetraplex real-time PCR, specific fluorescent probes	129	1/46: Apricot (1.2%)	10–50 mg/kg almond	Spiked sample: Rice cookies
Brazil nut	2009	72	Sulfur-rich seed protein	Ligation-dependent probe amplification	124	0/48	No data	No data
Brazil nut	2010	84	Ber e 2 11 S globulin	Real-time PCR; specific fluorescent probe	65	0/36	10 pg Brazil nut DNA 1,000 mg/kg	Spiked samples: Nut pastes with Brazil nut (50–1,000,000 mg/kg)
Cashew	2003	87	5S RNA	Conventional PCR, gel	~160	0/13	No data	Mixtures of tea, bamboo and cashew
Cashew	2006	88	Ana o 3 2S albumin	Real-time PCR; specific fluorescent probe	67	0/8	5 pg DNA 100 mg/kg cashew	Chocolate cookie spiked with cashew (1–1,000 mg/kg)
Cashew	2007	76	Ana o 3 2S albumin	Real-time PCR; specific fluorescent probe	67	0/17	1.25 pg DNA (2.5 genome equivalents) 100 mg/kg cashew	Spiked samples: Pistachio nougat with cashew (100–100,000 mg/kg)

ALLERGENS IN TREE NUTS, SESAME SEEDS, MUSTARD, AND CELERY

Food	Year	Ref	Target	Method			Detection limit	Samples
Cashew	2008	89	Ana o 3 2S albumin	Real-time PCR; specific probe	103	0/56	0.5 pg DNA (10 template copies) 2 mg/kg cashew	Spiked samples: Pesto samples with cashew (1–100 mg/kg)
Cashew	2009	72	Ana o 3 2S albumin	Ligation-dependent probe amplification	92	0/48	5 mg/kg cashew	Spiked samples: Pesto samples with cashew (1–100 mg/kg)
Hazelnut	2000	58	Cor a 1.03, major hazelnut allergen	Conventional PCR, gel	182	0/32	Less than 10 mg/kg hazelnut, corresponding to less than 1 mg/kg hazelnut protein	Spiked and incurred samples at low milligram/kilogram level: Cookies, cereals, chocolate, potato snack
Hazelnut	2002	67	Cor a 1.04, major hazelnut allergen	PCR-ELISA, specific probe	152	0/35	2 pg hazelnut DNA; less than 10 mg/kg hazelnut, corresponding to less than 1 mg/kg hazelnut protein	Spiked and incurred samples at low milligram/kilogram level: Cookies, cereals, chocolate
Hazelnut	2003	63	Nad 1, mitochondrial	Conventional PCR, gel	294	4/32: Carpinus sp., Ostrya carpinifolia	10 mg/kg hazelnut	Spiked sample: Chocolate
Hazelnut	2005	61	Cor a 1.03, major hazel pollen allergen	PCR-HPLC, specific PNA probe	156	0/14	5 pg hazelnut DNA	Incurred samples at the % level: Cereals, wafer, biscuit, chocolate
Hazelnut	2006	71	Cor a 1.03, major hazel pollen allergen	PCR-array, specific PNA probe	156	No data	50 pg hazelnut DNA	Incurred samples at unknown amount of hazelnut
Hazelnut	2007	100	Cor a 1.04, major hazelnut allergen	Real-time PCR; specific fluorescent probe	82	0/14	100 pg hazelnut DNA	Incurred samples at the 5–20% level
Hazelnut	2008	66	Hsp 1, heat shock protein	Real-time PCR; specific fluorescent probe	100	0/19	13 pg hazelnut DNA; 100 mg/kg hazelnut	Incurred samples: Pastry down to 100 mg/kg hazelnut

Continued

Table 4.4 (Continued) Published DNA-Based Methods for the Detection of Tree Nuts, Sesame, Mustard, and Celery (as of April 2010)

Allergenic Food	Year	Ref.	Target Gene Coding for	Method	Amplicon Size (bp)	Cross-Reactivity/Tested Foods	Sensitivity	Recovery Studies in Spiked/Incurred Matrices
Hazelnut	2009	73	Cor a 8, lipid transfer protein	Real-time PCR; SYBR Green; melting curve	78	0/18	10 pg hazelnut DNA; 10 mg/kg hazelnut	Spiked wheat flour down to 10 mg/kg hazelnut
Hazelnut	2009	72	Cor a 1.0401	Ligation-dependent probe amplification	104	0/48	5–100 mg/kg hazelnut	Spiked samples: Chocolate Incurred samples Walnut cookie
Hazelnut	2009	60	Cor a 1.03, major hazel pollen allergen	Duplex real-time PCR; SYBR Green, and specific fluorescent probe	109	0/25	50 pg hazelnut DNA; 50 mg/kg hazelnut	Spiked samples: Cookies
Hazelnut	2010	101	Cor a 1.03, major hazel pollen allergen	Tetraplex real-time PCR, specific fluorescent probes	145	1/46: Peach (10%)	10–50 mg/kg hazelnut	Spiked sample: Rice cookies
Hazelnut	2010	75	Not specified	Hexaplex real-time PCR, SYBR Green; melting curves	54	No data	5 pg hazelnut DNA	No data
Macadamia	2009	104	Vicilin precursor	Real-time PCR; specific fluorescent probe	73	0/16	1.45 pg DNA 200 mg/kg pecan	Incurred samples: Pastry with pistachio (10–100,000 mg/kg)
Macadamia	2009	72	Vicilin precursor	Ligation-dependent probe amplification	112	0/48	1000 mg/kg macadamia	Incurred samples: Walnut cookie
Pecan	2008	77	Vicilin-like seed storage protein	Real-time PCR; specific fluorescent probe	89	0/40	1 pg DNA (1.2 template copies) 100 mg/kg pecan	Incurred samples: Pastry with pecan (100–100,000 mg/kg)
Pecan	2009	72	Vicilin-like protein	Ligation-dependent probe amplification	96	0/48	No data	No data

ALLERGENS IN TREE NUTS, SESAME SEEDS, MUSTARD, AND CELERY

Food	Year	Ref	Target	Method	Amplicon	Specificity	Sensitivity	Sample
Pistachio	2006	70	Dehydrin	Conventional PCR, gel	280 + 391 + Third one	0/18	100 mg/kg pistachio	Incurred sample: Mortadella with pistachio (40+100 mg/kg)
Pistachio	2008	69	Internal transcribed spacer between 18S and 5.8S ribosomal RNA (multicopy)	Real-time PCR; specific fluorescent probe	64	0/26	0.012 pg DNA (1.2 template copies) 4 mg/kg pistachio	Incurred samples: Pastry with pistachio (4–100,000 mg/kg)
Pistachio	2009	72	Dehydrin	Ligation-dependent probe amplification	100	0/48	No data	No data
Walnut	2006	106	Jug r 2 Vicilin seed storage protein	Real-time PCR; specific fluorescent probe	85	0/24 (Pecan after 35 cycles)	100 mg/kg walnut/ 240 pg walnut DNA	Incurred samples: Pastry with walnut (100–100,000 mg/kg)
Walnut	2007	107	Maturase (chloroplast)	Conventional PCR, gel	120	1/14: Pecan	0.5 pg walnut DNA (denoted as 10 mg/kg walnut equivalency)	DNA mixtures: genomic salmon DNA samples containing walnut DNA
Walnut	2009	72	Vicilin precursor	Ligation-dependent probe amplification	120	0/48	No data	No data
Walnut	2009	108	Jug r 2 vicilin seed storage protein	Real-time PCR; specific fluorescent probe	88	0/14	1.25 pg walnut DNA 10 mg/kg walnut	Spiked samples: Wheat powder with walnut (10–100,000 mg/kg)
Sesame	2007	65	2S albumin allergen	Real-time PCR; specific fluorescent probe	66	0/8	5 pg sesame seed DNA, 100 mg/kg sesame	Spiked sample: Cracker
Sesame	2007	62	Ses i 1, 2S albumin allergen	Real-time PCR; specific fluorescent probe	117	0/16	50 pg sesame seed DNA, 500 mg/kg sesame seed	Spiked sample: Crisp bread
Sesame	2008	109	2S albumin allergen	Tripleplex Real-time PCR; specific fluorescent probe	64	0/14	50 mg/kg sesame seed	Spiked sample: Barbeque spice, wheat flour

Continued

Table 4.4 (Continued) Published DNA-Based Methods for the Detection of Tree Nuts, Sesame, Mustard, and Celery (as of April 2010)

Allergenic Food	Year	Ref.	Target Gene Coding for	Method	Amplicon Size (bp)	Cross-Reactivity/ Tested Foods	Sensitivity	Recovery Studies in Spiked/ Incurred Matrices
Sesame	2009	60	Ses i 1, 2S albumin allergen	Duplex real-time PCR; specific fluorescent probe	117	0/25	10 pg sesame seed DNA, 50 mg/kg sesame seed	Spiked sample: Cookie
Sesame	2009	72	7S globulin	Ligation-dependent probe amplification	108	0/48	No data	No data
Sesame	2010	75	Not specified	Hexaplex real-time PCR, SYBR Green; melting curves	100	No data	0.5 pg sesame seed DNA	No data
Sesame	2010	101	Oleosin	Tetraplex real-time PCR; specific fluorescent probes	145	0/46	10–50 mg/kg sesame	Spiked sample: Rice cookies
Mustard	2008	109	Sin a	Tripleplex Real-time PCR; specific fluorescent probe	170–180	1/14: Radish	50 mg/kg mustard	Spiked sample: Barbeque spice, wheat flour

Celery	2004	112	Api g 1	Real-time PCR; specific fluorescent probe	145	Spices, no details	30 pg celery seed DNA	No data
Celery	2004	64	Mannitol dehydrogenase	Conventional PCR, gel	279	0/16	490–1530pg DNA, 1000 mg/kg celery	Incurred samples: Meat pâtés (100–10,000 mg/kg)
Celery	2007	59	Mannitol dehydrogenase	Real-time PCR; specific fluorescent probe	101	0/60	5–10 mg/kg celery seed	Incurred samples: Emulsion-type sausage (1–1,000 mg/kg)
Celery	2008	109	Mannitol dehydrogenase	Tripleplex real-time PCR; specific fluorescent probe	151	0/14	All matrices 10 mg/kg celeriac powder, except 50 mg/kg in wheat/maize flour	Spiked samples: Vegetable burger, barbeque spice, wok vegetables, raw minced beef, wheat/maize flour
Celery	2010	101	Mannitol dehydrogenase	Tetraplex real-time PCR, specific probes	145	0/46	No data	No data

Another approach to specifically detect an allergenic food is to detect a specific sequence stretch of its genetic information, the DNA. Making use of DNA as a specific marker for the presence of an allergenic food is thus based on the assumption that the DNA and protein fraction are not separated by food technological processes. Several studies have demonstrated good correlation between protein-based and DNA-based methods in the detection of allergenic foods at the low milligram/kilogram level (summarized in Holzhauser, Stephan, and Vieths, S [40]). The most popular methodology of DNA-based detection of allergenic food is the polymerase chain reaction (PCR), of which the so-called real-time PCR with real-time verification of an amplified DNA sequence is state-of-the-art technology. PCR for the detection of allergenic foods has become popular because of several advantages, such as high selectivity and specificity, the ability to design specific detection, a fully reproducible chemistry, and a sensitivity that is similar to that of ELISA for a large number of allergenic foods. Once published, the method may be reproduced depending on laboratory skills, in contrast to antibody-based methods, which require the availability of the antibody. However, there are also limitations in PCR methodology, such as occasional matrix susceptibility that may result in higher limits of detection (LODs).

Finally, less common are immunoblotting or immunoprecipitation techniques, antibody-based biosensors, or the MS detection of allergenic foods. The last technique is less evolved for the detection of allergens but has promising potential.

All described analytical techniques are in principle applicable for verification of obligatory labeling requirements that do not refer to a certain component like protein or DNA but to the entire allergenic food. No matter which method is chosen for allergen detection, it needs to reliably detect the food component with allergenic potential at a level at which severe allergic reactions are avoided in the majority of food-allergic subjects. Taking into account published data on eliciting thresholds and typical serving sizes, such level of sensitivity should be in the low milligram/kilogram range and depend on the allergenic food, such as 1–100 mg/kg, as summarized by Poms et al.[41] and in this chapter.

So far, particular ELISA and PCR methods have been developed to detect tree nuts and seeds such as sesame, mustard, and celery. Several of those applications allow detecting or quantifying the allergenic food of interest in a variety of relevant food matrices and with a sensitivity that is suitable to protect allergic subjects from severe allergic reactions. None of these tests may fulfill all analytical criteria, but some have been shown to cover most of the relevant analytical scenarios. Whereas ELISA methods are sensitive and generally quantitative, PCR is based on reproducible chemistry and is highly specific. Moreover, quantitative PCR is technically feasible but has not been published. Hence, the choice of a suitable method depends on a variety of factors that have to be taken into account: (1) method availability, (2) required sensitivity, (3) required specificity, (4) matrix ruggedness, (5) quantitative features if required, and (6) the available laboratory equipment and technical capability.

Comparable numbers of protein-based (Table 4.3) and DNA-based (Table 4.4) methods have been developed. Approximately 70 methods for the detection of tree nuts, sesame seeds, mustard, and celery are summarized and reviewed next.

SAMPLE PREPARATION

For Protein Detection

Sample preparation for antibody-based techniques is rather simple because of the high binding affinity of antibodies, allowing separation of the analyte from other components of a food sample extract, especially if the detection occurs in solid-phase-type assays, such as microtiter plate-based ELISA, blotting membranes, or biosensor surfaces. The food sample preparation mainly consists of grinding, extraction, and clarification, without further steps of protein purification. Referenced examples of the many published methods for allergenic seeds discussed in this chapter were selected to highlight the range of conditions chosen for protein extraction prior to immunochemical detection.

Usually, food samples are first ground in a blender for homogenization. Aliquot sample weights between 0.5 and 10 g are subsequently extracted in suitable buffers at ratios between 1:4 and 1:20 (w/v for solid samples and v/v for liquid samples).[42–46] In most cases, phosphate-buffered saline (PBS)[44,47,48] or Tris-buffered saline (TBS)[42,49,50] are used for extraction at a neutral to slightly alkaline environment. Saline is usually around 150 mM; occasionally, high-salt buffers having 1M sodium chloride are used for stabilization of seed storage proteins.[44] Some use commercial extraction buffers of unknown composition.[45,51] For acidic food samples, Lee et al.[48] also adjusted the sample pH between 6.0 and 8.0 with 1N NaOH. In some cases, detergents such as Tween or Triton are added, usually around 0.1–0.5%.[44,47] For better recovery of target proteins, some investigators add irrelevant proteins or protein mixtures such as fish gelatin[52,53] or skim milk powder[45,47,53] at around 1–10%.

The protein extraction is usually accomplished after a few minutes and up to 1 or 2 h[42,43] and at ambient temperature[43] or elevated temperatures up to 60°C.[46] Some researchers reduce extraction time to 2 min using ultrahomogenization devices, such as UltraTurrax.[50] Food sample extracts are usually centrifuged or filtered for clarification prior to analysis in ELISA or biosensor methods.

Protein standards, which are made from seeds for determination of LOD or quantitative evaluation, are usually processed accordingly. The ground seeds might be defatted[54,55] or applied as full-fat seed flour[42,43] to protein extraction.

Sample preparation for MS analysis has only been described for hazelnut[56] and celery[57] within this group of allergenic foods. It requires MS-compatible chemistry for extraction (e.g., the avoidance of detergents) and, depending on the MS technique, the digestion of protein samples into peptides using suitable proteases. For further details, please refer to the work of Weber et al.[56] and Faeste et al.,[57] and Chapters 3, 5, and 6.

For Nucleic Acid Detection

Nucleic acids, especially DNA, that are used for PCR detection of allergens need to be of high purity to avoid a disadvantageous influence on PCR efficiency. PCR is based on numerous repetitive and identical amplification reactions. Each matrix effect that results in a lowering of efficiency in the amplification reaction multiplies within each cycle of this sequence and may finally result in insufficient amplification of target DNA below detectability. Thus, it is critical to avoid PCR inhibitors (i.e., food matrix components) that substantially decrease amplification efficiency. The purified DNA is finally concentrated for increased sensitivity.

The major steps of sample preparation for PCR analysis are (1) grinding, (2) extraction, (3) purification, and (4) concentration of the nucleic acids. The range of conditions for extraction and purification of DNA from foods of this chapter are summarized, and selected references are given.

First, food samples are ground in a blender for homogenization. Usually, aliquot sample weights between 0.1 and 5 g are extracted in suitable buffers: DNA is extracted in the presence of detergents and proteases, which break up cell and nuclear membranes, and at neutral to slightly alkaline pH. Classic protocols apply proteinase K as a protease and detergents such as cetyltrimethylammoniumbromide (CTAB)[58–60] or sodium dodecyl sulfate in the presence of guanidine hydrochloride or guanidine thiocyanate.[61] The extraction is usually done at elevated temperature, such as 65°C, and within 30 to 90 min. Lipids are often removed by chloroform.[58,59,61,62] Occasionally, ribonucleases (RNases) are applied to remove RNA. The DNA purification is usually done by precipitation of DNA with CTAB[60] or alcohol[58,59] or by selected DNA binding to silica in the presence of chaotropic salts. Alternatively, commercial kits for DNA extraction and silica-based single-round purification have been popular for such reasons as reduced hands-on time, easy handling, and avoidance of harmful compounds.[63–66] However, the detection sensitivity in PCR appears to be inferior compared to classic DNA extraction protocols that involve either two rounds of DNA precipitation with CTAB and isopropanol[60] or a combination of DNA precipitation and final cleanup with commercial silica particles as emulsions[58] or solid-phase membranes.[59] Moreover, Holzhauser and colleagues[67] applied two rounds of DNA purification with commercial silica columns as an alternative to DNA precipitation and achieved DNA quality and PCR sensitivity at the low milligram/kilogram level that is also known for the described classic protocols. Purified DNA that is bound to silica surface is usually eluted at low volume (50–100 µl), or purified precipitated DNA is dissolved in a low volume of neutral to slightly alkaline Tris buffer.

DETECTION AND QUANTIFICATION

Protein Detection

Except for two publications with preliminary data on the potential of MS detection of allergenic hazelnut[56] or celery,[57] all other protein detection methods are antibody based (Table 4.3). The great majority of antibody-based methods for allergen detection discussed in this chapter are ELISA tests. Surface plasmon resonance biosensor, immunoblot, or rocket immunoelectrophoresis techniques have inferior impact. By the number of published methods, sandwich ELISA, which binds the target antigen between two specific antibodies, appears to be twice as popular as competitive ELISA tests. Nonetheless, there are nine competitive ELISA tests, of which the indirect competitive format was exclusively chosen. In indirect competitive ELISA, antigen from standard preparation or food sample extracts competes with solid-phase coated antigen for a limited number of specific antibodies. By contrast to sandwich ELISA, the measurable signal decreases with increasing amount of antigen in the standard or food sample. Indirect competitive ELISA tests are quicker in development because only one antiserum source is necessary, and usually antibodies do not need to be purified from the antiserum. However, competitive formats, in contrast to sandwich ELISA, may give rise to false-positive results at the LOD if matrix components interfere with the maximal antibody binding to the solid-phase antigen in the absence of antigen from the food sample. Most ELISA tests make use of polyclonal antisera or antibodies purified from them; the great majority are rabbit antibodies, followed by sheep and goat antibodies, and hen's egg IgY. Some authors also performed immunoabsorption or affinity purification of antibodies. Mouse monoclonal antibodies have only been used in two cases for the detection and quantification of hazelnut with ELISA[45] and biosensor,[51] respectively. Usually, enzymes for colorimetric staining are either directly coupled to the allergen-specific detection antibody or introduced by conjugates with specificity to the animal species of the allergen detection antibody. Except for one ELISA protocol with fluorescent europium-labeled hazelnut-specific antibody,[68] all other ELISA tests use horseradish peroxidase (HRP) or alkaline phosphatase (AP) as the enzymatic marker for colorimetric detection of the specific antibody binding. The fluorescence detection of hazelnut did not result in additional increase of sensitivity when compared to classic ELISA with HRP and colorimetric detection of hazelnut protein.[42,52]

Nucleic Acid Detection

The sensitive detection of nucleic acids requires the exponential amplification of a specific DNA sequence in PCR. The primer sequences that define the length of the amplified sequence need to be specific for the species of the allergenic food of interest. This amplicon should be rather short and between 50 and 150 bp in length because food technological processing results in truncated DNA stretches. Depending on the extent of processing, the DNA might be shortened below 200 bp. The DNA-based methods that are summarized in Table 4.4 generally take into account this aspect and amplify DNA products with a mean amplicon size of 134 ± 76 bp (median 113 bp). However, there are also few examples of primers that amplify sequences of up to 391 bp. More than half of the reviewed PCR methods in this chapter amplify DNA sequences of genes for single food allergens, even though this is not a specific requirement from the analytical point of view. Only one method for pistachio detection amplifies a multicopy gene.[69]

Conventional PCR relies on the specificity of the primer pair only, and amplicons are separated by size in agarose gel electrophoresis with fluorescence detection after incorporation of DNA intercalating dyes, such as ethidium bromide. Highly specific conventional PCR tests have been described.[58,64,70] However, the detection of amplicons in agarose gel electrophoresis is not sequence specific, and coamplification of unknown cross-reactive DNA sequences to products of similar size may not be discriminated. Therefore, it is state of the art to verify the sequence of amplicons.[40] This can be done after PCR with sequence-specific probes in so-called PCR-ELISA (i.e., microwell) format,[67] by high-performance liquid chromatographic (HPLC) analysis,[61] by array technology,[71] or by capillary electrophoresis.[72] However, post-PCR manipulation of amplicons is cumbersome and potentially prone to cross contaminate future PCR experiments with amplifiable DNA. Thus, the most popular and sophisticated development is the verification of the amplicon sequence by fluorescent probes in real time. The real-time PCR with fluorescent and sequence-specific probes is thus the most frequently applied technique, as is summarized in Table 4.4. Real-time PCR may also be done with DNA intercalating dyes, such as SYBR® Green, instead of probes.[73–75] However, this type of amplicon detection is not sequence specific, and even melting curve analysis cannot replace the high specificity of amplicon-specific probes. The combination of highly specific primers and additional sequence verification with specific probes in real-time PCR offers unparalleled specificity and low risk of cross contamination of future PCR runs.[59,60,76,77]

POTENTIAL AND LIMITATIONS OF PUBLISHED METHODS

Almond

In 1999, Acosta et al.[78] applied polyclonal antibodies from rabbits raised against the purified primary storage protein of almond (almond major protein, AMP) in a noncompetitive ELISA. That format was used to test the impact of pH and different heating methods on immunogenicity of the almond protein and to test the response of different cultivars. Depending on thermal treatment, the immunoreactivity of the antibodies was reduced to 13% in comparison to untreated AMP protein. Immunogenicity was best at pH 7.0 and was only slightly reduced in a pH range of 4.0–11.5 but decreased strongly at higher and lower pH values. The antibodies were also used for a competitive almond ELISA. Cross-reactivity was seen with other nuts and legumes. Botanically closely related species were not included in cross-reactivity studies, and spiked food matrices were not evaluated. Roux et al.[79] published an updated competitive ELISA format using the same antibody. This time, heat treatment was tested with two cultivars, and the detection level was improved. They also tested the recovery from five food matrices spiked with AMP. Depending on the food matrix, almond could be detected between 5 and 37 mg/kg. Cross-reactivity studies were not performed. In 2002, the same group published a third article, again dealing with effects of heat treating on antigenicity of almond proteins. Venkatachalam et al.[80] compared the effects of heating by analysis with the established inhibition ELISA and also with a new sandwich ELISA format. The sandwich ELISA consisted of polyclonal antibodies from rabbit and goat both raised against unprocessed nonpareil almond protein. No validation information was given for the sandwich ELISA. The statistical analysis of the effects of heat processing, expressed by the ratios of

IC_{50} processed almond/IC_{50} unprocessed almond, did not show a significant difference in immunogenicity in most cases.

Hlywka et al.[81] published the development of a sandwich ELISA for the specific detection of almond. They used sheep and goat polyclonal antibodies that were raised against roasted almonds. Cross-reactivity was tested with more than 40 foods, and some reactivity was seen with sesame seed, black walnut, Brazil nut, macadamia, hazelnut, and pistachio. Cross-reactivity ranged between 56.7 and 17.8 mg/kg, calculated from the published data. Kernels from phylogenetically closely related peach or almond were not tested. The recovery of spiked almond was similar for spiked and incurred milk chocolate samples and ranged between 86% and 100%. The detection limit of the ELISA was at 1 mg/kg almond; the response to different cultivars was not checked. A retail survey of 20 brands of cereals did not detect unlabeled almond protein. An unexpected result was that although stated as an ingredient, almond could not be detected in some products. The authors explained this as the possibility that the manufacturers could most probably not exclude the possibility of cross contamination and applied precautionary labeling.[81]

A real-time PCR method for the detection of almond was published by Pafundo et al..[74] They presented the validation of two SYBR® Green PCR methods. One primer pair targeted a sequence of a multicopy gene coding for chloroplastic ribulose 1,5-bisphosphate carboxylase. Cross-reactivity experiments performed with only eight different foods gave false-positive results with six foods, and the primer combination was thus not applicable for the detection of almond. Another primer pair targeted a sequence of the gene coding for an 11S globulin. However, the sequence of this primer pair was not published. Cross-reactivity was not seen in any of the eight tested foods. However, cross-reactivity was not checked in most relevant foods of closely related species like apricot, peach, or plum. Furthermore, no practical detection limit has been investigated in different almond-spiked matrices. Sensitivity experiments were performed with serial dilutions of genomic DNA and plasmid DNA containing targeted sequences. According to the results, even one copy of target sequence could be detected reproducibly.

Brazil Nut

Blais et al.[54] developed a sandwich ELISA for the detection of Brazil nut in food. They used egg yolk antibodies (IgY) raised against Brazil nut protein by immunizing a hen with purified Brazil nut protein. The detection antibody was produced by labeling the anti-Brazil nut antibody with biotin. The specificity was examined with only five foods, and no cross-reactivity was seen. The sensitivity was investigated with 10 different food matrices spiked with Brazil nut in a range of 0.13 to 10 mg/kg. The detection limit, depending on the food matrix, was between 0.25 and 1 mg/kg. Since only values for mean absorbance were given, no results for the recovery can be concluded.[54]

In 2004, a competitive ELISA was published by Clemente et al.[82] The authors used purified 2S albumin protein from Brazil nut for immunizing rabbits and raising antibodies against the 2S albumin protein. The authors developed a competitive

ELISA test since the sandwich ELISA did not detect the 2S albumin well. The working range of the assay was deduced from the precision profile and ranged between 1 and 100 µg/ml Brazil nut 2S protein. The practical applicability of the test was not proven with any food matrices spiked with Brazil nut. The specificity was assessed with other nuts and legumes (eight foods) without showing positive signals. The analysis of retail products, some of which carried Brazil nut labeling, provided positive or negative results in correspondence to the labeling.[82]

Girdhari et al.[83] developed another competitive ELISA for the detection of Brazil nut. In contrast to Clemente et al.,[82] the competitive ELISA applied antibodies raised against the whole protein fraction of Brazil nut. Rabbit immunization was done with defatted Brazil nut protein extract. The specificity of the assay was tested against 66 different food components; only cinnamon exhibited a significant interference of 1.36%, which is equivalent to a false-positive signal of 13,600 mg/kg Brazil nut. From investigations with different types of heat treatment, it was concluded that the immunogenic stability of Brazil nut protein does not change. The detection range of the standard curve was 10–90 ng/ml Brazil nut protein. The sensitivity of the ELISA was investigated with four different food matrices, which were spiked with 1 and 10 mg/kg of soluble Brazil nut protein or 10 to 100 mg/kg of defatted Brazil nut flour. The recovery of defatted Brazil nut ranged depending on the matrix and the spiked agent between 63% and 315%.[83]

Brežná et al.[84] published the first PCR method dealing with the detection of Brazil nuts in food in 2010. They developed a specific Taqman® real-time PCR method targeting a 65-bp sequence on the gene coding for Ber e2, an 11S globulin. Sensitivity experiments were performed with model nut pastes of defined Brazil nut that ranged from 50 to 1 million mg/kg in a mixture with walnut. The practical detection limit was deduced from the reproducible detection of the smallest sample spike (1,000 mg/kg Brazil nut). There were 36 other tested plant and animal foods that did not cross-react. The authors stated that this method was one or two orders of magnitude less sensitive than required by expert groups of allergologists.

Cashew

The first ELISA method for the detection of cashew was published in 2003. Wei et al.[85] raised polyclonal antibodies in a goat against all water-soluble protein of unheated cashew and in rabbits against purified anacardein, the major soluble cashew protein. Antibodies from both animals were immunoadsorbed with cross-reactive proteins of a variety of plant foods, identified in Western blotting prescreens. Thereafter, the formerly cross-reactive foods did not cross bind except for sunflower seed (0.0023%), pistachio (0.002%), walnut (0.0018%), and pecan (0.004%). The recovery rate in seven different food matrices spiked with 0.1 to 100 mg/100 mg (equivalent to 5–5,000 mg/kg defatted cashew) anacardein ranged from 50% to 136%. The coefficient of variation depended on the matrix and spiking level, and ranged for milk chocolate spiked with cashew from 13.3% at the highest spiking level to 40% at the lowest level. Comparable data for recovery rates were obtained for defatted cashew flour spikes. The LOD was not given, but a mean standard curve detection range from 0.01 to 0.15 mg/kg anacardein was noted. Wei et al. also tested the influence of four different heating methods on the antigenicity of anacardein. The recovery rates after four different heat treatment procedures in comparison to anacardein of unprocessed cashew were as follows: roasting (18%), autoclaving (44%), microwaving (89%), and blanching (57%).[85]

An abstract about a validated ELISA for cashew detection was published by Gaskin et al.[86] They developed an ELISA using polyclonal antibodies from sheep and rabbit raised against the protein fraction of roasted cashews. Among 99 foods, cross-reactivity was only detected with hazelnut and pistachio. The mean recovery rates from the following food matrices was ice cream 103% ± 5.8%, cookies 75% ± 6.9%, and milk chocolate 102% ± 3.4%. The investigation of 59 retail samples detected cashew in 4 out of 5 samples with cashew labeling as an ingredient, in 5 of 36 carrying precautionary labeling, and in none of the 18 samples for which cashew was not labeled.[86]

The first qualitative PCR method for cashew detection was published by Dhiman and Singh.[87] The conventional PCR method with agarose gel electrophoresis of amplicons was originally intended for the detection of cashew in adulterated tea and relied only on the specificity of the primer pair. The target of the PCR was a sequence of approximately 160 bp on the spacer region between 5S ribosomal RNA (rRNA) genes. Specificity was checked with bamboo, 12 different tea cultivars, 9 different plant species, and genomic DNA from animal, human, and bacterial genomes. The sensitivity of the method was not investigated.[87]

Several real-time methods for detection of cashew have been published. The first was published in 2006 by Brzezinski.[88] A Taqman® real-time PCR was developed, targeting a 67-bp long sequence on the cashew 2S albumin (Ana o 3). The DNA was extracted with a commercial extraction kit. Experiments performed with raw and roasted cashew nut did not show remarkable different cycle threshold (C_T) values. The sensitivity of the method was investigated with a "chocolate chip cookie" spiked with cashew in the range of 1–1,000 mg/kg. Results were only given for spiking levels down to 100 mg/kg, and a remark was made that 1 mg/kg did not give any positive signal. The authors calculated a theoretical detection limit of 50 mg/kg, which was deduced from experiments with purified cashew DNA. However, the practical detection limit from spiking experiments was 100 mg/kg. The cross-reactivity studies comprised four tree nuts and three different varieties of peanuts, and no positive signal was observed. The author did not include pistachio, a close relative of cashew, in cross-reactivity testings.

Piknová and Kuchta[76] published results of a Taqman® PCR in 2007. They used the published primers and the probe of Brzezinski.[88] A slightly different PCR program with increased annealing temperatures was used for amplification. In summary, there were no remarkable new data available except for some more foods tested in cross-reactivity studies. The practical detection limit of the method was determined with spiked pistachio nougat and was in concordance with the investigations of Brzezinski[88]: 0.01%. This study included pistachio in cross-reactivity studies, and no false positive was observed.[76]

The third Taqman® real-time PCR method was published by Ehlert et al.,[89] and the method also targeted the gene coding the allergenic 2S albumin. The sequence length was 103 bp. DNA extraction was performed with the CTAB method. In contrast to former publications, extensive in-house validation data for the method were published. Specificity of the method was investigated with DNA from 56 plant and animal foods, and none gave a positive signal. Response to four cashew samples was given without closer data. The sensitivity of the method was validated with pesto samples spiked with cashew in a range of 1 to 100 mg/kg. The practical detection limit was 2 mg/kg. The advantage of the new method is improved specificity and demonstrated sensitivity in comparison to the other real-time PCR methods. The authors stated that they obtained false-positive signals with the real-time PCR method from Piknová and Kuchta[76] with five different pistachio DNA extracts and pink pepper, whereas their real-time PCR method did not give false-positive signals. Twenty retail samples were checked for correct labeling of cashew, and cashew was only detected positively in samples declaring cashew as an ingredient.

Hazelnut

The importance of hazelnut as an allergenic food is reflected in the numerous published methods for hazelnut detection (Tables 4.3 and 4.4). In the 1980s, several immunoassays, especially immunoprecipitation and ELISA techniques, for the detection and quantification of hazelnut as a quality ingredient were published; however, these were without an appropriate sensitivity to identify relevant traces of allergenic hazelnut (summarized in Holzhauser and Vieths[42]). The first method to verify contamination or mislabeling of hazelnut was a rocket immunoelectrophoresis (RIE) method that detected nondeclared hazelnut protein. The method was shown to detect between 0.002% and 0.3% hazelnut protein in various matrices.[49,90] However, validation data were basically lacking.

In 1999, Holzhauser and Vieths[42] described the detection of hazelnut by a sandwich ELISA test that applied a rabbit polyclonal antiserum as a source of hazelnut protein-specific capture antibodies and a sheep polyclonal antiserum as a source of hazelnut protein-specific detector antibodies. The rabbit antiserum was immunoabsorbed against walnut and pumpkin seed extract, which were identified as the most critical cross-reactive foods in a prescreening. Extensive testing of characteristic food components for potential cross-reactivity ($n = 39$) revealed only pumpkin seed, walnut, and cashew as potential food components that would give false-positive signals of 6, 4, and 2 mg/kg hazelnut protein, respectively. All other tested foods did not give signals at or above 1 mg/kg hazelnut protein. Further, 10% pumpkin seed, 20% walnut, or 50% cashew as components in complex foods would not give a false-positive signal, equivalent to less than 1 mg/kg hazelnut protein. The highly specific ELISA displayed a statistical LOD, based on the analysis of blank food extracts, of 0.03–0.4 mg/kg hazelnut. In six different blank samples of milk and dark and white chocolate, the mean statistical LOD was 0.1 mg/kg hazelnut protein (59% coefficient of variation [CV]). Hazelnut that was spiked into coconut cookie, cereal bar, almond chocolate bar, and milk chocolate at levels of 10 to 1,000 mg/kg was recovered at 104% (17.8% CV). The systematic investigation of six native and two toasted (each at 140°C and 20, 30, and 40 min) hazelnut samples revealed, on the basis of the applied sample extraction procedure, a mean correlation factor of 13.2 (28.5% CV) between detectable hazelnut protein and full-fat hazelnut. In 12/28 commercial retail food samples without labeling or declaration of hazelnut components, between 2 and 421 mg/kg hidden hazelnut protein were identified and quantified. In subsequent studies, the ELISA successfully identified samples with hazelnut protein below 1 mg/kg.[58,67] Further, the ELISA was successfully applied to identify critical control points and to monitor the efficiency of cleaning procedures in the allergen sanitation of both pilot plant and industrial manufacture of cookies, with special regard to the avoidance of cross contamination at or below 1 mg/kg hazelnut protein.[91,92]

Koppelman et al.[43] published a similar but more cross-reactive ELISA for hazelnut in which 100% portions of walnut, cashew, almond, and Brazil nut resulted in a false-positive signal of 787, 34, 28, and 28 mg/kg hazelnut, respectively. By contrast to Holzhauser et al.,[42] the authors used raw hazelnut protein as the immunogen for antibody production and as a standard for quantification. Nonetheless, the antibodies detected raw and roasted hazelnut protein at a comparable extent, with a slightly less-sensitive response to roasted hazelnut. No data were given on the accuracy of hazelnut quantification in either spiked or incurred samples. The ELISA successfully quantified hazelnut in undeclared consumer products but without validation data on recovery. Based on details about sample preparation and ELISA sensitivity, the LOD was 0.1 mg/kg hazelnut protein in food samples.

Blais and Phillippe[47] published a sandwich ELISA but used hazelnut-specific hen's egg IgY. The testing of various spiked samples demonstrated comparable sensitivity, but only limited data on specificity and no data on accuracy were given. A qualitative sandwich-type ELISA on dipstick surface was presented by Stephan et al.[52] The use of a chromogenic precipitating dye on the surface of the dipstick allowed hazelnut detection without further need for microplate reader or washer. The sensitivity was around 0.2–1 mg/kg hazelnut protein. Cross-reactivity was only observed for walnut. Thirty-eight retail food samples were analyzed by immunodipstick and the previously published ELISA[42] there was complete correlation of results, and the intensity of colorimetric detection by immunodipstick increased gradually with increasing amounts of hazelnut. Even though only marginally quicker than ELISA, the immunodipstick allowed sensitive and specific hazelnut detection with low-end laboratory equipment. Ben Rejeb and colleagues[44] applied rabbit antibodies in competitive ELISA and achieved sensitivity comparable to other hazelnut-specific ELISA tests. Recoveries between 64% and 97% were found for 1–10 mg/kg hazelnut protein spiked into milk chocolate, cookies, breakfast cereals, and ice cream. Another competitive ELISA with hazelnut-specific hen's egg IgY was developed by Drs et al.[93] However, the ELISA showed extensive cross-reactivity to characteristic food components at the percentage level. Kiening et al.[45] have been the only ones so far who applied monoclonal antibodies for hazelnut detection in a sandwich-type ELISA. The hands-on time of only 30 min allowed rapid testing for hazelnut with a sensitivity comparable to other ELISA tests.[42,43] The ELISA was highly specific, with walnut giving the highest rate of cross-reactive detection of 12 mg/kg hazelnut equivalent. Recoveries of hazelnut spiked into cookie, cereals, ice cream, and milk and dark chocolate at the level of 1–10 mg/kg ranged from 86% to 127%. However, the authors applied artificial spikes with preextracted hazelnut protein bound to carboxymethylcellulose. Retail food samples tested positively at the low milligram/kilogram level. Fæste et al.[68] presented a sandwich ELISA with europium-labeled detector antibody. The sensitivity was again comparable, but the specificity appeared improved over previously published ELISAs: Only walnut of 26 tested food commodities gave a false-positive signal equivalent to 1 mg/kg hazelnut protein. Recoveries between 50% and 123% at the 1- to 150-mg/kg spike level were achieved, but spikes were done with preextracted hazelnut protein, which does not reflect a realistic situation. Blais et al.[94] and Ben Rejeb et al.[95] published immunochemical multiallergen screening methods that included hazelnut as one of the allergenic foods. The details are given here in the section "Tree Nuts Multiplex Assays."

Several methods, other than ELISA, for the protein-based detection of hazelnut were published.

Scheibe et al.[95] applied rabbit antibodies in immunoblot analysis to detect 5 mg/kg hazelnut protein in chocolate. In comparison to published ELISA, the sensitivity was lower, and the study lacked adequate validation data on specificity, reproducibility, and accuracy. Jonsson and Hellenäs[97] first applied polyclonal anticorylin antibodies in a surface plasmon resonance biosensor analysis of food samples. Their detection limit was 10 mg/kg hazelnut protein, but validation data are basically lacking. In 2006, Malmheden Yman et al.[46] also published a surface plasmon resonance biosensor protocol to detect hazelnut in a multiallergen mode in addition to sesame, milk, egg, peanut, and shellfish. The sensitivity was around 10 mg/kg, but it is unclear whether this was for hazelnut or hazelnut protein. No details about recovery in food matrix or specificity details are given. Bremer et al.[51] presented another biosensor test to detect and quantify hazelnut protein in olive oil, both as allergenic cross contact and for olive oil adulterations; 0.1 mg/kg hazelnut protein was detectable with high specificity by a monoclonal antibody. The advantage of the method was propagated for high-speed analysis for a limited number of food samples.

Finally, MS methods were suggested for the detection of hazelnut. Monaci and Visconti[98] reviewed current literature on MS for allergen detection with a special focus on peanut, milk, and gluten. MS was also suggested for hazelnut, but no specific data were shown. Weber et al.[56] described the various MS techniques used to characterize food allergens using hazelnut as an example: The known allergens Cor a 1, Cor a 8, Cor a 9, and Cor a 11 were identified. However, the preliminary study lacked data about sensitivity and specificity regarding the unequivocal detection of hazelnut in complex food matrices.

A range of qualitative PCR tests was published for the detection of hazelnut. Holzhauser et al.[58] were the first to publish a PCR method to specifically detect, for this purpose, an allergenic food (i.e. hazelnut) at the low milligram/kilogram level. This conventional PCR with agarose gel electrophoresis of amplicons relied on the specificity of the primer pair only; no cross-reactivity was observed in any of the 35 tested food ingredients. The PCR successfully detected 10 mg/kg hazelnut spiked into cookie, cereal bar, almond chocolate, and milk and dark chocolate. The comparative analysis of 27 retail food commodities with PCR and ELISA[42] showed excellent correlation; dark chocolate having as little as 0.6 mg/kg hazelnut protein tested positive in PCR. In 2002, Holzhauser et al.[67] improved their previous PCR test with special regard to sequence verification of the amplicons and toward optimized primers for increased robustness in a microwell-based detection of amplicons. This PCR-ELISA was again highly specific without any observed cross-reactivity to numerous investigated characteristic food ingredients. The comparative testing of 41 commercial retail foods with PCR-ELISA and hazelnut-specific protein ELISA[42] demonstrated that the PCR-ELISA test was able to detect hazelnut in food commodities having less than 1 mg/kg hazelnut protein. Discrepancy was found in only 3/41 samples having either less than 1 mg/kg hazelnut protein or hazelnut protein below the LOD of ELISA but with a positive result in PCR-ELISA. The PCR was adapted to be run as a real-time PCR with a sequence-specific fluorescence probe and has been published in the official method collection of the German food and feed code of law (LFBG, Lebensmittel-, Bedarfsgegenstände- und Futtermittelgesetzbuch [Lebensmittel- und Futtermittelgesetzbuch]) after positive ring trial evaluation.[99]

Herman et al.[63] developed another conventional PCR based on a mitochondrial gene and achieved a sensitivity of 10 mg/kg hazelnut in chocolate. Germini et al.[61] combined PCR with a sequence-specific anion exchange HPLC utilizing a peptide nucleic acid (PNA) probe for post-PCR sequence verification of amplicons; no cross-reactivity was seen in 14 different foods. The sensitivity was 5 pg hazelnut DNA, but data on sensitivity in food samples are lacking. Rossi et al.[71] developed a duplex PCR for peanut and hazelnut and implied PNA probe detection of amplicons on an array for simultaneous hazelnut and peanut detection. The sensitivity was 50 pg hazelnut DNA. Except for peanut versus hazelnut, no data on specificity are given. Neither spiked nor incurred samples with known amounts of hazelnut were analyzed to further characterize the method. Arlorio et al.[100] first published a hazelnut-specific real-time PCR with a gene-specific probe. Unfortunately, sensitivity data (100 pg hazelnut DNA) are scarce, and recovery was studied in incurred cream and chocolate at only high levels (5–20%) of hazelnut.

Piknová et al.[66] published another real-time PCR with a gene-specific probe. Their sensitivity was 100 mg/kg hazelnut incurred in pastry. D'Andrea et al.[73] applied melting curve analysis in real-time PCR and successfully detected 10 mg/kg hazelnut in wheat flour. Schöringhumer et al.[60] performed real-time PCR with a gene-specific probe and detected 50 mg/kg hazelnut spiked into cookie. Köppel et al.[101] detected hazelnut in a tetraplex real-time PCR with amplicon-specific probe; in an interlaboratory validation of spiked rice cookies, 50 mg/kg hazelnut were detectable in 25/26 analyses and 10 mg/kg in 21/26 analyses. Pafundo et al.[75] presented another hazelnut detection within a hexaplex real-time PCR and SYBR® Green detection of amplicons. Unfortunately, sensitivity studies with DNA mixtures were preliminary, and specificity data are lacking.

Pecan

The first quantitative, but unvalidated, method for the detection of pecan nut was published by Venkatachalam et al.[102] They used rabbit polyclonal antibodies that were immunized with unprocessed defatted pecan flour protein for use in Western blots and inhibition ELISA with a detection range from 32 to 800 ng/ml pecan protein.

Since this ELISA was a tool for determining the effects of thermal treatment and in vitro digestion to antigenicity of pecan protein, no validation of cross-reactivity was performed. Interestingly, pecan proteins were antigenetically stable toward heat treatment and digestion.[102]

A competitive ELISA has been described by Polenta et al.[103] They used polyclonal antibodies from rabbits, raised against a protein extract of pecan. In comparison to the work of Venkatachalam et al.,[102] the sensitivity of the method was increased 40-fold. To improve reproducibility, the competition step was performed at a 10-fold concentration prior to dilution and addition to the plate. The detection range of the calibration curve was 0.8 to 50 ng/ml pecan protein. The sensitivity of the method in food was evaluated with pecan protein-spiked milk chocolate samples at three different concentrations (10, 100, and 200 mg/kg). The recovery was between 86% and 107%. Walnut was the only cross-reactive ingredient, with a signal equivalent to 7.8%. Western blot experiments revealed much higher LOD, ranging between 100 and 500 mg/kg.[103]

Brežná and Kuchta[77] in 2008 published the first PCR method dealing with the detection of pecan nuts in food. They developed a genus-specific Taqman® real-time PCR method targeting a sequence of 89 bp on the gene coding for an allergenic vicilin-like seed storage protein. Sensitivity experiments were performed with incurred model pastry samples with pecan contents ranging from 0.01% to 10%. The practical detection limit was deduced from the reproducible detection of the smallest sample spike (0.01% pecan). A sample containing 0.002% was only detected in 2/3 parallels. Cross-reactivity was not observed with DNA from 10 varieties of the close relative *Juglans regia* or from 5 species of the genus *Juglans*. Also, 25 other tested plant and animal foods did not cross-react. The response was similar for 10 different varieties of pecan nut and 5 species from the same genus carya.[77]

Pistachio

The first DNA-based qualitative detection method for the detection of pistachio was published in 2006 by Barbieri and Frigeri.[70] They developed three primer pairs for a conventional PCR and detected the amplicons post-PCR with agarose gel electrophoresis. These conventional PCR relied on the specificity of the primer pair only. Primer pairs 1 and 2 targeted a sequence on the COR gene coding for the dehydrin family. The sensitivity of the method was tested with incurred mortadella samples with pistachio of 40 and 100 mg/kg and a cross-contaminated product resulting from shared production equipment. The third primer pair showed cross-reactivity and amplified sequences from different nuts. The second primer pair was less sensitive than primer pair 1, and three bands were seen in agarose gel electrophoresis with higher DNA concentrations. For the most promising primer pair, two specific bands were expected, but three were seen. This pair was able to detect at least 100 mg/kg. Cross-reactivity was tested with six tree nuts, peanut, and some spices used for mortadella production. Although the authors did not investigate other food matrices or other potential cross-reactive foods, the method was suggested for the application to various food matrices, like confectionary products.[70]

Brežná et al.[69] in 2008 published another method dealing with the detection of pistachio in food. They developed a pistachio-specific Taqman real-time PCR method targeting a multicopy sequence of 64 bp on the internal transcribed spacer between 18S rRNA and 5.8S rRNA genes. Response to DNA from leaves (11 pistachio cultivars) and nuts (4 independent market samples) tested positive without further information. Sensitivity experiments were performed with incurred model pastry samples with pistachio ranging from 0.0004% to 10%. The practical detection limit was deduced from the reproducible detection of the smallest sample spike (0.0004% or 4 mg/kg pistachio). The method demonstrated high specificity to pistachio since not 1 of the 26 tested plant and animal species gave positive signals. They checked 44 commercially available food samples for pistachio, and 7 of them contained undeclared pistachio.[69]

Macadamia

Brežná et al.[104] published the only macadamia-specific method dealing with the detection of macadamia nut in food. They developed a macadamia nut-specific Taqman® real-time PCR method targeting a sequence of 73 bp on the gene coding for a vicilin-like protein. Response to two nut cultivars was positive without further information. Sensitivity experiments were performed with incurred model pastry samples having macadamia nut between 0.001% and 10%. The practical detection limit was denoted as 0.02% macadamia and was deduced from the reproducible detection of the smallest sample spike (0.02% macadamia). The method demonstrated high specificity to macadamia since none of the 16 tested plant and animal species gave positive signals; 14 commercially available food samples were checked for macadamia, and 7 of them contained undeclared pistachio.[104]

Walnut

A short abstract for walnut detection was published in 2003 by Niemann and Hefle.[105] The sandwich ELISA consisted of polyclonal antibodies from rabbits and sheep, and the sensitivity, which was investigated with incurred samples, was as low as 1 mg/kg walnut. The specificity of the ELISA was examined with more than 50 foods, and some cross-reactivity was observed with hazelnut, pecan, and sesame seed.[105]

A walnut-specific ELISA was published by a Japanese group in 2008. Doi et al.[55] developed a sandwich ELISA by raising polyclonal antibodies in rabbits against purified 2S albumin from the roasted walnut variety *Chandler*. These anti-2S albumin antibodies were used as capture and as HRP-labeled detection antibodies. The authors compared the response of four different walnut varieties (raw and roasted) to the walnut variety *Chandler* that was used for immunization. The other varieties were detected between 82.1% to 125% (ratio to *Chandler* [raw]). The recovery of 10 mg/kg walnut protein in seven different incurred food matrices ranged between 83.4% and 123%, and the intra- and interassay precision expressed via the coefficient of variation was less than 7.2% and 8.2%, respectively. The limit of detection (LOD) and limit of quantification (LOQ) were 0.156 and 0.312 mg/kg walnut protein, respectively. In cross-reactivity studies of more than 150 food ingredients, a positive signal was seen with pecan nut (0.01%) and hazelnut (0.0001%). From 41 commercially processed foods, walnut was detected in 12 samples, in accordance with labeling.[55]

In 2009, Niemann et al. published a walnut-specific sandwich ELISA.[53] Polyclonal antibodies from sheep and rabbit raised against a mixture of roasted English walnut varieties were used as capture and detection antibodies, respectively. For the final detection, an AP-labeled goat antirabbit IgG was used. Several spiked matrices were tested, with an extensive focus on muffins. The authors also tested the response of spiked and incurred samples of milk chocolate matrix and obtained comparable results. The recovery of 10 mg/kg walnut in milk chocolate was 9.5 mg/kg (SD [standard deviation] 1.31), and the interassay coefficient of variation was 13.7%. The LOQ was denoted with 1 mg/kg walnut. In the matrix butter cookie, the response to the walnut variety "black walnut" was approximately 43%. The lower detectability was reflected by an inferior LOQ for black walnut, which was denoted with 5 mg/kg after improving the extraction protocol. Cross-reactivity studies with more than 80 foods, including other tree nuts, did not show any cross-reactivity. In contrast to the earlier reported ELISA in 2003, sesame seed did not cross-react. Hazelnut, mentioned as cross-reactive food in the former study, was not mentioned at all. Pecan, a close botanical relative, still showed some cross-reactivity. A cross-reactivity of approximately 2.5% was calculated from a figure comparing the optical density (OD) value of vanilla ice spiked with pecan or walnut. In an investigation of 40 retail food samples, partially carrying walnut labeling, advisory statements, or no declaration of walnut, walnut was only detected at levels of below 50 mg/kg in samples with precautionary labeling and in all samples that contained labeling of walnut as ingredient.[53]

Brežná et al.[106] developed a Taqman® real-time PCR method. This assay was based on the detection of an 85-bp DNA sequence from the walnut gene jug r 2, which codes for a vicilin-like seed storage protein. The DNA was isolated using a commercially available kit that was based on chaotropic solid-phase extraction. To avoid false-positive results for pecan nut, the PCR ended after cycle 35. None of the 24 tested characteristic foods gave positive results, whereas 8 different varieties of walnut tested positive, without further information about the response. Sensitivity experiments were performed with incurred model pastry samples, with walnut ranging from 0.01% to 10%. The practical detection limit was determined at 0.01%, which is near the cutoff cycle number. The investigation of 13 commercial food samples gave positive results for 4 samples, of which 2 were not adequately labeled.[106]

In 2007, a conventional PCR method using post-PCR detection of amplicons after agarose gel electrophoresis was published by Yano et al.[107] An additional endonuclease digestion of post-PCR products was used to discriminate between walnut and pecan, which was 100% cross-reactive. The detection limit obtained from unrealistic DNA mixtures of salmon genome DNA with walnut or pecan nut DNA was 10 mg/kg. The authors did not perform spiking experiments with relevant food matrices but claimed that trace amounts can be detected. A PCR study with 10 purchased samples detected walnut in 2 cases, for which one was not labeled.[107]

In 2009, another real-time PCR method was published, targeting the walnut gene jug r 2; Wang et al.[108] used the primer and probe sequences of Brežná et al.[106] with some slight modifications. The forward primer was extended by one base of cytosine at the 5′ end, and the reverse primer was extended by two bases, one base adenine and one base guanine at the 5′ end, resulting in an amplicon length of 88 bp. The probe was altered by reducing the original sequence of one base at the 5′ and the 3′ end, respectively. The cycling conditions were the same except for the denaturation temperature, which was raised from 94°C to 95°C. These minor changes in the primer sequences were sufficient to avoid the formerly obtained false-positive signal for pecan nut. Specificity testing with 14 different plant foods, including pecan and seven other tree nuts did not show any cross-reactivity. Sensitivity experiments were performed with wheat powder spiked with walnut in a range of 0.001% (10 mg/kg) to 10%, and even the lowest amount was reproducibly detected. The practical detection limit of the method was increased 10 times in comparison to the results of Brežná et al.[106]

Tree Nuts Multiplex Assays

In 2003, Blais et al.[94] published a visual analyzable enzyme immunoassay for the simultaneous detection of peanut, Brazil nut, and hazelnut allergens in foods. The assay principle was based on a reverse dot blot enzyme immunoassay, and the antibodies were immobilized on a strip of polyester cloth. The antibodies raised against the different targets were produced in chicken egg yolks. Anti-Brazil nut and antipeanut antibodies were produced by immunization of the hen with the whole protein fraction, whereas the antihazelnut antibodies were raised using the globulin fraction from hazelnut protein. The detection antibody was the same as the capture antibody but was also labeled with biotin to allow final detection with a commercially available streptavidin peroxidase conjugate. The sensitivity of this qualitative test was investigated with three target allergen spiked food matrices (oatmeal cookies, ice cream, and chocolate in a range of 0–10 mg/kg). All three allergens could be detected in a spike level of at least 1 mg/kg. Incurred chocolate samples in the 1- to 10-mg/kg range were only available for peanut and hazelnut and tested positive. Cross-reactivity of single antibodies to other foods were not described, except for Brazil nut IgY, which was used in a Brazil nut-specific sandwich-ELISA.

Ben Rejeb et al.[95] published a screening assay based on a competitive indirect format for the detection of peanut, hazelnut, almond, cashew, and Brazil nut. Specific antibodies were raised by immunizing rabbits with one of the allergenic proteins. In general, cross-reactivities to beef, almond, egg, and lobster were described. Most of these false-positive signals were claimed to be matrix effects that disappeared at a dilution of 1/100. Only the almond-specific antibody was truly cross-reactive to cashew, and the authors did not test all foods that are known to be potentially cross-reactive to almond in comparable tests. Sensitivity experiments were focused on chocolate matrices as a characteristic food for undeclared traces of investigated allergens. The signal was judged positive if the OD value of the sample was less than 80% of the OD from the blank value because some the chocolate matrix gave signals between 80% and 100% of the blank OD. The range of chocolate spiked into one or two of the allergens was 1–10 mg/kg. No false positives were detected, and all spike levels were detectable.[95]

Ehlert et al.[72] published a ligation-dependent probe amplification for simultaneous detection of 10 allergenic foods: peanut, cashew, pecan, pistachio, hazelnut, sesame seed, macadamia, almond, walnut, and Brazil nut. The technique was based on the amplification of a DNA product formed by ligation of bipartite hybridization probes with flanking primer-binding sites equal for all target molecules. The final post-PCR detection was dependent on the length of polymorphisms of the different DNA constructs. Specificity for the ligation probe target sequences was verified with 48 different foods, whereas the almond-specific probe could not differentiate between botanically closely related species like peach, plum, or apricot. The LOD for single allergens in different foods was denoted with a 5-mg/kg range. But, the spiking with single allergens was only prepared for peanut in cookies, for peanut and hazelnut in chocolate, and for cashew in pesto. Spiking experiments with almond, pecan, macadamia, pistachio, sesame seed, walnut, and Brazil nut were not mentioned; therefore, the general conclusion that the LOD was in the low milligram/kilogram range is questionable. The detection of unequal proportions of allergenic compounds, simulated by cookies containing up to 25% walnut, reduced the detection limit of the method to 1,000 mg/kg for peanut, pecan, and macadamia and to 100 mg/kg hazelnut.[72]

Köppel et al.[101] published two tetraplex real-time PCRs for the detection and quantification of DNA from eight allergens in food. Tetraplex system 1 was designed to detect simultaneously hazelnut, peanut, celery, and soy, and tetraplex system 2 was designed to detect sesame, milk, almond, and egg. Most of the primers and probes were taken from published singleplex PCR methods. Specificity of both methods was investigated with 46 different foods, and cross-reactivity above 1% was seen in two PCR systems. Peach led to a strong false-positive signal of 10% in the hazelnut system and apricot to a signal of 1.2% in the almond system. Sensitivity was investigated with DNA extracts diluted in herring sperm DNA down to 0.0032%, and all systems tested positive for the lowest concentration. Rice cookies were produced to contain 10 and 50 mg/kg of peanut, hazelnut, almond, sesame, and soy. The practical detection limit was investigated with both spike levels and unspiked rice cookie in an interlaboratory validation study. The detection limit was estimated in the range of 10–50 mg/kg, although several spiked samples tested negative. Detection limits for the other allergens were not investigated. The authors investigated by PCR 40 retail samples for traces of almond in comparison to an almond-specific ELISA. All samples detected positive by PCR were detected positive by ELISA.

Sesame Seeds

Malmheden Yman et al.[46] applied polyclonal rabbit IgG and hen's egg IgY antibodies in a biosensor and detected sesame seed protein at a level of 10 mg/kg. However, detailed data about specificity or protein recovery in various food matrices are missing.

In 2007, Brzezinski first published[65] a real-time PCR making use of a sequence-specific fluorescent probe to verify the 66-bp amplicon derived from a gene of the sesame seed 2S albumin. On the basis of sesame seed spiked in crackers, the method was sensitive for detection of 100 mg/kg sesame seed. No cross-reactivity was observed in a limited number of investigated food commodities.

In 2007, Schöringhumer and Cichna-Markl[62] published another sesame-specific real-time PCR with a sequence-specific fluorescent probe to verify the identity of a 117-bp amplicon from the gene of Ses I 1, the 2S albumin allergen. The PCR proved to be sensitive to sesame; no cross-reactivity to 16 selected foods was observed. In crisp bread, 500 mg/kg sesame seed spiked to the matrix were detectable. The same primer pair but a different fluorescent probe were applied in a duplex real-time PCR for the simultaneous detection in 2009 of sesame and hazelnut[60]; 50 mg/kg sesame seed spiked into cookies were successfully detected. Cross-reactivity studies were extended to 25 foods and further proved specificity to sesame without cross-sensitivity to any other tested food.

Mustorp and colleagues[109] detected sesame seeds at a level of 50 mg/kg that were spiked into both barbeque sauce and wheat flour. In their tripleplex real-time PCR, sesame was simultaneously detected with celery and mustard. A 64-bp amplicon of a gene of a 2S albumin was verified by a sequence-specific fluorescence probe. No cross-reactivity was observed with 14 foods other than sesame seed.

An indirect competitive ELISA on the basis of hen's egg IgY specific for sesame seed protein was developed by Husain and colleagues.[50] Their ELISA was specific for sesame seed proteins and did not cross-react with various tree nuts, cereals, peanut, or honey. However, there was a remarkable cross-reactivity of 0.7% to chocolate, which would correlate to a signal of 7,000 mg/kg sesame seed protein. It is unclear if this cross-reactivity was due to chocolate matrix or specific antibody binding to chocolate ingredients or hidden sesame seed protein. The LOD was around 10 mg/kg sesame seed protein in characteristic matrices such as crackers, cereals, bread, and rolls. Most recovery experiments were unfortunately done with scarcely realistic spikes of pre-extracted sesame seed protein. Spikes of ground sesame seeds in muesli and cookie resulted in a threefold overquantification at a level of 10–50 mg/kg, whereas excellent recoveries of 100% were achieved at higher spike levels of 50 and 100 mg/kg sesame seed, respectively. Commercial foods were analyzed by both ELISA and a published real-time PCR by the same group.[62] Results of both methods were generally in good agreement and underlined the applicability of PCR and ELISA.

Pafundo et al.[75] published a sesame DNA-based detection of sesame that was part of a hexaplex real-time PCR with SYBR® Green fluorescence to detect six allergenic foods simultaneously. Only a few validation data were given, such as sensitivity testing on the basis of only DNA mixtures that resulted in an LOD of 0.5 pg sesame seed DNA. No specificity data were displayed.

Mustard

In 2007, Koppelman and colleagues[110] published an ELISA for mustard; a polyclonal rabbit antiserum was developed against a protein extract of *Brassica juncea* for use in a competitive-type format. The method was especially applied to mustard seed oil to determine residual protein. In this matrix, a sensitivity of 1.5 mg/kg was achieved. The crude antiserum revealed cross-sensitivity to several of 16 tested foods, of which soy, corn, and egg yolk were the most potent, with cross-reactivity ranging between 0.016% and 0.28%, corresponding to a false-positive signal of 160 to 2,800 mg/kg mustard protein. This should be taken into account when analyzing foods that contain these common ingredients. Rapeseed (*Brassica napus*, *Brassica campestris*) was not investigated; however, it might be even more cross-reactive because of its close phylogenetic relationship to mustard.

Lee et al.[48] published two sandwich-type ELISAs with a reciprocal combination of polyclonal rabbit and sheep antisera made against a mixture of yellow (*Sinapis alba*) and brown and oriental (*Brassica juncea*, *Brassica nigra*) mustard seeds. The limit of quantification was between 1 and 3 mg/kg mustard. Both formats were highly specific with only rapeseed, of more than 90 food ingredients tested, giving a false-positive signal of approximately 12,000–17,000 mg/kg (1.2–1.7%). With the sheep capture ELISA model, frankfurter sausages with between 1 and 1,000 mg/kg mustard flour were quantified with an average recovery rate of 95%. Recovery rates were superior over those obtained by comparative quantification with a commercially available ELISA kit. The ELISA was applied to several retail foods with good correlation between declared and detectable mustard. Some food items were identified as having considerable levels of undeclared mustard.

Shim and Wanasundara[111] developed polyclonal rabbit antibodies against Sin a 1, the 2S albumin allergen of yellow/white mustard. The purified antibodies were used in a sandwich-type ELISA to quantify the single allergen Sin a 1 in mustard. The potential to use this ELISA in complex food matrices, however, is unclear because no data about specificity and recovery of mustard in complex food matrices were shown.

Mustorp et al.[109] designed a triplex real-time PCR for the simultaneous detection of mustard, celery, and sesame seed. Multiple primers and probes were found to amplify sequences between 170 and 180 bp of yellow (*Sinapis alba*), black (*Brassica nigra*), and brown and oriental (*Brassica juncea*) mustard. There was successful detection of 50 mg/kg mustard spiked into barbeque spice and wheat flour. Only radish gave a false-positive result of 14 food ingredients tested. The level of cross-reactivity unfortunately was not further specified.

Celery

Several forms of celery are found in foods: Celery tuber (celeriac) is eaten as raw or cooked vegetable but is also used for production of celeriac powder as a spice. Celery seeds are also used as a spice, and celery stalks are eaten as a vegetable. One difficulty in the detection of celery results from the fact that celery extracts with potentially decreased amounts of detectable protein or DNA are used for flavoring purposes. Another difficulty is the close phylogenetic relationship between celery and other plant food species of the *Apiacea* family that are frequently used as food ingredients. Most of the published literature for celery detection does not specify which type of celery was investigated. Thus, validation data such as LOD are of unknown meaning if the type of celery is not specified.

Stephan et al.[112] developed a real-time PCR for the detection of celery to monitor the efficiency of an allergen sanitation procedure in the industrial production of flavors extracted from foods. The amplification of a 145-bp amplicon from the gene of the major allergen Api g 1 was verified by a sequence-specific fluorescent probe. Details about specificity were not displayed. However, the authors indicated observed cross-reactivity with other spices. Consequently, this method may not be applicable to complex foods in which phylogenetically closely related spices are present. Unfortunately, no data were given on the identity of the cross-reacting spices.

Dovičovičová et al.[64] aimed at detecting celery with a conventional end-point PCR and subsequent agarose gel electrophoresis of a 279-bp celery amplicon of mannitol dehydrogenase. A sensitivity of 1,000 mg/kg celery in model meat pâtés was demonstrated. Furthermore, no cross-reactivity was observed in 16 selected foods of meat and plant origin, including several phylogenetically closely related spices of the *Apiaceae* family. Even though not sensitive, the target gene was a promising candidate for specific detection of celery.

Hupfer et al.[59] based their celery-specific PCR on the findings of Dovičovičová et al.[64]: Their real-time PCR generated a 101-bp amplicon of mannitol dehydrogenase gene that was verified by a sequence-specific probe. An extensive cross-reactivity study with 60 different items demonstrated high specificity for celery without any false-positive signal. Interestingly, even the 12 investigated plant species of the *Apiaceae* family, such as dill, fennel, carrot, parsley, or coriander, did not give false-positive results. These findings underline the high specificity that can be obtained with sequence-specific detection methods such as PCR. Moreover, the authors demonstrated high sensitivity to detect celery seed in incurred emulsion-type sausages: The analysis of sausages having between 1 and 1,000 mg/kg celery seed revealed a sensitivity of 5–10 mg/kg. Even the lowest concentration of 1 mg/kg celery seed was detectable in approximately half of all PCR reactions (23/51). The method was further applied to 19 retail food items, such as seasonings, bouillon-based products, and sauces; there was a generally good correlation between detectable and declared celery. However, 5/14 samples with declared celery gave negative results, which the authors explained as a result of low DNA in celery flavors used as ingredients or of low pH of seasonings and sauces that might degrade detectable DNA. After positive ring-trial evaluation, the method[113] was published in the official method collection of the German food and feed code of law (LFBG)[114]; in 112 PCR reactions, 10 mg/kg celery seed in emulsion-type sausages were detected with a rate of positivity of 94%. For celeriac powder, the method was slightly less sensitive, with 50 mg/kg detected at a rate of positivity of 90% in 112 PCR reactions.

Mustorp et al.[109] detected celery simultaneously to mustard and sesame in a triplex real-time PCR with sequence-specific fluorescent probes. The method amplifies a 151-bp product of mannitol dehydrogenase gene and was specific for celery without false-positive signals for 14 other tested foods, including members of the *Apiacea* family. In a range of characteristic food matrices, such as vegetable burger, barbeque spice, minced beef, or Wok vegetables, the method was able to detect 10 mg/kg of spiked celeriac powder. In wheat and maize flour, the sensitivity was slightly higher, with a detection of 50 mg/kg celeriac powder.

Another multiplex real-time PCR also included primers and probe for celery detection on the basis of the mannitol dehydrogenase gene.[101] However, the authors did not present validation data such as that regarding sensitivity, specificity, or robustness in various matrices.

The first celery-specific ELISA was published in 2010 by Fæste et al.[57] Purified polyclonal rabbit antibodies against celeriac protein were used in a sandwich-type ELISA to detect and quantify celery. The ELISA was highly sensitive, with a theoretical LOD of 0.5 mg/kg celeriac protein. Recovery rates for celeriac protein at the low milligram/kilogram level in taco mix, sausage, dressing, and pasta sauce were good. However, the ELISA displayed extensive cross-reactivity with at least 18 of 60 tested foods. The antibody response to potato and carrot was even better than to celeriac, resulting in cross-reactivity of more than 100%. Other members of the *Apiacea* family, such as parsnip, parsley, and dill, cross-reacted in the 10–40% range. Several other foods cross-reacted in the percentage range. Thus, the authors suggested this ELISA for screening purposes, and any positive result would have to be verified by confirmatory methods, such as PCR or MS. The authors further suggested, on the basis of experimental MS data, protein sequences for the specific detection in MS.

Puff et al.[115] presented a sandwich-type ELISA with monoclonal antibodies raised against celery and selected to discriminate other *Apiacea* foods. Polyclonal antisera raised against the same immunogens turned out to be highly cross-reactive, similar to the results of Fæste et al.[68], and were thus not implied. The LOD of the monoclonal antibody-based ELISA was around 10 ng/ml celery protein, corresponding to approximately 20 mg/kg celeriac in food. Almost no cross-reactivity was observed with *Apiaceae* foods such as carrot, dill, or lovage. Some cross-reactivity was found with parsley and mustard at the low percentage level.

COMMERCIAL TEST KITS FOR ALLERGEN DETECTION

The comparison of published protein- and DNA-based tests for allergen detection helps to understand the potential and limitation of the techniques with special regard to the analyte of interest. By contrast to peer-reviewed published methods, validation data for commercial tests are usually limited, and users are advised to validate those test kits with special regard to their needs. Most commercial methods have not undergone competitive testing or ring-trial analysis. Röder et al.[116] compared three commercial rapid lateral flow device (LFD) tests for the detection of hazelnut and three commercial rapid LFD tests for the detection of peanut. All commercial test kits were developed for qualitative analysis. The competitive performance testing involved the analysis of cross-reactivity and of the detectability of hazelnut or peanut that were spiked into chocolate and cookie dough matrix between 1 and 25 mg/kg. Some cross-reactivities with other foods were observed, and each two of three test kits successfully detected hazelnut or peanut at or below 10 mg/kg in both matrices.

Table 4.5 Companies Offering Commercial Test Kits for Allergenic Foods Discussed in This Chapter

Manufacturer/Supplier	URL
Neogen	http://www.neogen.com/
R-Biopharm	http://www.r-biopharm.com/
ifp	http://www.produktqualitaet.com
bioavid/R-Biopharm	http://www.bioavid.de
InCura	http://www.incura.it
Congen	http://www.congen.de
ELISA Systems	http://www.elisasystems.net/

Most of the manufacturer data were confirmed, but some discrepancy was found, especially about statements on sensitivity by one test kit manufacturer.

Garber and Perry[117] investigated the performance of three commercial sandwich ELISA test kits for the detection of hazelnuts and almonds. Hazelnuts and almonds were spiked into cooked oatmeal, dipping chocolate, and baked muffins. The authors observed LODs between 1 and 38 mg/kg and recoveries between 10% and 170%. Obviously, a suitable LOD and accurate quantification are prerequisites for the correct interpretation of analysis data for unknown food samples. General instructions and validation data supplied by manufacturers should thus be handled with care. This further underlines the necessity to independently validate commercial test kits with special regard to personal requirements. Further, harmonized protocols on the validation and the availability of reference material are necessary for the standardization of commercial allergen test kits. Because of the limited number of independent peer-reviewed performance data, commercial allergen detection test kits are not reviewed in detail here.

There are a vast and continuously increasing number of commercial test kits for allergen detection. A review of rapid commercial immunoanalytical tests was published.[118] However, a complete review of these tests is beyond the scope of this chapter. Potential users are thus advised to directly contact the manufacturers for more information. Some manufacturers are summarized without selection, priority, or claim of completeness in Table 4.5.

SUMMARY AND CONCLUSION

More than 20 potentially allergenic tree nuts are listed in Table 4.1 in addition to sesame seed, mustard, and celery, each of which requires obligatory labeling in several countries. Therefore, methods have been developed and published for eight tree nuts, sesame seed, mustard, and celery, which appear to be the most relevant from the clinical point of view (Figure 4.1). Approximately 70 methods are reviewed within this chapter, of which protein-based and DNA-based tests are equally represented. Starting with the 1992 RIE work of Eriksson and Malmheden Yman,[49,90] hazelnut was the first and so far most targeted allergenic tree nut, with more than one-third of

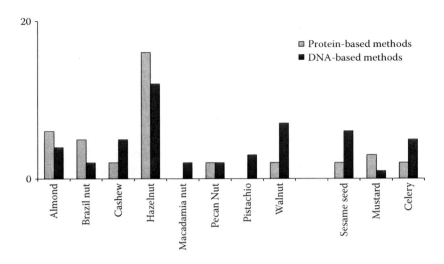

Figure 4.1 Comparison of protein- and DNA-based published methods of Tables 4.3 and 4.4 for the detection of tree nuts, sesame seed, mustard, and celery (as of April 2010).

all methods cited here. Several additional method developments are expected in the near future, especially for the detection of tree nuts other than hazelnut, as well as for sesame, mustard, and celery.

In this field, the ELISA technique has been by far the most popular protein-based technique, with steadily increasing numbers of publications since 1999.[42,43,78] At this time, detection of allergens mentioned in this chapter by PCR was a novelty, with the first PCR to detect hazelnut by Holzhauser et al. in 2000.[58] Until 2004, PCR was rarely applied for allergen detection; only since 2005 has the number of scientific contributions increased over four times compared to the prior years. Meanwhile, information on real-time PCR with verification of the amplicon sequence by specific fluorescent probes contributes the majority of published PCR techniques, and it is considered state-of-the-art technology. Both methods, ELISA and PCR, have specific benefits and limitations. Whereas ELISAs are generally quantitative and feature a sensitivity of approximately 1 mg/kg of the allergenic food, cross-reactivity to phylogenetically closely related foods, especially for some tree nuts and Apiaceae other than celery, might give false-positive results. By contrast, PCR generally features unparalleled specificity and is based on fully reproducible chemistry. DNA detection by PCR was demonstrated to correlate well with protein detection by ELISA, and sensitivities below 10 mg/kg were achieved with the first methods in the field.[58,67] Still, sample preparation is more tedious than for protein detection, and the choice of sample preparation is a crucial factor for sensitivity. Several multiplex PCR tests have been described that simultaneously detect different allergenic foods from the same sample DNA. Up to 10 allergenic foods were detectable in a ligation-dependent PCR.[72] Also, up to pentaplex detection of allergens with ELISA has been described,[95] and rapid antibody-based tests such as LFD are promising detection methods. Unfortunately, quantitative real-time PCR tests for allergenic foods are still lacking but are expected to be developed in the near future. No matter which specific benefits or limitations ELISA and PCR have, for both types of methods a suitable sensitivity can be achieved for the great majority of allergenic foods that have been discussed in this chapter. In addition, results obtained by ELISA and PCR are well correlated. Thus we believe that both protein- and DNA-based tests will be applied to increase food safety for food-allergic individuals. Also, MS methods may draw more attention in the future, but current developments are of preliminary status and have not been competitive enough in comparison to ELISA or PCR performance.

The harmonization of validation protocols, the availability of standard reference material, as well as ring-trial performance tests will be of particular importance to achieve comparable results between methods, whether based on protein or DNA detection or on published or commercial tests.

REFERENCES

1. Tariq, S.M., Stevens, M., Matthews, S., Ridout, S., Twiselton, R., and Hide, D.W. 1996. Cohort study of peanut and tree nut sensitisation by age of 4 years. *BMJ.* 313:514–517.
2. Sicherer, S.H., Muñoz-Furlong, A., and Sampson, H.A. 2003. Prevalence of peanut and tree nut allergy in the United States determined by means of a random digit dial telephone survey: A 5-year follow up study. *J Allergy Clin Immunol.* 112:1203–1207.
3. Zuidmeer, L., Goldhahn, K., Rona, R.J., et al. 2008. The prevalence of plant food allergies: a systematic review. *J Allergy Clin Immunol.* 121:1210–1218.
4. Flinterman, A.E., Akkerdaas, J.H., Knulst, A.C., van Ree, R., and Pasmans, S.G. 2008. Hazelnut allergy: from pollen-associated mild allergy to severe anaphylactic reactions. *Curr Opin Allergy Clin Immunol.* 8:261–265.
5. Burney, P., Summers, C., Chinn, S., Hooper, R., van Ree, R., and Lidholm J. 2010. Prevalence and distribution of sensitization to foods in the European Community Respiratory Health Survey: a EuroPrevall analysis. *Allergy.* Epub ahead of print.
6. Aaronov, D., Tasher, D., Levine, A., Somekh, E., Serour, F., and Dalal, I. 2008. Natural history of food allergy in infants and children in Israel. *Ann Allergy Asthma Immunol.* 101:637–640.
7. Rancé, F. 2003. Mustard allergy as a new food allergy. *Allergy.* 58:287–288.
8. Ballmer-Weber, B.K., Vieths, S., Lüttkopf, D., Heuschmann, P., and Wüthrich, B. 2000. Celery allergy confirmed by double-blind, placebo-controlled food challenge: a clinical study in 32 subjects with a history of adverse reactions to celery root. *J Allergy Clin Immunol.* 106:373–378.
9. Ballmer-Weber, B.K., Hoffmann, A., Wüthrich, B., et al. 2002. Influence of food processing on the allergenicity of celery: DBPCFC with celery spice and cooked celery in patients with celery allergy. *Allergy.* 57:228–235.
10. Pumphrey, R.S.H. and Stanworth, S.J. 1996. The clinical spectrum of anaphylaxis in north-west England. *Clin Exp Allergy.* 26:1364–1370.
11. Sampson, H.A. 1998. Fatal food-induced anaphylaxis. *Allergy.* 53:125–130.
12. Wüthrich, B. and Ballmer-Weber, B.K. 2001. Food-induced anaphylaxis. *Allergy.* 56:102–104.

13. Bock, S.A., Muñoz-Furlong, A., and Sampson, H.A. 2001. Fatalities due to anaphylactic reactions to foods. *J Allergy Clin Immunol.* 107:191–193.
14. Bock, S.A., Muñoz-Furlong, A., and Sampson, H.A. 2007. Further fatalities caused by anaphylactic reactions to food, 2001–2006. *J Allergy Clin Immunol.* 119:1016–1018.
15. Clark, A.T. and Ewan, P.W. 2005. The development and progression of allergy to multiple nuts at different ages. *Pediatr Allergy Immunol.* 16:507–511.
16. Wensing, M., Penninks, A.H., Hefle, S.L., et al. 2002. The range of minimum provoking doses in hazelnut-allergic patients as determined by double-blind, placebo-controlled food challenges. *Clin Exp. Allergy.* 32:1757–1762.
17. Morisset, M., Moneret-Vautrin, D.A., Kanny, G., Guénard, L., Beaudouin, E., Flabbée, J., and Hatahet, R. 2003. Thresholds of clinical reactivity to milk, egg, peanut and sesame in immunoglobulin E-dependent allergies: evaluation by double-blind or single-blind placebo-controlled oral challenges. *Clin Exp Allergy.* 33:1046–1051.
18. Ballmer-Weber, B.K., Holzhauser, T., Scibilia, J., et al. 2007. Clinical characteristics of soybean allergy in Europe: a double-blind, placebo-controlled food challenge study. *J Allergy Clin Immunol.* 119:1489–1496.
19. Taylor, S.L., Moneret-Vautrin, D.A., Crevel, R.W., et al. 2010. Threshold dose for peanut: Risk characterization based upon diagnostic oral challenge of a series of 286 peanut-allergic individuals. *Food Chem Toxicol.* 48:814–819.
20. 2003/89/EC. Commission Directive 2003/89/EC of 10 November 2003 amending Directive 2000/13/EC of the European Parliament and of the Council as regards certain food ingredients. *Off J EU.* L 308/15.
21. 2007/68/EC. Commission Directive 2007/68/EC of 27 November 2007 amending Annex IIIa to Directive 2000/13/EC of the European Parliament and of the Council as regards certain food ingredients. *Off J EU.* L 310/11.
22. 2000/13/EC. Directive 2000/13/EC of the European Parliament and of the Council of March 2000 on the approximation of the laws of the Member States relating to the labelling, presentation and advertising of foodstuffs. *Off J EU.* L109/29.
23. Verordnung des EDI vom 23. November 2005 über die Kennzeichnung und Anpreisung von Lebensmitteln (LKV) (Stand am 1. April 2010) SR-Nummer 817.022.21. Available at http://www.admin.ch/ch/d/sr/c817_022_21.html (accessed May 2010).
24. FALCPA. *U.S. Food Allergen Labeling and Consumer Protection Act of 2004.* Public Law No 108-282-Aug. 2, 2004. 118 Stat. 905.
25. FDA Homepage. Food Allergen Labeling: Question and Answer F10. Available at: http://www.fda.gov/food/guidancecomplianceregulatoryinformation/guidancedocuments/foodlabelingnutrition/foodlabelingguide/ucm064880.htm (accessed May 2010).
26. *Health Canada—Health Canada Reviews Comments Received on Regulatory Project 1220Enhanced Labelling for Food Allergens and Gluten Sources and Added Sulphites.* Available at http://hc-sc.gc.ca/fn-an/label-etiquet/allergen/proj/220-comment-enj.php (accessed August 2010).
27. *Australia New Zealand Food Standards Code.* Standard 1.2.3—Mandatory warning and advisory statements and declarations. Available at: http://www.foodstandards.gov.au/foodstandards/foodstandardscode/standard123mandatory4230.cfm (accessed May 2010).
28. *Australia New Zealand Food Standards Code.* Standard 1.4.2 Schedule 4. Available at http://www.foodstandards.gov.au/foodstandards/foodstandardscode/standard142maximumre4244.cfm (accessed May 2010).
29. MHLW home page. Available at http://www.mhlw.go.jp/english/topics/qa/allergies/al2.html (accessed February 2010).

30. Centre for Food Safety. Frequently asked questions. Available at http://www.cfs.gov.hk/english/faq/faq_12.html (accessed May 2010).
31. Radauer, C. and Breiteneder H. 2007. Evolutionary biology of plant food allergens. *J Allergy Clin Immunol.* 120:518–525.
32. Leduc, V., Moneret-Vautrin, D.A., Tzen, J.T., Morisset, M., Guerin, L., and Kanny, G. 2006. Identification of oleosins as major allergens in sesame seed allergic patients. *Allergy.* 61:349–356.
33. Akkerdaas, J.H., Schocker, F., Vieths, S., et al. 2006. Cloning of oleosin, a putative new hazelnut allergen, using a hazelnut cDNA library. *Mol Nutr Food Res.* 50:18–23.
34. Vieths, S., Scheurer, S., and Ballmer-Weber, B. 2002. Current understanding of cross-reactivity of food allergens and pollen. *Ann N Y Acad Sci.* 964:47–68.
35. van Ree, R. 2004. Clinical importance of cross-reactivity in food allergy. *Curr Opin Allergy Clin Immunol.* 4:235–240.
36. Mills, E.N. and Mackie, A.R. 2008. The impact of processing on allergenicity of food. *Curr Opin Allergy Clin Immunol.* 8:249–253.
37. Astwood, J.D., Leach, J.N., and Fuchs, R.L. 1996. Stability of food allergens to digestion in vitro. *Nat Biotechnol.* 14:1269–1273.
38. Schimek, E.M., Zwölfer, B., Briza, P., et al. 2005. Gastrointestinal digestion of Bet v 1-homologous food allergens destroys their mediator-releasing, but not T cell-activating, capacity. *J Allergy Clin Immunol.* 116:1327–1333.
39. Etesamifar, M. and Wüthrich B. 1998. IgE-vermittelte Nahrungsmittelallergie bei 383 Patienten unter Berücksichtigung des oralen Allergie-Syndroms. *Allergologie.* 21:451–457.
40. Holzhauser, T., Stephan, O., and Vieths, S. 2006. Polymerase chain reaction (PCR) methods for the detection of allergenic foods. In *Detecting allergens in food,* ed. Koppelman, S.J. and Hefle, S.L., pp. 125–143. Cambridge, UK: Woodhead.
41. Poms, R.E., Klein, C.L., and Anklam, E. 2004. Methods for allergen analysis in food: a review. *Food Addit Contam.* 21:1–31.
42. Holzhauser, T. and Vieths, S. 1999. Quantitative sandwich ELISA for determination of traces of hazelnut (*Corylus avellana*) protein in complex food matrices. *J Agric Food Chem.* 47:4209–4218.
43. Koppelman, S.J., Knulst, A.C., Koers, W.J., et al.1999. Comparison of different immunochemical methods for the detection and quantification of hazelnut proteins in food products. *J Immunol Methods.* 229:107–120.
44. Ben Rejeb, S., Abbott, M., Davies, D., et al.2003. Immunochemical-based method for detection of hazelnut proteins in processed foods. *J. AOAC Int.* 86:557–563.
45. Kiening, M., Niessner, R., Drs, E., et al.2005. Sandwich immunoassays for the determination of peanut and hazelnut traces in foods. *J Agric Food Chem.* 53:3321–3327.
46. Malmheden Yman, I., Eriksson, A., Johansson, M.A., and Hellenäs, K.-E. 2006. Food allergen detection with biosensor immunoassays. *J AOAC Int.* 89:856–861.
47. Blais, B.W. and Phillippe, L. 2001. Detection of hazelnut proteins in foods by enzyme immunoassay using egg yolk antibodies. *J Food Prot.* 64:895–898.
48. Lee, P.W., Hefle, S.L., and Taylor, S.L. 2008. Sandwich enzyme-linked immunosorbent assay (ELISA) for detection of mustard in foods. *J Food Sci.* 73:T62–T68.
49. Malmheden Yman, I., Eriksson, A., Everitt, G., Yman, L., and Karlsson, T. 1994. Analysis of food proteins for verification of contamination or mislabelling. *Food Agric Immunol.* 6:167–172.

50. Husain, F.T., Bretbacher, I.E., Nemes, A., and Cichna-Markl, M. 2010. Development and validation of an indirect competitive enzyme linked-immunosorbent assay for the determination of potentially allergenic sesame (*Sesamum indicum*) in food. *J Agric Food Chem.* 58:1434–1441.
51. Bremer, M.G., Smits, N.G., and Haasnoot, W. 2009. Biosensor immunoassay for traces of hazelnut protein in olive oil. *Anal Bioanal Chem.* 395:119–126.
52. Stephan, O., Moeller, N., Lehmann, S., Holzhauser, T., and Vieths, S. 2002. Development and validation of two dipstick type immunoassays for determination of trace amounts of peanut and hazelnut in processed foods. *Eur Food Res Technol.* 215:431–436.
53. Niemann, L., Taylor, S., and Hefle S. L. 2009. Detection of walnut residues in foods using an enzyme-linked immunosorbent assay. *J Food Sci.* 74:T51–T57.
54. Blais, B.W., Omar, M., and Phillippe, L. 2002. Detection of Brazil nut proteins in foods by enzyme immunoassay. *Food Agric Immunol.* 14:163–168.
55. Doi, H., Touhata, Y., Shibata, H., Sakai, S., Urisu, A., Akiyama, H., and Teshima, R. 2008. Reliable enzyme-linked immunosorbent assay for the determination of walnut proteins in processed foods. *J Agric Food Chem.* 56:7625–7630.
56. Weber, D., Polenta, G., Lau, B.P.-Y., and Benrejeb Godefroy, S. 2009. Detection and confirmation of food allergen using mass spectrometric techniques: characterization of allergens in hazelnut using ESI and MALDI mass spectrometry. In *Intentional and unintentional contaminants in food and feed,* ed. Al-Taher, F., Jackson, L., and DeVries, J.W., pp. 153–182. Washington, DC: American Chemical Society; distributed by Oxford University Press.
57. Fæste, C.K., Jonscher, K.R., Sit, L., Klawitter, J., Løvberg, K., and Moen, L.H. 2010. Differentiating cross-reacting allergens in the immunological analysis of celery (*Apium graveolens*) by mass spectrometry. *J AOAC Int.* 93:451–461.
58. Holzhauser, T., Wangorsch, A., and Vieths, S. 2000. Polymerase chain reaction (PCR) for detection of potentially allergenic hazelnut residues in complex food matrices. *Eur Food Res Technol.* 211:360–365.
59. Hupfer, C., Waiblinger, H.-U., and Busch, U. 2007. Development and validation of a real-time PCR detection method for celery in food. *Eur Food Res Technol.* 225:329–335.
60. Schöringhumer, K., Redl, G., and Cichna-Markl, M. 2009. Development and validation of a duplex real-time PCR method to simultaneously detect potentially allergenic sesame and hazelnut in food. *J Agric Food Chem.* 57:2126–2134.
61. Germini, A., Scaravelli, E., Lesignoli, F., Sforza, S., Corradini, R., and Marchelli, R. 2005. Polymerase chain reaction coupled with peptide nucleic acid high-performance liquid chromatography for the sensitive detection of traces of potentially allergenic hazelnut in foodstuffs. *Eur Food Res Technol.* 220:619–624.
62. Schöringhumer, K., and Cichna-Markl, M. 2007. Development of a real-time PCR method to detect potentially allergenic sesame (*Sesamum indicum*) in food. *J Agric Food Chem.* 55:10540–10547.
63. Herman, L., De Block, J., and Viane, R. 2003. Detection of hazelnut DNA traces in chocolate by PCR. *Int J Food Sci Technol.* 38:633–640.
64. Dovičovičová, L., Olexová, L., Pangallo, D., Siekel, P., and Kuchta, T. 2004. Polymerase chain reaction (PCR) for the detection of celery (*Apium graveolens*) in food. *Eur Food Res Technol.* 218:493–495.
65. Brzezinski, J. 2007. Detection of sesame seed DNA in foods using real-time PCR. *J Food Prot.* 70:1033–1036.

66. Piknova, L., Pangallo, D., and Kuchta, T. 2008. A novel real-time polymerase chain reaction (PCR) method for the detection of hazelnuts in food. *Eur Food Res Technol.* 226:1155–1158.
67. Holzhauser, T., Stephan, O., and Vieths, S. 2002. Detection of potentially allergenic hazelnut (*Corylus avellana*) residues in food: a comparative study with DNA PCR-ELISA and protein sandwich-ELISA. *J Agric Food Chem.* 50:5808–5815.
68. Faeste, C.K., Holden, L., Plassen, C., and Almli, B. 2006. Sensitive time-resolved fluoroimmunoassay for the detection of hazelnut (*Corylus avellana*) protein traces in food matrices. *J Immunol Methods.* 314:114–122.
69. Brežná, B., Dudásová, H., and Kuchta T. 2008. A novel real-time polymerase chain reaction method for the qualitative detection of pistachio in food. *Eur Food Res Technol.* 228:197–203.
70. Barbieri, G. and Frigeri, G. 2006. Identification of hidden allergens: detection of pistachio traces in mortadella. *Food Addit Contam.* 23:1260–1264.
71. Rossi, S., Searavelli, E., Germini, A., Corradini, R., Fogher, C., and Marchelli, R. 2006. A PNA-array platform for the detection of hidden allergens in foodstuffs. *Eur Food Res Technol.* 223:1–6.
72. Ehlert, A., Demmel, A., Hupfer, C., Busch, U., and Engel, K. 2009. Simultaneous detection of DNA from 10 food allergens by ligation-dependent probe amplification. *Food Addit Contam Part A.* 26:409–418.
73. D'Andrea, M., Coisson, J.D., Travaglia, F., Garino, C., and Arlorio, M. 2009. Development and validation of a SYBR-green in real-time PCR protocol to detect hazelnut (*Corylus avellana* L.) in foods through calibration via plasmid reference standard. *J Agric Food Chem.* 57:11201–11208.
74. Pafundo, S., Gullì, M., and Marmirol, N. 2009. SYBR®GreenER™ real-time PCR to detect almond in traces in processed food. *Food Chem.* 116:811–815.
75. Pafundo, S., Gulli, M., and Marmiroli, M. 2010. Multiplex real-time PCR using SYBR®GreenER™ for the detection of DNA allergens in food. *Anal Bioanal Chem.* 396:1831–1839.
76. Piknová, L. and Kuchta, T. 2007. Detection of cashew nuts in food by real time polymerase chain reaction. *J Food Nutr.* 46:101–1074.
77. Brežná, B. and Kuchta T. 2008. A novel real-time polymerase chain reaction method for the detection of pecan nuts in food. *Eur Food Res Technol.* 226:1113–1118.
78. Acosta, M.R., Roux, K.H., Teuber, S.S., and Sathe, S.K. 1999. Production and characterization of rabbit polyclonal antibodies to almond (*Prunus dulcis* L.) major storage protein. *J Agric Food Chem.* 47:4053–4059.
79. Roux, K. H., Teuber, S. S., Robotham, J. M., and Sathe, S. K. 2001. Detection and stability of the major almond allergen in foods. *J Agric Food Chem.* 49:2131–2136.
80. Venkatachalam, M., Teuber, S. S., Roux, K. H., and Sathe, S. K. 2002. Effects of roasting, blanching, autoclaving, and microwave heating on antigenicity of almond (*Prunus dulcis* L.) proteins. *J Agric Food Chem.* 50:3544–3548.
81. Hlywka, J.J., Hefle, S.L., and Taylor, S.L. 2000. A sandwich enzyme-linked immunosorbent assay for the detection of almonds in foods. *J Food Prot.* 63:252–257.
82. Clemente, A., Chambers, S.J., Lodi, F., Nicoletti, C., and Brett, G.M. 2004. Use of the indirect competitive ELISA for the detection of Brazil nut in food products. *Food Control.* 15:65–69.
83. Girdhari, S.M., Roux, K.H., and Sathe, S.K. 2009. A sensitive and robust competitive enzyme-linked immunosorbent assay for Brazil nut (*Bertholletia excelsa* L.) detection. *J Agric Food Chem.* 57:769–776.

84. Brežná, B., Dudásová, H., and Kuchta, T. 2010. A novel real-time polymerase chain reaction method for the detection of Brazil nuts in food. *J AOAC Int.* 93:197–201.
85. Wei, Y., Sathe, S.K., Teuber, S.S., and Roux, K.H. 2003. A sensitive sandwich ELISA for the detection of trace amounts of cashew (*Anacardium occidentale L.*) nut in foods. *J Agric Food Chem.* 51:3215–3221.
86. Gaskin, F.E., Niemann, L.M., Hefle, S.L., and Taylor, S.L. 2009. Validated enzyme-linked immunosorbent assay (ELISA) for detection of undeclared cashew nut residues in foods. *J Allergy Clin Immunol.* 123:s245.
87. Dhiman, B. and Singh, M. 2003. Molecular detection of cashew husk (*Anacrdium occidentale*) adulteration in market samples of dry tea (*camellia sinensis*). *Planta Med.* 69:882–884.
88. Brzezinski, J. 2006. Detection of cashew nut DNA in spiked baked goods using a real-time polymerase chain reaction method. *Food Comp Addit.* 89:1035–1038.
89. Ehlert, A., Hupfer, C., Demmel, A., Engel, K., and Busch, U. 2008. Detection of cashew nut in foods by a specific real-time PCR method. *Food Anal Methods.* 1:136–143.
90. Eriksson, A. and Malmheden Yman, I. 1992. Quantitative analysis of casein, egg proteins and hazelnut in food by rocket immunoelectrophoresis on PhastSystem™. In: *Food safety and quality assurance, applications of immunoassay*, pp. 65–68. Dordrecht, The Netherlands: Elsevier.
91. Röder, M., Ibach, A., Baltruweit, I., Gruyters, H., Janise, A., Suwelack, C., Matissek, R., Vieths, S., and Holzhauser, T. 2008. Pilot plant investigations on cleaning efficiencies to reduce hazelnut cross-contamination in industrial manufacture of cookies. *J Food Prot.* 71:2263–2271.
92. Röder, M., Baltruweit, I., Gruyters, H., Ibach, A., Mücke, I., Matissek, R., Vieths, S., and Holzhauser, T. 2010. Allergen sanitation in the food industry: A systematic industrial scale approach to reduce hazelnut cross-contamination of cookies. *J. Food Prot.* 73:1671–1679.
93. Drs, E., Baumgartner, S., Bremer, M. et al. 2004. Detection of hidden hazelnut protein in food by IgY-based indirect competitive enzyme-immunoassay. *Anal Chim Acta.* 520:223–228.
94. Blais, B. W., Gaudreault, M., and Phillippe, L. M. 2003. Multiplex enzyme immunoassay system for the simultaneous detection of multiple allergens in foods. *Food Control.* 14:43–47.
95. Ben Rejeb, S., Abbott, M., Davies, D., Cléroux, C., and Delahaut, P. 2005. Multi-allergen screening immunoassay for the detection of protein markers of peanut and four tree nuts in chocolate. *Food Addit Contam Part A.* 22:709–715.
96. Scheibe, B., Weiss, W., Rueff, F., Przybilla, B., and Gorg, A. 2001. Detection of trace amounts of hidden allergens: hazelnut and almond proteins in chocolate. *J Chromatography B.* 756:229–237.
97. Jonsson, H. and Hellenas, K.E. 2001. Optimizing assay conditions in the detection of food allergens with Biacore's SPR technology. *Biacor J.* 2:16–18.
98. Monaci, L. and Visconti, A. 2009. Mass spectrometry-based proteomics methods for analysis of food allergens. *Trends Anal Chem.* 28:581–591.
99. BVL L 44.00-8. 2010. *Technische Regel, Untersuchung von Lebensmitteln—Nachweis einer spezifischen DNA-Sequenz aus Haselnuss* (Corylus avellana) *in Schokolade mittels Real-time PCR*. Berlin: Beuth.
100. Arlorio, M., Cereti, E., Coisson, J.D., Travaglia, F., and Martelli, A. 2007. Detection of hazelnut (*Corylus* spp.) in processed foods using real-time PCR. *Food Control.* 18:140–148.

101. Koeppel, R., Dvorak, V., Zimmerli, F., Breitenmoser, A., Eugster, A., and Waiblinger, H.U. 2010. Two tetraplex real-time PCR for the detection and quantification of DNA from eight allergens in food. *Eur Food Res Technol.* 230:367–374.
102. Venkatachalam, M., Teuber, S. S., Peterson, W. R., Roux, K. H., and Sathe, S. K. 2006. Antigenic stability of pecan [*Carya illinoinensis* (Wangenh.) K. Koch] proteins: effects of thermal treatments and in vitro digestion. *J Agric Food Chem.* 54:1449–1458.
103. Polenta, G., Godefroy-Benrejeb, S., Delahaut, P., Weber, D., and Abbott, M. 2009. Development of a competitive ELISA for the detection of pecan (*Carya illinoinensis* (Wangenh.) K. Koch) traces in food. *Food Anal Methods.* Epub February 2009.
104. Brezna, B., Piknova, L., and Kuchta, T. 2009. A novel real-time polymerase chain reaction method for the detection of macadamia nuts in food. *Eur Food Res Technol.* 229:397–401.
105. Niemann, L. and Hefle, S.L. 2003. Validated ELISA for detection of undeclared walnut residues in food. *J Allergy Clin Immunol.* 109:s248.
106. Brežná, B., Hudecová, L., and Kuchta T. 2006. A novel real-time polymerase chain reaction (PCR) method for the detection of walnuts in food. *Eur Food Res Technol.* 223:373–377.
107. Yano, T., Sakai, Y., Uchida, K., et al. 2007 Detection of walnut residues in processed foods by polymerase chain reaction. *Biosci Biotechnol Biochem.* 71:51–57.
108. Wang, H., Yuan, F., Wu, Y., Yang, H., Xu, B., Liu, Z., and Chen, Y. 2009. Detection of allergen walnut component in food by an improved real-time PCR method. *J Food Prot.* 72:2433–2435.
109. Mustorp, S., Engdahl-Axelsson, C., Svensson, U., and Holck, A. 2008. Detection of celery (*Apium graveolens*), mustard (*Sinapis alba, Brassica juncea, Brassica nigra*) and sesame (*Sesamum indicum*) in food by real-time PCR. *Eur Food Res Technol.* 226:771–778.
110. Koppelman, S.J., Vlooswijk, R., Bottger, G., et al. 2007. Development of an enzyme-linked immunosorbent assay method to detect mustard protein in mustard seed oil. *J Food Prot.* 70:179–183.
111. Shim, Y.-Y. and Wanasundara, P.D. 2008. Quantitative detection of allergenic protein Sin a 1 from yellow mustard (*Sinapis alba* L.) seeds using enzyme-linked immunosorbent assay. *J Agric Food Chem.* 56:1184–1192.
112. Stephan, O., Weisz, N., Vieths, S., Weiser, T., Rabe, B.,. and Vatterott, W. 2004. Protein quantification, sandwich ELISA, and real-time PCR used to monitor industrial cleaning procedures for contamination with peanut and celery allergens. *J. AOAC Int.* 87:1448–1457.
113. BVL L08.00–56. 2008. *Technische Regel, Untersuchung von Lebensmitteln—Nachweis einer spezifischen DNA-Sequenz aus Sellerie* (Apium graveolens) *in Brühwürsten mittels Real-time PCR.* Berlin: Beuth.
114. LFBG. 2009. *Lebensmittel- und Futtermittelgesetzbuch in der Fassung der Bekanntmachung vom 24. Juli 2009 (BGBl. I S. 2205), geändert durch die Verordnung vom 3. August 2009 (BGBl. I S. 2630).* Bundesanzeiger Verlag, Zöln, Germany.
115. Puff, B., Reese, G., Vieths, S., and Holzhauser, T. 2009. Development of a novel immunoassay for the detection of celeriac as allergenic ingredient in compound food products. Xth International Conference on AgriFood Antibodies (ICAFA), Wageningen, The Netherlands, September 7–10.
116. Röder, M., Vieths, S., and Holzhauser, T. 2009. Commercial lateral flow devices for rapid detection of peanut (*Arachis hypogaea*) and hazelnut (*Corylus avellana*) cross-contamination in the industrial production of cookies. *Anal Bioanal Chem.* 395:103–109.

117. Garber, E.A.E. and Perry, J. 2010. Detection of hazelnuts and almonds using commercial ELISA test kits. *Anal Bioanal Chem.* 396:1939–1945.
118. Schubert-Ullrich, P., Rudolf, J., Ansari, P., Galler, B., Führer, M., Molinelli, A., and Baumgartner, S. 2009. Commercialized rapid immunoanalytical tests for determination of allergenic food proteins: an overview. *Anal Bioanal Chem.* 395:69–81.

CHAPTER 5

Allergens in Milk and Eggs

Mirva Steinhoff and Angelika Paschke-Kratzin

CONTENTS

Cow's Milk 129
    Isolation of Milk Allergens 134
    Detection of Milk Allergens 135
Hen's Egg Allergy 137
    Isolation of Hen's Egg Allergens 141
    Detection of Hen's Egg Allergens 143
References 145

COW'S MILK

Cow's milk contains many proteins that are considered antigenic and able to cause allergic reactions. Cow's milk contains 3–3.5% protein divided into two main groups: caseins (80%) and whey proteins (20%). The main allergic components within the whey fraction are the globular proteins β-lactoglobulin and α-lactalbumin, followed by smaller amounts of bovine serum albumin, lactoferrin, and immunoglobulin. An overview of the main characteristics of the milk proteins is presented in Table 5.1. Studies in the past indicated that the most abundant proteins in cow's milk β-lactoglobulin, α-lactalbumin, and the caseins were the major allergens.[1] Cow's milk allergens are classified using the following allergen nomenclature: *Bos d* (dedicated to the taxonomic name *Bos domesticus*) and a number that indicates the chronological order in which the allergen was identified as such. Bos d 1–3, as inhalant allergens, are not considered in this chapter because they are not involved in food allergies.

α-Lactalbumin is a monomeric protein of 123 amino acid residues with a molecular weight of 14.4 kDa and four disulfide bridges.[2] It occurs naturally in the form of a 36-kDa dimer, with each subunit corresponding to a 162-amino-acid polypeptide, and possesses two disulfide bridges and one free cysteine.[2] The whole casein

Table 5.1 Properties of Cow's Milk Allergens

Cow's Milk Proteins (100%)	Protein	Allergen Name	Allergenicity	Total Protein (%)	MW (kDa)	pI	Amino Acid Residues
Caseins (80%)	α_{s1}-Casein	Bos d 8	Major	32	23.6	4.9–5.0	199
	α_{s2}-Casein	—	—	10	25.2	5.2–5.4	207
	β-Casein	—	—	28	24.0	5.1–5.4	209
	γ_1-Casein	—	—	Traces	20.5	5.5	180
	γ_2-Casein	—	—	Traces	11.8	6.4	104
	γ_3-Casein	—	—	Traces	11.6	5.8	102
	κ-Casein	—	—	10	19	5.4–5.6	169
Whey proteins (20%)	α-Lactalbumin	Bos d 4	Major	5	14.2	4.8	123
	β-Lactoglobulin	Bos d 5	Major	10	18.3	5.3	162
	Immunoglobulins	Bos d 7	—	3	150	—	—
	BSA	Bos d 6	—	1	66.3	4.9–5.1	582
	Lactoferrin	—	—	Traces	80	8.7	703

Note: BSA = bovine serum albumin.

appears to be an association of four different proteins, α_{s1}-, α_{s2}-, β-, and κ-casein, in approximate proportions of 40%, 10%, 40%, and 10%, respectively.[3] Plasmin, the native milk protease, cleaves β-casein and generates the γ-casein fragments.[4] Milk only contains trace amounts of γ-caseins, while proteolytic ripened cheeses contain plentiful amounts of γ-caseins.[5] In some studies, β-lactoglobulin was found to be the fraction with the greatest sensitizing potential, while the α-lactalbumin fraction gave weaker positive reactions; casein was the least sensitizing of the fractions studied.[6] This view has not been completely confirmed because sensitivities to the various cow's milk proteins have been reported to be widely distributed.[7,8] Nevertheless, the majority of published studies reported that caseins as well as the whey proteins were major allergens. *Major allergens* generally are defined as proteins for which 50% or more of the allergenic patients studied have specific immunoglobulin (Ig) E. Cross-reactivity between cow's milk proteins and milk proteins from other species depends on phylogenetic relationship.[5] The highest homologies are observed between the milk proteins of cows and other bovidae, such as buffalo, and, less distinctive, sheep and goat. Homology of the amino acid sequence ranges from 84% for κ-casein and 96% for β-lactoglobulin.[9] Soy milk and milk of mares have been reported to be alternatives for patients with cow's milk allergy.[9]

It has rarely been applied to determine food allergy objectively in large, unselected population studies.[10,11] Moreover, most estimates of the occurrence of cow's milk allergy are based on other diagnostic measurements than the DBPCFC (double-blind, placebo-controlled food challenge) reported to be the "gold standard" of allergen diagnostic tests.[12] For example, self-reported questionnaires or skin prick tests were often used to assert the prevalence of milk allergy. Different methods applied to determine prevalence of the allergen in question render the comparing and combining almost impossible. Hence, comparison of different population-based studies results in a wide variation of estimated prevalence of cow's milk allergy. The exemplary studies on the prevalence of milk allergy given in Table 5.2 vary in unselected children between 0.8% and 2.8% and in adults between 0.3% and 3.0%. Reviews of studies since 2000 value the prevalence of cow's milk allergy to be 2–3% in unselected children and about 1% in adults.[1,4,13–15] Nevertheless, prevalence of milk allergy is strongly dependent on the age of patients. There are findings that the majority of children with milk allergy develop tolerance in early childhood.[16] Ninety-seven children with cow's milk allergy were reviewed after five years by Bishop et al.[17] The initial cohort study started with 100 children at the age of 16 months with a challenge-proven cow's milk allergy. In this study, tolerance of cow's milk was demonstrated in 28% of patients by 2 years of age, 56% by 4 years, and 78% by 6 years. Although milk allergy is normally outgrown by children during the first years of life, the sensitization to milk proteins is the most frequent food allergy in childhood. One of the reasons why allergy to cow's milk shows its highest prevalence in children is its early introduction into the diets of babies when breast-feeding is impossible. Because the only therapy for allergy is the avoidance of the regarding food, in particular nutrition of newborns with milk allergy is highly critical. Hypoallergenic infant formulas are produced from caseins or whey proteins by

Table 5.2 Prevalence of Cow's Milk Allergy

Determined Sensitivity (%)	Subjects	Diagnose Test	Country	Reference
1.0	969 unselected children aged 12 months	DBPCFC	United Kingdom	Venter et al. (2006)[114]
0.6	804 people of 4,093 persons answering a questionnaire	Skin prick test	Germany	Zuberbier et al. (2004)[115]
0.3	Adults	Not specified	United States	Sampson (2004)[10]
2.5	Young children			
1.8	1,537 unselected adults (averaged age 50 years)	Skin prick test	Germany	Schafer and Breuer (2003)[116]
2.0–3.0	Analysis of 229 articles on cow´s milk allergy for the years 1967 to 2001	Elimination/ challenge test	Developed countries	Host (2002)[117]
2.3	4,178 unselected adults (aged 25 – 74)	Skin prick test	Germany	Schafer at al. (2001)[118]
1.1	2,721 unselected children at the age of 2½ years	Various tests	Norway	Eggesbo et al. (2001)[78]
1.2	502 unselected adults (aged 20–44)	Specific and total IgE	Iceland	Gislason (1999)[119]
0.7	414 unselected adults (aged 20–44)	Specific and total IgE	Sweden	
2.0	Cohort study extrapolated to a random community population	Skin prick test	Australia	Hill et al. (1997)[120]
0.8	251 unselected 12-month-old children	Specific IgE	Estland	Julge et al. (1997)[121]
14.3	355 children (5.4 years) with allergic reactions to food	Specific IgE	Spain	Crespo et al. (1995)[122]
2.8	1,158 unselected newborns during first year of life	Elimination/ challenge test	Netherlands	Schrander et al. (1993)[123]
2.2	1,749 unselected newborns during the first 3 years of life	Elimination/ challenge test	Denmark	Host and Halken (1990)[16]

means of heat denaturation and enzymatic hydrolyses, sometimes in combination with ultrafiltration or high pressure to provide nutrition.[18]

In general, thermal processing of allergens can modify conformational epitopes, which might lose their binding capacity to specific antibodies, altering tertiary structure.[18] Linear epitopes are not affected by structural changes and maintain their allergenic properties after heating. Heat processing can have different impacts on the stability of the various individual milk proteins. Casein is often reported to be thermostable, whereas β-lactoglobulin is reported to be more thermolabile, but the influence of heating on the allergens strongly depends on temperature and heating duration.[1,13] A study with severe pasteurization conditions (15 min at 90°C) decreased the immunoreactivity of lactalbumin to 12.72% and lactoglobulin to 18.74%. The immunoreactivity was detected by indirect and competitive enzyme-linked immunosorbent assay (ELISA).[19]

In contrast, pasteurization and homogenization of whole milk was shown not to reduce allergenicity in skin prick tests or DBPCFCs.[20] Homogenization does not affect tolerance to milk even in individuals who tolerate untreated cow's milk but react to processed milk.[21] This may reflect the fact that, depending on the severity of the thermal treatment, a proportion of the milk proteins may remain in the native state, which may be sufficient for IgE reactivity to be retained. Nevertheless, it is reported that heating is not necessarily sufficient to reduce immunoreactivity of milk allergens. The persistence of allergenicity in heat-treated milk might be confirmed by the fact that sensitization to milk develops after consumption of heated products as the only kind that is available to the consumer.

Using mass spectroscopy, current reports analyzed the peptide profile of milk and its changes during thermal treatment and storage. This method allowed detection of a significantly increased peptide in ultrahigh-temperature milk stored at room temperature.[22] This peptide was identified as the N-terminus of α_{s1}-casein. Monaci and van Hengel[23] observed a modification of β-lactoglobulin mass spectra caused by lactosylation after heating of milk samples. During heating in the presence of reducing sugars, proteins are submitted to the Maillard reaction. In this reaction, first sugars are covalently fixed on the amino groups of lysosyl residues, followed by condensation and polymerization reactions. Taheri-Kafrani et al.[24] showed that glycation of β-lactoglobulin in the early stage of the Maillard reaction has a small effect on its recognition by IgE, whereas a high degree of glycation has a masking effect on the recognition of epitopes. Moreover, the influence on antigenicity depends not only on temperature and time of heating but also on possible interactions within the food matrix.[1] Especially, cross-linking of proteins often results in important changes in the chemical and functional properties of the molecule. In this case, the term *cross-linking* in proteins is used to describe the covalent bonding of a protein to itself or to another protein.[25] Singh et al.[25] overviewed several reaction of proteins during food processing (Figure 5.1). Cross-linking reactions may dramatically influence molecular weight, shape, and charging of the surface of the molecule and the accessibility of epitopes. In terms of analytical detection of allergens, these modifications influence extractability and antigenicity.

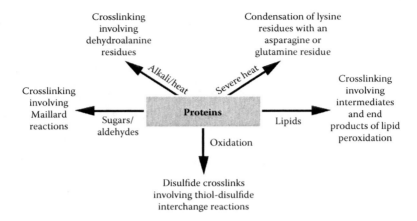

Figure 5.1 Crosslinking reactions of proteins that may occur during food processing. (According to Singh (1991). *Trends Food Sci. Technol.*, 2, 196–200.)

Isolation of Milk Allergens

Many studies have presented the isolation of the whey proteins from cow's milk via preliminary precipitation of casein in liquid milk samples by acidification. The supernatant that includes the whey proteins has then mostly been analyzed using gel electrophoresis,[26–28] high-performance liquid chromatography (HPLC),[29–34] or capillary electrophoresis (CE).[26,27,35,36] For example, separation of casein and whey fractions was achieved by acidic precipitation of proteins from skimmed milk using hydrochloric acid.[37–39] Titration of milk to pH 4.6 causes the precipitation of casein as a coagulum, while whey proteins remain soluble in milk serum. Adjacent whey proteins can be precipitated in the supernatant brought to pH 6.5, adding acetone, and centrifuging at −15°C for 4 h.

Bobe et al.[33] described a method for separation and quantification of bovine milk proteins by reversed-phase (RP-HPLC). This method was used to separate κ-casein, α_{S1}-casein, α_{S2}-casein, β-casein, α-lactalbumin, and β-lactoglobulin using a silica-based C-18 RP-HPLC column and acetonitrile, trifluoroacetic acid, and water as the mobile phase. Highly purified α-lactalbumin, β-lactoglobulin, and casein were prepared from raw milk by anion exchange chromatography using an ÄKTA system (Amersham Biosciences).[40] After purification, characterization of the structure of the prepared proteins was carried out using ELISA, MALDI-TOF-MS (matrix-assisted laser desorption/ionization-time of flight-mass spectrometry), and nuclear magnetic resonance (NMR) analysis.

In contrast, Naoe et al.[41] investigated a liquid-liquid extraction method of α-lactalbumin using reverse micelles composed of a tensid and isooctane to separate milk proteins. Reverse micelles are spontaneous aggregates of amphiphilic molecules in nonpolar media and are capable of solubilizing water and hydrophilic protein. The extraction percentage was almost 100%, and the α-lactalbumin was recovered from the micellar organic phase without structural damage.

CE was used as an efficient and sensitive method to determine α-lactalbumin in milk powders.[42] In this study, an acetic acid buffer was utilized to extract the whey proteins, which were then analyzed by CE using an electrokinetic injection onto an uncoated column. The separation was done rapidly within 5 min and displayed a detection limit of 0.01 mg/L of α-lactalbumin.

Fairise and Cayot[43] used CE as well to separate milk proteins. But, in this investigation the method was based on the micellar electrokinetic chromatography principle, which is a combination of classical CE and hydrophobic interaction chromatography, resulting in the use of surfactant included in the electrophoretic media. Yoshida[44] separated some minor milk proteins between 250 and 100 kDa in acid whey. The estimated protein fraction received according to molecular size by gel filtration chromatography was first separated in albumins and globulins. Then, each protein group was isolated by diethylaminoethyl ion exchange chromatography and hydrophobic interaction chromatography. Isolated proteins were bovine serum albumin (67 kDa), lactoferrin (87 kDa), and xanthine oxidase (150 kDa) for example. There are also several methods that especially target allergenic milk proteins in hypoallergenic infant formulas.[45,46]

Detection of Milk Allergens

Compared to the many techniques available for the analysis of milk proteins in milk or dairy products, there were fewer studies targeting detection of allergenic cow's milk proteins in processed food products. Hence, the literature referring to detection of traces of milk proteins in food products is relatively sparse. The analytical detection of trace amounts of allergenic ingredients is usually more complicated because of the presence of other, often abundant, components of the food matrix that can mask the allergen, which has an impact on the recovery of food allergens.[47] Some examples of released studies concerning detection of milk allergens are given in Table 5.3. Most of them were developed to distinguish cow's milk from sheep's or goat's milk or soymilk.[48–50] Other studies determined the residual allergenicity of hypoallergenic infant formulas or milk substitutes.[51,52]

In the case of analytical detection of allergens in food, the extraction principally is the determining step. If the isolation of the allergen is incomplete, false-negative results can be the consequence. Optimum extractability of allergens essentially depends on the extraction solution, and no single buffer is appropriate for use as a universal extractant for different allergens in diverse foods.[53] Nevertheless, for many foods, extraction with phosphate-buffered saline (PBS) is sufficient.

Hefle and Lambrecht[54] developed a validated sandwich ELISA for detection of undeclared casein in food; their study was based on extraction with $0.01M$ PBS using monoclonal antibodies. Non-milk-containing products such as fruit juices, fruit juice bars, sorbets, and dark and kosher-labeled chocolate were analyzed. In this investigation, the ELISA had a detection limit of less than 0.5 ppm of casein, and the content in the foods ranged from less than 0.5 ppm to more than 40,000 ppm casein. The majority of immunoassay methods use the ELISA format for the detection of milk allergens.

Table 5.3 Detection of Cow's Milk Allergens

Assayed Substance	Method	Matrix	Detection Limit	Reference
β-Lactoglobulin	ELISA (sandwich)	Sausages, bread, pâté	0.04 ppm	De Luis et al. (2008)[55]
Cow DNA	Real-time TaqMan PCR	Raw cow's/sheep's milk mixtures	0.4%	Lopez-Calleja et al. (2007)[48]
		Cow's/sheep's milk mixtures	0.48%	
Caseins	ELISA	Various foods	0.5 ppm	Hefle and Lambrecht (2004)[54]
β-Casein	Optical immunosensor	Bovine cheese	85 ng/ml	Muller-Renaud et al. (2004)[56]
α-Lactalbumin	Biosensor	Heat-treated milk	Not specified	Dupont et al. (2004)[57]
Whey proteins	ELISA	Cow's milk	13–20 µg/L	Karamonova et al. (2003)[124]
Whey proteins	Western blotting	Soy milk	0.1%	Molina et al. (1998)[50]
Caseins	Immunoblotting	Milk protein hydrolyzed formulae	Not specified	Restani et al. (1996)[51]
β-Lactoglobulin	ELISA	Hypoallergenic milk	0.08 µg/L	Mariager et al. (1994)[125]
Caseins	RIE	Various foods	25–100 mg/L	Malmheden et al. (1994)[126]
Caseins	ELISA	Ovine cheese	0.5–25%	Rodriguez et al. (1993)[49]
β-Lactoglobulin	ELISA	Infant formulas, human milk	0.002 µg/L	Makinen-Kiljunen and Palosuo (1992)[52]

Note: RIE = rocket immunoelectrophoresis.

Currently available ELISA methods for detecting milk allergens in food are generally based on the detection of β-lactoglobulin or caseins. Mäkinen-Kiljunen and Palosuo[52] developed a sensitive ELISA with a detection limit of 0.002 µg/L for determination of bovine β-lactoglobulin in infant feeding formulas and in human milk. The estimated recovery rates of β-lactoglobulin were 127% from the diluting buffer and 97% from human breast milk. Likewise, a sandwich ELISA was successfully developed for the detection of defined amounts of cow's milk in ewe's milk and cheese.[49] The mixtures of milk and cheese samples were each homogenized in PBS with a mechanical blender and analyzed after appropriate dilution. The method allows detection and quantification of 0.5–15% bovine milk in ovine milk and 0.5–25% of bovine cheese in ovine cheese.

De Luis et al.[55] evaluated competitive and sandwich ELISA tests to determine β-lactoglobulin and ovomucoid in processed foods. In this study, sausages, bread, and pâté as model processed foods containing low-heat skimmed milk powder and egg powder as allergic ingredients were prepared following standard manufacturing processes. After sample extraction with PBS, ELISA tests were performed, and for the sandwich format, samples were positive for β-lactoglobulin at percentages of added milk of 0.005% and 0.05% for sausages and bread, respectively. In the case of the pâté samples, both ELISA formats gave positive results at 0.25% of milk addition. The results underline the fact that the determination of proteins in food products is greatly influenced by the particular ELISA format used as well as heat processing conditions applied to the food products.

A Western blotting method for the detection of whey milk proteins in commercial soy milks was applied to assess food safety by Molina et al.[50] According to the generally lower detection limit of the blotting method compared to ELISA, in this investigation 0.1% bovine protein in soy protein was detectable. Likewise, Restani et al.[51] used the blotting method to evaluate the residual antigenic activity of milk protein hydrolyzed formulas because some hydrolysates have been reported to induce serious allergic reactions in sensitive children. The appraisal resulted in verification that residual intact cow's milk proteins or polypeptidic material with conserved allergic potential are present in such products.

β-Casein was quantified in milk and cheese, using an optical immunosensor, based on surface plasmon resonance measurement.[56] The assay consisted of a two-step sandwich strategy, with two anti-β-casein antibodies each directed against the extremity of the casein; only native β-casein is quantified and not any degradation product. The method was applied to raw milk and cheese to quantify intact β-casein and to follow the proteolysis of β-casein during ripening process. Also, a biosensor was used by Dupont et al.[57] to follow the denaturation process of α-lactalbumin in milk after heating with the aim to control the quality of drinking milk or to control the heating systems.

Several methods do not target the allergen but rather a marker indicative of the presence of the offending food. In DNA-based methods, DNA is targeted for this purpose. A real-time polymerase chain reaction (PCR) based on the amplification of a fragment of the mitochondrial 12S ribosomal RNA gene was developed and evaluated for the detection and quantification of cow's milk in raw and heated mixtures of cow's and sheep's milk.[48] In this study, experimental raw and heat-treated binary mixtures were analyzed, demonstrating the specificity and sensitivity of the assay for detection and quantification of cow's milk in the range of 0.5–10%.

HEN'S EGG ALLERGY

The chemical composition of eggs of hens (*Gallus domesticus*) has been extensively investigated. Reports document that the major egg allergens are mainly proteins in egg white.[58] Major allergenic egg proteins are ovalbumin (Gal d 2), conalbumin (syn. Ovotransferrin; Gal d 3), ovomucoid (Gal d 1), and lysozyme (Gal d 4).[58] These proteins make up 80% of the total protein content of egg white.[59,60] Regarding the allergenic potency of these proteins, different results have been reported. First, ovomucoid was found to be the most allergenic protein in raw and boiled eggs.[61] Later, studies established that ovalbumin and conalbumin were the major egg allergens.[62,63] In middle of the 1990s Bernhisel-Broadbent et al.[64] announced that the use of commercially pure ovalbumin to evaluate the allergenic potential has led to the impression that ovalbumin is the immunodominant allergen in egg white protein. Commercial reagent-grade purified ovalbumin contains significant quantities of contaminating ovomucoid, which may have led to erroneous interpretation of results. All in all, ovomucoid seems to be the most potential hen's egg allergen.[65] Ovomucin is a minor egg white allergen with a molecular mass of about 165 kDa.[66]

Proteins from egg yolk have received little attention as allergens, although they bind specific IgE in the sera of allergic patients.[58] In the yolk, the protein α-livetin (Gal d 5) is of interest because it is involved in the bird-egg syndrome, by which sensitization might occur by inhalation during contact with birds.[67] The proteins apovitellenin I and IV and phosvitin are reported to be minor allergens of egg yolk.[68] In addition, a large range of proteins from hen's eggs are shown to bind IgE from egg-allergenic patients but with lower prevalence.[58,69,70] In the case of food allergy, less-significant proteins are macroglobulin, avidine, and several different enzymes.

Today, the primary structure, number of amino acid residues, and the molecular masses of the hen's egg allergens are already known.[71–77] The molecular and allergenic characteristics of hen's egg allergens are presented in Table 5.4. Egg and milk are among the most frequent causes of allergic reactions in children,[70] but estimates of the total prevalence of allergy to egg vary considerably. Eggesbo et al.[78] estimated the prevalence in Norwegian children to be 1.6%, while the corresponding report regarding German children indicated a prevalence of 2.8%.[79] The exemplary studies on egg allergy given in Table 5.5 varied in unselected children between 0.8% and 3.6% and in adults between 0.2% and 3.2%. Mine and Yang[80] estimated in their comprehensive review the prevalence of hen's egg allergy to vary between 1.6% and 3.2%. The difficulties in determining the prevalence of hen's egg allergy are caused by the fact that the majority of children develop an oral tolerance as they age. Several studies estimated the outgrowing of egg allergy and demonstrated that this allergy usually resolves by school age.[81–83] Savage et al.[84] also demonstrated that a majority of patients with egg allergy will develop egg tolerance, although the rate of tolerance development seems to be slower than described in earlier reports. In this study, more than 50% of the 12-year-old patients did not tolerate the consumption of concentrated egg. The prevalence of the bird-egg syndrome is still uncertain, but it is less common than food allergy to egg and more widespread in adults than in young children.[67,85]

Processing procedures may modulate the allergenic properties of many kinds of proteins. Generally, allergenicity of egg white proteins may be reduced by heat treatment. Hoffmann[63] demonstrated that boiled eggs exhibited decreased, but still significant, allergenicity. A later study reported that IgE binding of egg white proteins decreased about 58% in RAST after heating to 90°C for 10 min.[58] Urisu et al.[86] compared the allergenicities of heated and ovomucoid-depleted egg white, freeze-dried egg white, and heated egg white in a DBPCFC in egg-allergic subjects. In this study, the heated and ovomucoid-depleted egg white preparations were less allergenic than the other preparation (the freeze-dried egg white). Similar results were obtained by Mine and Zhang[87] when examining the influence on allergenicity and antigenicity of the four major egg allergens on physical and chemical manipulation. In this study, it was found that thermal treatment caused a decrease in human IgG-binding capacity

ALLERGENS IN MILK AND EGGS

Table 5.4 Properties of Hen's Egg Allergens

Liquid Hen's Egg (100%); Protein Content 11.5–12.4%	Protein	Allergen Name	Allergenicity	Fraction Proteins (100%)	MW (kDa)	pI	Amino Acid Residues
Egg white (69.6%); Protein content 9.7–10.6%	Ovalbumin	Gal d 2	Major	54	42.7	4.5	385
	Ovomucoid	Gal d 1	Major	11	28	4.1	186
	Conalbumin (syn. ovotransferrin)	Gal d 3	Major	12–13	77	6.1	686
	Lysozyme	Gal d 4	Major	3.4–3.5	14	10.4	129
	Ovomucin	—	Minor	1.5–3.5	165	4.5–5.0	580
	Others	—	Minor	15–18.1	—	—	—
Egg yolk (30.4%); Protein content 15.7–16.6%	α-Livetin	Gal d 5	Minor	(Livetins 9.3)	65–70	05.31	589
	Phosvitin	—	Minor	13.4	35	—	—
	Apovitellenins I	—	Minor	Apovitellenin (I–VI) 37.3	9.5	—	—
	Apovitellenins VI	—	Minor		170	—	—
	Others	—	Minor	40	—	—	—

Table 5.5 Prevalence of Hen's Egg Allergy

Determined Sensitivity (%)	Subjects	Diagnose Test	Country	Reference
0.8	969 unselected children aged 12 months	DBPCFC	United Kingdom	Venter et al. (2006)[114]
0.8	804 people of 4,093 persons answering a questionnaire	Skin prick test	Germany	Zuberbier et al. (2004)[115]
0.2	Adults	Not specified	United States	Sampson (2004)[10]
1.3	Young children			
0.4	1,537 unselected adults (average age 50 years)	Skin prick test	Germany	Schafer and Breuer (2003)[116]
1.6	2,721 unselected children aged 2½ years	DBPCFC		Eggesbo et al. (2001)[78]
1.9	4178 unselected adults (aged 25–74)	Skin prick test	Germany	Schafer at al. (2001)[118]
0.4	502 unselected adults (aged 20–44)	Specific and total IgE	Iceland	Gislason (1999)[119]
0.2	414 unselected adults (aged 20–44)	Specific and total IgE	Sweden	
73.0	196 food-allergic children	DBPCFC, RAST	United States	Sampson and Ho (1997)[127]
3.2	Cohort study extrapolated to a random community population	Skin prick test	Australia	Hill et al. (1997)[120]
3.6	251 unselected 12-month-old children	Specific IgE	Estland	Julge et al. (1997)[121]
20.1	355 children (mean age 5.4 years) with allergic reactions to food	Specific IgE	Spain	Crespo et al. (1995)[122]
26.0	180 food-allergic children	DBPCFC	United States	Bock and Atkins (1990)[70]

of all examined allergens, whereas only the IgE-binding capacity of ovomucoid and ovalbumin was influenced by heating.

It has been shown that heat treatment of egg white proteins resulted in an increase in degree of hydrolysis with pepsin and chymotrypsin.[88] Denaturation renders proteins more accessible to enzymatic digestion with these enzymes. In the same study, the digest with trypsin was not influenced by the heat treatment of egg proteins. A combination of heating and enzymatic digestion was reported to reduce the allergenicity of pasteurized egg successfully without a significant change in texture and flavor of the foods.[89]

There are many reports about reducing the allergenicity of hen's egg and hen's egg products using high pressure, enzymatic digestion, heating, or combined use of these processing procedures.[90–93] There are many ways in which the antigenicity of proteins can be changed during processing, especially when this processing takes place in the complex milieu of a food, with so many other ingredients available to participate in complex physical and chemical reactions.[94] When heated in the presence of wheat flour, ovomucoid becomes insoluble by undergoing intermolecular disulfide protein-polysaccharide polymerization, making the molecule less extractable and antigenic.[95,96]

Isolation of Hen's Egg Allergens

The major source of allergens is usually the raw unprocessed food itself. In the case of egg allergens, ovalbumin, ovomucoid, and lysozyme, for example, generally are successfully isolated from raw hen's egg. For immunological examination, hen's egg antigen solutions were often prepared by stirring crude egg with an equal volume of extraction solution for hours at room temperature followed by centrifugation. In these works, physiological saline,[62,97] PBS,[64] or $0.1M$ acetate buffer,[98] for example, were applied to isolate egg allergens from liquid egg. Salt is known to play an important role in the solubility characteristics of proteins via influencing protein-protein and protein-solvent interactions.

Hildebrandt et al.[99] modified and compared in their work six different extraction methods for the analysis of egg allergens. For the appraisal, protein content and the allergenic potential of the extracts were studied. In this work, PBS was the most qualified extractant for the isolation of hen's egg allergens among the six extraction solutions tested. In contrast, urea ($8M$) has the ability to reduce the allergenicity of hen's egg allergens and is therefore not qualified as an extractant for the analysis of egg allergens.

Different methods have been developed for purifying major egg white proteins, including protein precipitation by salts or by ionic strength reduction and liquid chromatography. Most investigations use anion exchange chromatography for purification of isolated proteins due to the presence of coprecipitated proteins. Owing to its high negative charge density, ovalbumin drives other egg white proteins from the anion exchange column progressively. Once the contaminant protein is separated from the protein of interest, a high-salt buffer is used to get the desired protein to elute from the column.

Awade et al.[76] published a two-step chromatography procedure for the purification of hen's egg white ovomucin, lysozyme, ovotransferrin, and ovalbumin followed by characterization of purified proteins. As a first step, purification of ovomucin and lysozyme was carried out by gel permeation chromatography on a Superose 6 prep-grade column. In the second step, anion exchange chromatography on Q-Sepharose Fast Flow (Q-Sepharose FF, Pharmacia, Sweden) led to the isolation of ovotransferrin and ovalbumin from a gel permeation chromatographic peak. For preparation of large quantities of nonaltered ovalbumin, anion exchange chromatography also was used.[100] With an isocratic elution program using $0.14M$ sodium chloride aqueous solution and Q-Sepharose FF gel, ovalbumin with a purity rate of 94% was recovered.

The egg proteins ovomucoid, ovalbumin, ovotransferrin, lysozyme, and α-livetin were purified with the aim of further characterization of the proteins.[75] In this study, ovomucoid, ovalbumin, and lysozyme were also purified by anion-exchange chromatography on Q-Sepharose FF gel according to Ebbehoej et al.[101] In another study, Awade and Efstathiou[66] reported a comparison of gel permeation chromatography, RP-HPLC, and anion exchange HPLC for egg white protein analysis. These three liquid chromatographic methods appeared to be complementary for rapid egg white protein analysis in this investigation. Anion exchange chromatography offered the more complete analysis, although gel permeation should be recommended for ovomucin separation. RP-HPLC would be preferable for an accurate estimation of lysozyme and ovotransferrin since with anion exchange chromatography these proteins are slightly contaminated with other minor proteins. Due to the presence of coprecipitated proteins, mainly ovalbumin and lysozyme, preparation of pure ovomucin remains a challenge. The other egg albumins can hardly be removed by washing procedures, and gel filtration chromatography that is mostly used to purify ovomucin is not suitable for large-scale production.

Thus, the effect of different salt concentrations on the extractability of ovomucin was analyzed by gel filtration chromatography and sodium dodecyl sulfate polyacrylamide gel electrophoresis (SDS-PAGE).[102] At increasing sodium chloride concentration, the ovalbumin rate increased, whereas the corresponding lysozyme rate decreased. An increasing salt concentration also caused a slight decrease of the ovomucin content. In this study, the protein compositions of ovomucin extracts were significantly affected by the salt concentration. Sodium iodide and sodium pyrophosphate were also found to be salting-in compounds that changed the character of the solvent in a manner similar to that of SDS, enhancing the solubility of egg white proteins.[103]

Not only ionic strength can be of use for isolation of egg white proteins but also change of pH. In 2000, an easy method for separation of lysozyme from chicken egg white by reductants and thermal treatment was reported.[104] By adding ascorbic acid to the fresh chicken egg white to reduce the pH to about 4.0 and then heating the mixture to $70 \pm 1°C$ until no further precipitation occurred, crude lysozyme solution was obtained.

Of course, recovery rates are strongly dependent on the source used for protein isolation. Hiidenhovi et al.[105] compared different egg albumin fractions as sources of ovomucin. For this purpose, ovomucin was fractionated from whole egg albumin, thick egg albumin, liquid egg albumin, and a liquid egg albumin filtration by-product

ALLERGENS IN MILK AND EGGS

by using the isoelectric precipitation method. There was great variation between the ovomucin contents of the different albumen fractions. In conclusion, both the filtration by-product and the liquid egg appeared to be potential alternatives to whole egg albumin and thick egg albumin as sources of ovomucin.

Detection of Hen's Egg Allergens

Egg-derived components are often added to processed food for many different purposes (e.g., as emulsifiers or gelling agents). In the past, several methods for the detection of egg in foods have been developed, mostly immunological techniques using anti-egg white antibodies. Plenty of studies have been published using the ELISA technique for detection of egg proteins in food. These methods are generally based on the detection of ovalbumin or ovomucoid. Some examples of previously released studies about detection of egg allergens using different analytical methods in various foods are given in Table 5.6. In 1988, immunochemical identification and quantification of ovalbumin additive in canned mushrooms was reported.[106] Addition of either egg white or ovalbumin in canned mushrooms during blanching or before autoclaving increases the apparent weight of drained mushrooms up to 20%. Mushrooms are purchased by their drained weight, so the amount of added

Table 5.6 Detection of Hen's Egg Allergens

Assayed Substance	Method	Matrix	Detection Limit	Reference
Ovomucoid	ELISA (sandwich)	Sausages, bread, pâté	0.19 ppm	De Luis et al. (2008)[55]
Ovalbumin	ELISA (competitive)	Commercially purified ovalbumin	0.041 ng/ml extract	Li et al. (2008)[111]
Ovalbumin	Immunoblotting	Surimi-derived products	0.5 ng/μl extract	Romero-Rodriguez et al. (2002)[128]
Egg proteins	Dipstick immunoassay	Butter biscuits, garlic dressing	0.02 ppm	Baumgartner et al. (2002)[113]
Ovalbumin	ELISA (sandwich)	Pasta	1 ppm	Hefle et al. (2001)[109]
Egg proteins	ELISA (competitive)	Ice cream, meatballs, bread, wieners, pasta, maple syrup	0.02 ppm	Yeung et al. (2000)[107]
Egg white proteins	ELISA (direct)	Raw and pasteurized pork meat pastes	300 ppm	Leduc et al. (1999)[108]
		Sterilized pork meat pastes	1,250 ppm	
Ovalbumin	Immunoblotting	Milk, cheese, yogurt, ice cream	50,000 ppm	Turin and Bonomi (1994)[129]
Lysozyme	ELISA (sandwich)	Fruit juices, salad dressing, wine, beer	1–12 ng/ml[a]	Rauch et al. (1990)[130]
Ovalbumin	ELISA (competitive)	Canned mushrooms	20 ppm	Breton et al. (1988)[106]

[a] Determination range.

egg protein must be regulated. Briefly, the mushrooms were treated with ovalbumin, heated, extracted with PBS, and analyzed via ELISA. In this study, 10 ng/ml ovalbumin could be detected in mushroom extracts, equating to 20 ppm ovalbumin in drained mushrooms.

Compared to these results, the work of Yeung et al.[107] resulted in a more sensitive determination method for egg proteins in food products. Ice cream, meatballs, bread, wieners, pasta, and maple syrup were artificially contaminated with whole egg protein with the aim to determine recovery rates. Recoveries, ranging from 67% to 96%, were obtained relating to the foods mentioned, and the detection limit was found to be 0.2 ppm. Leduc et al.[108] also applied the ELISA technique to determine the content of egg white proteins in meat products. Experimental pork meat pastes containing defined amounts of egg white underwent pasteurization and sterilization. Samples were extracted with PBS and analyzed with direct ELISA experiments. The detection limit of egg white antigens was 0.03% of dry powder in raw and pasteurized products and 0.125% in sterilized products. Hence, this study highlighted the fact that food proteins added in processing may retain allergic potential.

A relevant study reporting the development of a sandwich ELISA method for the detection of undeclared egg residues in pasta products was published by Hefle et al.[109] Reference pasta standards and 20 brands of egg-free pasta were extracted, then clarified by centrifugation and analyzed via ELISA. The detection limit of the assay was 1 ppm spray-dried whole egg. Of the egg-free pasta samples, 55% (22 samples) tested positive for the presence of undeclared egg residues, with values ranging from 1 to more than 100,000 ppm. In 2008, an evaluation of indirect competitive and double-antibody sandwich ELISA test to determine ovomucoid as well as β-lactoglobulin in model processed foods was published.[55] In this study, sausages, bread, and pâté as model processed foods containing low percentages of milk and egg as allergic ingredients were prepared following standard manufacturing processes. For the sandwich format, samples were positive for ovomucoid at percentages of added egg powder of 0.005% for sausages and of bread and at 0.05% of added egg for both formats. For the pâté samples, only the indirect competitive assay could detect ovomucoid powder at 0.25% of egg addition.

To determine if acidic matrices such as salad dressings had an effect on the detection of allergenic protein residues by ELISA, the detection of egg, milk, and gluten in salad dressings was investigated using commercial ELISA test kits. The authors of this study mentioned that the ability of ELISA tests to accurately detect the allergenic protein residues in salad dressings might be compromised by the acidic conditions, probably due to the decrease in the solubility of the allergenic proteins.[110] In contrast, measurement of ovalbumin, not in foods but in commercially purified ovalbumin, resulted in an extremely low detection limit of 0.041 ng/ml extract.[111]

These studies demonstrated that the choice of extraction buffer, type of processing and matrix composition have a major impact on the extraction efficiency and the detecting limit of the allergenic proteins. From a theoretical point of view, ELISA methods are quantitative, but for the same reasons as the detection limit, results can only be semiquantitative or qualitative unless the method is validated appropriately. As for many other allergens, ELISAs for detection of egg proteins are marketed in kit format, although there is often widely differing results for allergen detection using different test kits.

Faeste et al.[112] tested the performance of three commercially available kits for quantitative egg analysis using six model heat-processed foods. Stirred egg as non-processed food, scrambled egg, batter, pasta, minced meat, and mayonnaise were prepared containing defined amounts of egg proteins and analyzed via test kits of R-Biopharm (Ridascreen®), Tepnel (BioKits®), and Morinaga Institute of Biological Science (Morinaga®). Although the egg content of the model foods was determined correctly in the nonprocessed samples (except pasta samples analyzed with Ridascreen), the data derived for heat-treated foods diverged. The authors concluded that these big differences in egg protein detectability resulted most probably from the different extraction strategies used in the kits. In contrast to the other assays, the denaturing-reducing conditions of the Morinaga extraction resulted in much more of the egg protein being solubilized and available for detection, particularly in the samples exposed to higher heat or those containing wheat.

Other antibody-based techniques in addition to the ELISA technique have also been examined. Baumgartner et al.[113] reported an approach to the development of a dipstick assay for the determination of egg proteins in food. Compared to other techniques, dipstick tests are inexpensive, portable, and rapid and do not require technical skills to perform. Although this approach did not allow quantitation, detection of about 20 µg/kg (0.02 ppm) egg protein in butter biscuits and garlic dressing was possible.

REFERENCES

1. Wal, J. M. (2004): Bovine milk allergenicity, *Ann Allergy Asthma Immunol*, 93, S2–S11.
2. Wal, J. M. (1998): Allergy review series II: an update on allergens: cow's milk allergens, *Allergy*, 53, 1013–1022.
3. Elsayed, S., Hill, D. J., and Do, T. V. (2004): Evaluation of the allergenicity and antigenicity of bovine-milk as1-casein using extensively purified synthetic peptides, *Scand J Immunol*, 60, 486–493.
4. Monaci, L., Tregoat, V., van Hengel, A. J., and Anklam, E. (2006): Milk allergens, their characteristics and their detection in food: a review, *Eur Food Res Technol*, 223, 149–179.
5. Restani, P., Ballabio, C., Di Lorenzo, C., Tripodi, S., and Fiocchi, A. (2009): Molecular aspects of milk allergens and their role in clinical events, *Anal Bioanal Chem*, 395, 47–56.
6. Sharma, S., Kumar, P., Betzel, C., and Singh, T. P. (2001): Structure and function of proteins involved in milk allergies, *J Chromatogr B Biomed Sci Appl*, 756, 183–187.
7. Walker-Smith, J. (2003): Cow's milk allergy: a new understanding from immunology, *Ann Allergy Asthma Immunol*, 90, 81–83.
8. Wal, J. M. (2001): Structure and function of milk allergens, *Allergy*, 56 Suppl 67, 35–38.
9. Jäger, L. and Vieths, S. (2008): Nahrungsmittelallergene. In: Jäger, L., Wüthrich, B., Ballmer-Weber, B., and Vieths, S., eds.: *Nahrungsmittelallergien und-intoleranzen*, 111–220. Elsevier, Munich, Germany.

10. Sampson, H. A. (2004): Update on food allergy, *J Allergy Clin Immunol*, 113, 805–819.
11. Wood, R. A. (2003): The natural history of food allergy, *Pediatrics*, 111, 1631–1637.
12. Keil, T. (2007): Epidemiology of food allergy: what's new? A critical appraisal of recent population-based studies, *Curr Opin Allergy Clin Immunol*, 7, 259–263.
13. Host, A. (1994): Cow's milk protein allergy and intolerance in infancy. Some clinical, epidemiological and immunological aspects, *Pediatr Allergy Immunol*, 5, 1–36.
14. Skripak, J. M., C., M. E., Mudd, K., and Wood, R. A. (2007): The natural history of IgE-mediated cow's milk allergy, *J Allergy Clin Immunol*, 120, 1172–1177.
15. Chatchatee, P., Jarvinen, K.-M., Bardina, L., Beyer, K., and Sampson, H. A. (2001): Identification of IgE- and IgG-binding epitopes on as1-casein: differences in patients with persistent and transient cow's milk allergy, *J Allergy Clin Immunol*, 107, 379–383.
16. Host, A. and Halken, S. (1990): A prospective study of cow milk allergy in Danish infants during the first 3 years of life. Clinical course in relation to clinical and immunological type of hypersensitivity reaction, *Allergy*, 45, 587–596.
17. Bishop, J. M., Hill, D. J., and Hosking, C. S. (1990): Natural history of cow milk allergy: clinical outcome, *J Pediatr*, 116, 862–867.
18. Besler, M., Steinhart, H., and Paschke, A. (2001): Stability of food allergens and allergenicity of processed foods, *J Chromatogr B Biomed Sci Appl*, 756, 207–228.
19. Wroblewska, B. and Jedrychowski, L. (2001): Changes of immunoreactive properties of cow milk proteins as a result of technological processing, *Biotechnologia*, 189–201.
20. Host, A., Husby, S., and Osterballe, O. (1988): A prospective study of cow's milk allergy in exclusively breast-fed infants. Incidence, pathogenetic role of early inadvertent exposure to cow's milk formula, and characterization of bovine milk protein in human milk, *Acta Paediatr Scand*, 77, 663–670.
21. Paajanen, L., Tuure, T., Poussa, T., and Korpela, R. (2003): No difference in symptoms during challenges with homogenized and unhomogenized cow's milk in subjects with subjective hypersensitivity to homogenized milk, *J Dairy Res*, 70, 175–179.
22. Meltretter, J., Schmidt, A., Humeny, A., Becker, C.-M., and Pischetsrieder, M. (2008): Analysis of the peptide profile of milk and its changes during thermal treatment and storage, *J Agric Food Chem*, 56, 2899–2906.
23. Monaci, L. and van Hengel, A. J. (2007): Effect of heat treatment on the detection of intact bovine beta-lactoglobulins by LC mass spectrometry, *J Agric Food Chem*, 55, 2985–2992.
24. Taheri-Kafrani, A., Gaudin, J.-C., Rabesona, H., Nioi, C., Agarwal, D., Drouet, M., Chobert, J.-M., Bordbar, A.-K., and Haertle, T. (2009): Effects of heating and glycation of beta-lactoglobulin on its recognition by IgE of sera from cow milk allergy patients, *J Agric Food Chem*, 57, 4974–4982.
25. Singh, H. (1991): Modification of food proteins by covalent crosslinking, *Trends Food Sci Technol*, 2, 196–200.
26. Kinghorn, N. M., Norris, C. S., Paterson, G. R., and Otter, D. E. (1995): Comparison of capillary electrophoresis with traditional methods to analyze bovine whey proteins, *J Chromatogr A*, 700, 111–123.
27. Shieh, P. C. H., Hoang, D., Guttman, A., and Cooke, N. (1994): Capillary sodium dodecyl sulfate gel electrophoresis of proteins. I. Reproducibility and stability, *J Chromatogr A*, 676, 219–226.
28. Chen, W. L., Hwang, M. T., Liau, C. Y., Ho, J. C., Hong, K. C., and Mao, S. J. T. (2005): beta-Lactoglobulin is a thermal marker in processed milk as studied by electrophoresis and circular dichroic spectra, *J Dairy Sci*, 88, 1618–1630.

29. Parris, N. and Baginski, M. A. (1991): A rapid method for the determination of whey protein denaturation, *J Dairy Sci*, 74, 58–64.
30. Parris, N., White, A. E., and Farrell, H. M., Jr. (1990): Identification of altered proteins in nonfat dry milk powder prepared from heat-treated skim milk, *J Agric Food Chem*, 38, 824–829.
31. Bican, P. and Spahni, A. (1991): Reversed phase high performance liquid chromatography of whey proteins, *J High Resolut Chromatogr*, 14, 287–289.
32. De Frutos, M., Cifuentes, A., Amigo, L., Ramos, M., and Diez-Masa, J. C. (1992): Rapid analysis of whey proteins from different animal species by reversed-phase high-performance liquid chromatography, *Z Lebensm Unters Forsch*, 195, 326–331.
33. Bobe, G., Beitz, D. C., Freeman, A. E., and Lindberg, G. L. (1998): Sample preparation affects separation of whey proteins by reversed-phase high-performance liquid chromatography, *J Agric Food Chem*, 46, 1321–1325.
34. Elgar, D. F., Norris, C. S., Ayers, J. S., Pritchard, M., Otter, D. E., and Palmano, K. P. (2000): Simultaneous separation and quantitation of the major bovine whey proteins including proteose peptone and caseinomacropeptide by reversed-phase high-performance liquid chromatography on polystyrene-divinylbenzene, *J Chromatogr A*, 878, 183–196.
35. Chen, F. T. A. and Zang, J. H. (1992): Determination of milk proteins by capillary electrophoresis, *J AOAC Int*, 75, 905–909.
36. De Block, J., Merchiers, M., and Van Renterghem, R. (1999): Capillary electrophoresis of the whey protein fraction of milk powders. A possible method for monitoring storage conditions, *Int Dairy J*, 8, 787–792.
37. Bleumink, E. and Young, E. (1968): Identification of the atopic allergen in cow milk, *Int Arch Allergy Appl Immunol*, 34, 521–543.
38. Lee, S. H., Jeon, W. M., Kim, Y. K., Lee, S. U., and Jeong, S. Y. (1991): Electrophoretic analysis of major proteins in bovine milk, *Hanguk Chuksan Hakhoe Chi*, 33, 392–398.
39. Maubois, J. L. and Ollivier, G. (1997): Extraction of milk proteins, *Food Sci Technol*, 80, 579–595.
40. Blanc, F., Herve, B., Alessandri, S., Bublin, M., Paty, E., Leung, S. A., Patient, K. A., and Wal, J.-M. (2008): Update on optimized purification and characterisation of natural milk allergens, *Mol Nutr Food Res*, 52, 166–175.
41. Naoe, K., Noda, K., Konishi, T., Kawagoe, M., and Imai, M. (2004): Liquid-liquid extraction of a-lactalbumin using reverse micellar organic solvent, *BioFactors*, 22, 347–351.
42. Gutierrez, J. E. N. and Jakobovits, L. (2003): Capillary electrophoresis of alpha-lactalbumin in milk powders, *J Agric Food Chem*, 51, 3280–3286.
43. Fairise, J.-F. and Cayot, P. (1998): New ultrarapid method for the separation of milk proteins by capillary electrophoresis, *J Agric Food Chem*, 46, 2628–2633.
44. Yoshida, S. (1988): Isolation of some minor milk proteins, distributed in acid whey from approximately 100,000 to 250,000 daltons of particle size, *J Dairy Sci*, 71, 1–9.
45. Docena, G., Rozenfeld, P., Fernandez, R., and Fossati, C. A. (2002): Evaluation of the residual antigenicity and allergenicity of cow's milk substitutes by in vitro tests, *Allergy*, 57, 83–91.
46. Niggemann, B., Binder, C., Klettke, U., and Wahn, U. (1999): In vivo and in vitro studies on the residual allergenicity of partially hydrolysed infant formulae, *Acta Paediatr*, 88, 394–398.
47. Poms, R., Emons, H., and Anklam, E. (2006): Reference materials and method validation in allergen detection, In S. J. Kopelman and S. L. Hefle, Eds., *Detecting Allergens in Food*, 348–356. Woodhead Publishing, Cambridge, UK.

48. Lopez-Calleja, I., Gonzalez, I., Fajardo, V., Martin, I., Hernandez, P. E., Garcia, T., and Martin, R. (2007): Real-time TaqMan PCR for quantitative detection of cows' milk in ewes' milk mixtures, *Int Dairy J*, 17, 729–736.
49. Rodriguez, E., Martin, R., Garcia, T., Gonzalez, I., Morales, P., Sanz, B., and Hernandez, P. E. (1993): Detection of cows' milk in ewes' milk and cheese by a sandwich enzyme-linked immunosorbent assay (ELISA), *J Sci Food Agric*, 61, 175–80.
50. Molina, E., Amigo, L., and Ramos, M. (1998): Detection of bovine milk proteins in soymilk by Western blotting, *J Food Prot*, 61, 1691–1694.
51. Restani, P., Plebani, A., Velona, T., Cavagni, G., Ugazio, A. G., Poiesi, C., Muraro, A., and Galli, C. L. (1996): Use of immunoblotting and monoclonal antibodies to evaluate the residual antigenic activity of milk protein hydrolyzed formulas, *Clin Exp Allergy*, 26, 1182–1187.
52. Mäkinen-Kiljunen, S., and Palosuo, T. (1992): A sensitive enzyme-linked immunosorbent assay for determination of bovine beta-lactoglobulin in infant feeding formulas and in human milk, *Allergy (Copenhagen)*, 47, 347–352.
53. Pastorello, E. A. and Trambaioli, C. (2001): Isolation of food allergens, *J Chromatogr B Analyt Technol Biomed Life Sci*, 756, 71–84.
54. Hefle, S. L. and Lambrecht, D. M. (2004): Validated sandwich enzyme-linked immunosorbent assay for casein and its application to retail and milk-allergic complaint foods, *J Food Prot*, 67, 1933–1938.
55. de Luis, R., Mata, L., Estopanan, G., Lavilla, M., Sanchez, L., and Perez, M. D. (2008): Evaluation of indirect competitive and double antibody sandwich ELISA tests to determine beta-lactoglobulin and ovomucoid in model processed foods, *Food Agric Immunol*, 19, 339–350.
56. Muller-Renaud, S., Dupont, D., and Dulieu, P. (2004): Quantification of beta-casein in milk and cheese using an optical immunosensor, *J Agric Food Chem*, 52, 659–664.
57. Dupont, D., Rolet-Repecaud, O., and Muller-Renaud, S. (2004): Determination of the heat treatment undergone by milk by following the denaturation of alpha-lactalbumin with a biosensor, *J Agric Food Chem*, 52, 677–681.
58. Anet, J., Back, J. F., Baker, R. S., Barnett, D., Burley, R. W., and Howden, M. E. H. (1985): Allergens in the white and yolk of hen's egg. A study of IgE binding by egg proteins, *Int Arch Allergy Appl Immunol*, 77, 364–371.
59. Osuga, D. T. and Feeney, R. E. (1968): Biochemistry of the egg-white proteins of the ratite group, *Arch Biochem Biophys*, 124, 560–574.
60. Kovacs-Nolan, J., Phillips, M., and Mine, Y. (2005): Advances in the value of eggs and egg components for human health, *J Agric Food Chem*, 53, 8421–8431.
61. Bleumink, E. and Young, E. (1969): Atopic allergen in hen egg. I. Identification of the skin-reactive fraction in egg white, *Int Arch Allergy Appl Immunol*, 35, 1–19.
62. Langeland, T. (1982): A clinical and immunological study of allergy to hen's egg white. III. Allergens in hen's egg white studied by crossed radio-immunoelectrophoresis (CRIE), *Allergy*, 37, 521–530.
63. Hoffmann, D. R. (1983): Immunochemical identification of the allergens in egg white, *J Allergy Clin Immunol*, 71, 481–486.
64. Bernhisel-Broadbent, J., Dintzis, H. M., Dintzis, R. Z., and Sampson, H. A. (1994): Allergenicity and antigenicity of chicken egg ovomucoid (Gal d III) compared with ovalbumin (Gal d I) in children with egg allergy and in mice, *J Allergy Clin Immunol*, 93, 1047–1059.
65. Kreft, D., Bauer, R., and Goerlich, R. (1995): *Nahrungsmittelallergene—Charakteristika und Wirkungsweisen*, de Gruyter Verlag, Berlin.

66. Awade, A. C. and Efstathiou, T. (1999): Comparison of three liquid chromatographic methods for egg-white protein analysis, *J Chromatogr B Biomed Sci Appl*, 723, 69–74.
67. Quirce, S., Maranon, F., Umpierrez, A., De Las Heras, M., Fernandez-Caldas, E., and Sastre, J. (2001): Chicken serum albumin (Gal d 5*) is a partially heat-labile inhalant and food allergen implicated in the bird-egg syndrome, *Allergy*, 56, 754–762.
68. Walsh, B. J., Barnett, D., Burley, R. W., Elliott, C., Hill, D. J., and Howden, M. E. H. (1988): New allergens from hen's egg white and egg yolk. In vitro study of ovomucin, apovitellenin I and VI, and phosvitin, *Int Arch Allergy Appl Immunol*, 87, 81–86.
69. Langeland, T. (1983): A clinical and immunological study of allergy to hen's egg white. VI. Occurrence of proteins cross-reacting with allergens in hen's egg white as studied in egg white from turkey, duck, goose, seagull, and in hen egg yolk, and hen and chicken sera and flesh, *Allergy*, 38, 399–412.
70. Bock, S. A. and Atkins, F. M. (1990): Patterns of food hypersensitivity during sixteen years of double-blind, placebo-controlled food challenges, *J Pediatr*, 117, 561–567.
71. Blake, C. C., Koenig, D. F., Mair, G. A., North, A. C., Phillips, D. C., and Sarma, V. R. (1965): Structure of hen egg-white lysozyme. A three-dimensional Fourier synthesis at 2 angstrom resolution, *Nature*, 206, 757–761.
72. Kato, I., Schrode, J., Kohr, W. J., and Laskowski, M., Jr. (1987): Chicken ovomucoid: determination of its amino acid sequence, determination of the trypsin reactive site, and preparation of all three of its domains, *Biochemistry*, 26, 193–201.
73. Nisbet, A. D., Saundry, R. H., Moir, A. J. G., Fothergill, L. A., and Fothergill, J. E. (1981): The complete amino acid sequence of hen ovalbumin, *Eur J Biochem*, 115, 335–345.
74. Williams, J., Elleman, T. C., Kingston, I. B., Wilkins, A. G., and Kuhn, K. A. (1982): The primary structure of hen ovotransferrin, *Eur J Biochem*, 122, 297–303.
75. Jacobsen, B., Hoffmann-Sommergruber, K., Have Tilde, T., Foss, N., Briza, P., Oberhuber, C., Radauer, C., Alessandri, S., Knulst, A. C., Fernandez-Rivas, M., and Barkholt, V. (2008): The panel of egg allergens, Gal d 1-Gal d 5: their improved purification and characterization, *Mol Nutr Food Res*, 52 Suppl 2, S176–S185.
76. Awade, A. C., Moreau, S., Molle, D., Brule, G., and Maubois, J. L. (1994): Two-step chromatographic procedure for the purification of hen egg white ovomucin, lysozyme, ovotransferrin and ovalbumin and characterization of purified proteins, *J Chromatogr A*, 677, 279–288.
77. Imoto, T., Okazaki, K., Yamada, H., Fujita, K., Yamato, T., and Koga, D. (1981): Identification of residue 103 in hen egg-white lysozyme, *J Biochem*, 90, 991–995.
78. Eggesbo, M., Botten, G., Halvorsen, R., and Magnus, P. (2001): The prevalence of allergy to egg: a population-based study in young children, *Allergy*, 56, 403–411.
79. Schafer, T., Kramer, U., Dockery, D., Vieluf, D., Behrendt, H., and Ring, J. (1999): What makes a child allergic? Analysis of risk factors for allergic sensitization in preschool children from East and West Germany, *Allergy Asthma Proc*, 20, 23–7.
80. Mine, Y. and Yang, M. (2008): Recent advances in the understanding of egg allergens: basic, industrial, and clinical perspectives, *J Agric Food Chem*, 56, 4874–4900.
81. Heine, R. G., Laske, N., and Hill, D. J. (2006): The diagnosis and management of egg allergy, *Curr Allergy Asthma Rep*, 6, 145–152.
82. Teuber, S. S., Beyer, K., Comstock, S., and Wallowitz, M. (2006): The big eight foods: clinical and epidemiological overview, *Food Allergy*, 49–79.
83. Boyano-Martinez, T., Garcia-Ara, C., Diaz-Pena, J. M., and Martin-Esteban, M. (2002): Prediction of tolerance on the basis of quantification of egg white-specific IgE antibodies in children with egg allergy, *J Allergy Clin Immunol*, 110, 304–309.

84. Savage, J. H., Matsui, E. C., Skripak, J. M., and Wood, R. A. (2007): The natural history of egg allergy, *J Allergy Clin Immunol*, 120, 1413–1417.
85. Szepfalusi, Z., Ebner, C., Pandjaitan, R., Orlicek, F., Scheiner, O., Boltz-Nitulescu, G., Kraft, D., and Ebner, H. (1994): Egg yolk alpha-livetin (chicken serum albumin) is a cross-reactive allergen in the bird-egg syndrome, *J Allergy Clin Immunol*, 93, 932–942.
86. Urisu, A., Ando, H., Morita, Y., Wada, E., Yasaki, T., Yamada, K., Komada, K., Torii, S., Goto, M., and Wakamatsu, T. (1997): Allergenic activity of heated and ovomucoid-depleted egg white, *J Allergy Clin Immunol*, 100, 171–176.
87. Mine, Y. and Zhang, J. (2002): Comparative studies on antigenicity and allergenicity of native and denatured egg white proteins, *J Agric Food Chem*, 50, 2679–2683.
88. Odani, S., Awatuhara, H., and Kato, Y. (1997): Antigenic change of native and heat-denatured ovalbumin digested with pepsin, trypsin, or chymotrypsin, *Nippon Kasei Gakkaishi*, 48, 717–722.
89. Hildebrandt, S., Kratzin, H. D., Schaller, R., Fritsche, R., Steinhart, H., and Paschke, A. (2008): In vitro determination of the allergenic potential of technologically altered hen's egg, *J Agric Food Chem*, 56, 1727–1733.
90. Matsuda, T., Tsuruta, K., Nakabe, Y., and Nakamura, R. (1985): Reduction of ovomucoid immunogenic activity on peptic fragmentation and heat denaturation, *Agric Biol Chem*, 49, 2237–2241.
91. Gremmel, S. and Paschke, A. (2007): Reducing allergens in egg and egg products. In C. Mills, H. F. Wichers, and K. Hoffmann-Sommergruber, Eds., *Managing Allergens in Food*, 178–189. Woodhead Publishing, Cambridge, UK.
92. Joo, K. and Kato, Y. (2006): Assessment of allergenic activity of a heat-coagulated ovalbumin after in vivo digestion, *Biosci Biotechnol Biochem*, 70, 591–597.
93. Lopez-Exposito, I., Chicon, R., Belloque, J., Recio, I., Alonso, E., and Lopez-Fandino, R. (2008): Changes in the ovalbumin proteolysis profile by high pressure and its effect on IgG and IgE binding, *J Agric Food Chem*, 56, 11809–11816.
94. Davis, P. J., Smales, C. M., and James, D. C. (2001): How can thermal processing modify the antigenicity of proteins? *Allergy*, 56 Suppl 67, 56–60.
95. Kato, Y., Oozawa, E., and Matsuda, T. (2001): Decrease in antigenic and allergenic potentials of ovomucoid by heating in the presence of wheat flour: dependence on wheat variety and intermolecular disulfide bridges, *J Agric Food Chem*, 49, 3661–3665.
96. Kato, Y., Suginohara, K., and Fujiwara, M. (2001): A novel and simple method of insolubilization of ovomucoid in cookies prepared from batter containing egg white, *Food Sci Technol Res*, 7, 35–38.
97. Langeland, T. (1982): A clinical and immunological study of allergy to hen's egg white. II. Antigens in hen's egg white studied by crossed immunoelectrophoresis (CIE), *Allergy*, 37, 323–333.
98. Hirose, J., Kitabatake, N., Kimura, A., and Narita, H. (2004): Recognition of native and/or thermally induced denatured forms of the major food allergen, ovomucoid, by human IgE and mouse monoclonal IgG antibodies, *Biosci Biotechnol Biochem*, 68, 2490–2497.
99. Hildebrandt, S., Steinhart, H., and Paschke, A. (2008): Comparison of different extraction solutions for the analysis of allergens in hen's egg, *Food Chem*, 108, 1088–1093.
100. Croguennec, T., Nau, F., Pezennec, S., and Brule, G. (2000): Simple rapid procedure for preparation of large quantities of ovalbumin, *J Agric Food Chem*, 48, 4883–4889.
101. Ebbehoej, K., Dahl, A. M., Froekiaer, H., Noergaard, A., Poulsen, L. K., and Barkholt, V. (1995): Purification of egg-white allergens, *Allergy*, 50, 133–141.

102. Omana, D. A. and Wu, J. (2009): A new method of separating ovomucin from egg white, *J Agric Food Chem*, 57, 3596–3603.
103. Kakalis, L. T. and Regenstein, J. M. (1986): Effect of pH and salts on the solubility of egg white protein, *J Food Sci*, 51, 1445–1447, 1455.
104. Chang, H.-M., Yang, C.-C., and Chang, Y.-C. (2000): Rapid separation of lysozyme from chicken egg white by reductants and thermal treatment, *J Agric Food Chem*, 48, 161–164.
105. Hiidenhovi, J., Maekinen, J., Huopalahti, R., and Ryhaenen, E.-L. (2002): Comparison of different egg albumen fractions as sources of ovomucin, *J Agric Food Chem*, 50, 2840–2845.
106. Breton, C., Phan Thanh, L., and Paraf, A. (1988): Immunochemical identification and quantification of ovalbumin additive in canned mushrooms, *J Food Sci*, 53, 226–230.
107. Yeung, J. M., Newsome, W. H., and Abbott, M. A. (2000): Determination of egg proteins in food products by enzyme immunoassay, *J AOAC Int*, 83, 139–143.
108. Leduc, V., Demeulemester, C., Polack, B., Guizard, C., Le Guern, L., and Peltre, G. (1999): Immunochemical detection of egg-white antigens and allergens in meat products, *Allergy (Copenhagen)*, 54, 464–472.
109. Hefle, S. L., Jeanniton, E., and Taylor, S. L. (2001): Development of a sandwich enzyme-linked immunosorbent assay for the detection of egg residues in processed foods, *J Food Prot*, 64, 1812–1816.
110. Lee, P. W., Niemann, L. M., Lambrecht, D. M., Nordlee, J. A., and Taylor, S. L. (2009): Detection of mustard, egg, milk, and gluten in salad dressing using enzyme-linked immunosorbent assays (ELISAs), *J Food Sci*, 74, T46–T50.
111. Li, Y., Song, C., Zhang, K., Wang, M., Yang, K., Yang, A., and Jin, B. (2008): Establishment of a highly sensitive sandwich enzyme-linked immunosorbent assay specific for ovomucoid from hen's egg white, *J Agric Food Chem*, 56, 337–342.
112. Faeste, C. K., Loevberg, K. E., Lindvik, H., and Egaas, E. (2007): Extractability, stability, and allergenicity of egg white proteins in differently heat-processed foods, *J AOAC Int*, 90, 427–436.
113. Baumgartner, S., Steiner, I., Kloiber, S., Hirmann, D., Krska, R., and Yeung, J. (2002): Towards the development of a dipstick immunoassay for the detection of trace amounts of egg proteins in food, *Eur Food Res and Technol*, 214, 168–170.
114. Venter, C., Pereira, B., Grundy, J., Clayton, C. B., Arshad, S. H., and Dean, T. (2006): Prevalence of sensitization reported and objectively assessed food hypersensitivity amongst six-year-old children: A population-based study, *Pediatr Allergy Immunol*, 17, 356–363.
115. Zuberbier, T., Edenharter, G., Worm, M., Ehlers, I., Reimann, S., Hantke, T., Roehr, C. C., Bergmann, K. E., and Niggemann, B. (2004): Prevalence of adverse reactions to food in Germany—A population study, *Allergy*, 59, 338–345.
116. Schafer, T. and Breuer, K. (2003): Epidemiology of food allergies, *Hautarzt*, 54, 112–120.
117. Host, A. (2002): Frequency of cow's milk allergey in childhood, *Ann Allergy Asthma Immunol*, 89, 33–37.
118. Schafer, T., Bohler, E., Ruhdorfer, S., Weigl, L., Wessner, D., Heinrigh, J., Filipiak, B., Wichmann, H. E., and Ring, J. (2001): Epidemiology of food allergy/food intolerance in adults: Associations with other manifestations of atopy, *Allergy*, 56, 1172–1179.
119. Gislason, D., Bjornsson, E., Gislason, T., Jamson, C., Sjoberg, O., Elfman, L., and Boman, G. (1999): Sensitization to airborne and food allergens in Reykjavik (Iceland) and Uppsala (Sweden)—A comparative study, *Allergy*, 54, 1160–1167.

120. Hill, D. J., Hosking, C. S., Zhie, C. Y., Leung, R., Baratwidja-ja, K., Iikura, Y., Iyngkaran, N., Gonzalez-Andaya, A., Wah, L. B., and Hsieh, K. H. (1997): The frequency of food allergy in Australia and Asia, *Environ Tox Pharm*, 4, 101–110.
121. Julge, K., Vasar, M., and Bjorksten, B. (1997): The development of atopic sensitization in Estonian infants, *Acta Paediatr*, 86, 1188–1194.
122. Crespo, J. F., Pascual, C., Burks, A. W., Helm, R. M., and Esteban, M. M. (1995): Frequency of food allergy in a pediatric population from Spain, *Pediatr Allergy Immunol*, 6, 39–43.
123. Schrander, J. J., van den Bogart, J. P., Forget, P. P., Schrander-Stumpel, C. T., Kuijten, R. H., and Kester, A. D. (1993): Cow's milk protein intolerance in infants under 1 year of age: A prospective epidemiological study, *Eur J Pediatr*, 152, 640–644.
124. Karamonova, L., Fukal, L., Kodicek, M., Rauch, P., Mills, C. E. N., and Morgan, M. R. A. (2003): Immunoprobes for thermally-induced alterations in whey protein structure and their application to the analysis of thermally-treated milks, *Food Agric Immunol*, 15, 77–91.
125. Mariager, B., Soelve, M., Eriksen, H., and Brogren, C.-H. (1994): Bovine beta-lactoglobulin in hypoallergenic and ordinary infant formulas measured by an indirect competitive ELISA using monoclonal and polyclonal antibodies, *Food Agric Immunol*, 6, 73–83.
126. Malmheden, Y. I., Eriksson, A., Everitt, G., Yman, L., and Karlsson, T. (1994): Analysis of food proteins for verification of contamination or mislabeling, *Food Agric Immunol*, 6, 167–172.
127. Sampson, H. A. and Ho, D. G. (1997): Relationship between food-specific IgE concentrations and the risk of positive food challenges in children and adolescents, *J Allergy Clin Immunol*, 100, 444–451.
128. Romero-Rodriguez, M. A., Barcia-Vieitez, R., and Vazquez-Oderiz, M. L. (2002): An immunochemical technique for the detection of ovalbumin in surimi-derived products, *J Sci Food Agric*, 82, 1614–1616.
129. Turn, L. and Bonomi, F. (1994): Immunochemical detection of ovalbumin in dairy-based foods, *J Sci Food Agric*, 64, 39–45.
130. Rauch, P., Hochel, I., and Kas, J. (1990): Sandwich enzyme immunoassay of hen egg lysozyme in foods, *J Food Sci*, 55, 103–105.

CHAPTER **6**

Detection of Allergens in Cereals

Dimosthenis Kizis and George Siragakis

CONTENTS

Introduction 154
   Allergenic Food and Allergens 154
   Legislation 154
   Cereals as Allergens and with Regard to Celiac Disease 155
   Egg Allergens 156
   Milk Allergens 157
   Soy Allergens 157
   Sesame Seed Allergens 158
   Celery as Allergen 158
   RASFF Reports 158
Methods for Allergen Detection in Cereals 158
   Enzyme-Linked Immunosorbent Assay 162
   Polymerase Chain Reaction 164
Detection of Food Allergens and Potentially Allergenic Food Constituents in Cereal Food Products 164
   Detection of Cereal Allergens in Cereal Food Products 164
   Detection of Other Allergens in Cereals 168
      Egg Detection 168
      Detection of Whey Proteins and Caseins 169
      Soy Detection 170
      Sesame Protein Detection 170
References 171

INTRODUCTION

Allergenic Food and Allergens

Over 160 food materials have been identified as allergenic. Only eight of them involve more than 90% of all food allergies.[1] for the allergic consumer, it is particularly important to have full information about potential allergens contained in a food product. Practically all known food allergens that can cause an immunological reaction are proteins. Allergenic proteins are normally heat resistant, withstand food-manufacturing processes, and are unaffected by low pH and enzymes in the gastrointestinal tract. It is estimated that the causes of the majority of all food allergies are proteins in common foods such as milk; eggs; fish; crustaceans; legumes (e.g., peanuts, soybeans, peas, lupine seeds); nuts (e.g., hazelnuts, walnuts, pecans, cashews, pine nuts, pistachios, macadamia nuts, almonds, apricot kernels); seeds (e.g., sesame seeds, sunflower seeds, poppy seeds, mustard seeds); cereals (wheat, rye, barley, oats); corn; and buckwheat. However, many other foods can also cause allergies, although reactions to these are less common. Due to many serious reactions to celery, reported in particular from central and southern Europe, celery is included among the foods that must always be declared.

Legislation

Legislation in the European Union has been modified regarding food labeling to ensure derogations to the obligatory declaration of food ingredients are not applicable to those ingredients that may induce food allergies or food intolerances (Annex IIIa of Directive 2007/68/EC[2]). This pertains to cereals containing gluten, crustaceans, eggs, fish, peanuts, soybeans, milk, and dairy products including lactose, nuts, sesame seeds, celery, mustard, and sulfite at a concentration of 10 mg/kg and above. There are no established standards for any residual levels of allergens in products labeled as "free from" those allergens. However, there is a Codex Alimentarius Standard for Gluten Free Products that are produced from gluten-containing cereals, and this permits a maximum of 200 mg/kg gluten in the finished product and allows for a cereal-derived product to be labeled gluten free if it does not exceed that limit. This codex standard does not apply to products made from ingredients that naturally do not contain gluten, for which a maximum content of 20 mg/kg gluten is proposed. The figure of 20 mg/kg is not selected as a threshold limit below which consumption is proven to be safe, but in the absence of formally validated methods of analysis, it is a best practice analytical figure for the level of quantification at which reliable results should be expected in most product matrices. Directive 2007/68/EC, which has replaced Directive 2005/26/EC, Foodstuffs for particular nutritional uses that have been specially formulated, processed, or prepared to meet the dietary needs of people intolerant to gluten and marketed as such should be labeled either as "very low gluten" or "gluten free" in accordance with the provisions laid down in this regulation. These provisions can be achieved by the use of foodstuffs that have been specially processed to reduce the gluten content of one or more gluten-containing ingredients or foodstuffs in which the gluten-containing ingredients have been substituted by other ingredients naturally free of gluten. Commission Directive 2006/141/EC on infant formulas and follow-on formulas, amending Directive 1999/21/EC, prohibits the use of ingredients containing gluten in the manufacture of such foodstuffs. Therefore, the use of the terms *very low gluten* or *gluten free* on the labeling of such products should be prohibited given that, pursuant to the present regulation, this labeling is used for indicating a content of gluten not exceeding 100 mg/kg.

The most recent commission Regulation EC No 41/2009 refers specifically to the composition and labeling of foodstuffs suitable for people intolerant to gluten. This regulation shall apply from January 1, 2012; however, foodstuffs that at the date of entry into force of the present regulation already comply with the provisions of the regulation may be placed on the market in the community. The regulation sets a certain threshold for the gluten content of foodstuffs consisting of or containing one or more ingredients made from wheat, rye, barley, oats, or their crossbred varieties that have been especially processed to reduce gluten. These shall not contain a level of gluten exceeding 100 mg/kg in the food as sold to the final consumer and must be labeled using the term *very low gluten*. They may bear the term *gluten free* if the gluten content does not exceed 20 mg/kg in the food as sold to the final consumer. A further notification is made for oats contained in foodstuffs for people intolerant to gluten. The final gluten content in such oats must not exceed 20 mg/kg and must have been specially produced, prepared, or processed in a way to avoid contamination by wheat, rye, or barley. The same threshold level of 20 mg/kg gluten content also applies to ingredients that substitute wheat, rye, barley, oats, or their crossbred varieties in gluten-free labeled foodstuffs.

In general terms, it can be stated that all allergens and products thereof mentioned can cause adverse health effects, and in some cases, exposure to these can be fatal. These are the most common food allergens that are generally resistant to food processing, and they have the capacity to trigger an allergic reaction in an allergic consumer if they are added to foods. Processing can influence allergenicity of the foods, as does the food matrix in which the allergens are presented to the consumer. In addition, individuals who suffer from allergies to the same food may react to different components of that foodstuff. Some of these allergens are widely distributed throughout Europe, while others, such as mustard and celery, are more geographically restricted. Numerous other food allergens have been identified, including fruits, vegetables, and latex. Among the allergens included in Annex IIIa of Directive 2003/89/EC regarding a summary assessment of allergenic foods, the ones that are commonly tested in cereals are mainly gluten itself, soybean, sesame seed, and celery, followed by egg and milk allergens in processed cereal products. A short discussion of these factors as allergens and how they can cause allergy follows.

Cereals as Allergens and with Regard to Celiac Disease

Cereals like wheat, rye, barley, oats, and rice can provoke food allergy after ingestion or inhalation, with wheat the most common cause. According to the Structural Classification of Proteins (SCOP) database, the major allergenic proteins of cereals belong to the prolamin superfamily, which includes the major storage proteins of seed grains (except for oats and rice) and several low molecular weight cysteine-rich proteins. A further classification of these allergens situates these proteins into two groups, the α-amylase/protease inhibitors and cereal prolamins. Allergens of the first group are found in most of the cereals as monomers or polymers formed of small subunits (12–16 kDa) and are inhibitors of trypsin and α-amylase. The tetrameric CM16 inhibitor from wheat, the homologous CMb inhibitor from barley, and the α-amylase/trypsin inhibitors Sec c1, RDAI-1, and RDAI-3 are some representative allergenic proteins of this prolamin superfamily group.[3] The cereal prolamins group includes the gluten protein component of wheat flour, which consists of the polymeric glutenin-type and monomeric gliadin-type proteins, which give different physical properties to dough. Glutenins are found as low molecular mass (LMM) and high molecular mass (HMM) glutenins, and gliadins are classified into α-, β-, γ-, and ω-fractions according to their mobility in electrophoresis. Gliadins, together with rye secalins and barley hordeins, are the major endosperm storage proteins in cereals. Principal allergens of this group are the LMM glutenin and α-, γ-, and ω-5-gliadin fractions from wheat, γ-35- and γ-70 rye secalins, and γ-3 hordein from barley.[3]

Allergy to cereals in general is not frequent as few cases are reported. Cereals are considered as allergenic factors mainly with regard to celiac disease. Celiac disease (gluten intolerance) is an immunologically based disease that is not mediated by immunoglobulin (Ig) E antibodies and is caused by gluten protein. Celiac disease affects 1 in every 200 people of the European population[4] and about 1 in every 250 in the United States.[5] A local immunological response to gluten or gluten equivalents takes place in the small intestine, causing inflammation and damage to the small intestinal mucosa, which can further lead to nutritional deficiency. Even 100 mg of gliadin can cause clinical symptoms to a sensitized individual. The disease is apparently triggered mostly by specific toxic peptides of the gliadin fraction of wheat gluten.[4,6] Recovery of such an intestinal injury can take several months. The diet of an individual genetically predisposed to the disease should exclude products containing wheat, rye, barley, and oats, although it can be based on cereals with reduced levels of gluten, such as wheat starch, and naturally gluten-free products like corn, rice, millet, or buckwheat.[7] There is a continuous effort of industries to find alternative raw materials to produce gluten-free products.[8] The current Codex Alimentarius limit for gluten-free foods sets a threshold dose of 200 mg gluten/kg food for celiac patients; however, this may not be the rule for all celiac patients since insufficient data exist for the tolerance of such amounts.

Egg Allergens

Egg proteins are frequent triggers of allergic reactions. Hen's eggs is one of the most frequent causes of adverse reactions to foods in children.[9] There are possible clinical cross-reactivities between hen's eggs and eggs from other species. Heat denaturation and other food-processing treatments do not reliably reduce the allergenicity. Doses reported to trigger allergic reactions in clinical studies range from microgram to low-milligram levels of egg proteins. Threshold doses between 1 and

200 mg egg (0.13–20 mg egg protein) were determined by several oral challenge studies with egg-allergic individuals.[10]

There are several allergens that have been identified in egg, with the ovomucoid Gal d 1, ovalbumin Gal d 2, ovotransferrin Gal d 3, and lysozyme Gal d 4 representing the major allergens in egg white and chicken albumin (a-livetin) in egg yolk. Egg white was shown to be more frequently responsible for allergic reactions in egg-allergic individuals than egg yolk.[11] Egg or egg components are used in many different food products and may not be easily identified as such, especially when they are listed according to their functions (e.g., as binder, emulsifier, or coagulant). Egg may be an ingredient in noodles, or it is used to give pretzels, bagels, and other baked goods their shiny appearance. The most frequent matrix for egg contamination in packed foods is pasta. Other foods that may contain egg are creams, soups, dressings, sauces, processed meat products, breakfast cereals, or drinks. Egg-derived products such as lecithin (emulsifier), provitamin A (colorant), or lysozyme (preservative)—an allergen per se—are sources of potential allergens for egg-sensitive individuals.

Milk Allergens

Most cow's milk proteins are potential food allergens. Numerous milk allergens have been identified, and some remain active during food preparation and during digestion. The major cow's milk allergens are caseins and whey proteins β-lactoglobulin, and α-lactalbumin.[12] Data available show that a substantial proportion of allergic individuals react to low (in the range of micrograms) amounts of allergens, but the data are insufficient to establish validated threshold doses or to derive a level of exposure that could protect allergic consumers against a reaction to milk products present in their food in trace amounts. These considerations may be applied to milk of species other than cows, such as buffaloes, goats, and ewes. Apparently, cow's milk allergens are stable, and they retain their allergenicity after common industrial treatments.[13] Cow's milk allergens could be present in breast milk, infant formulas, milk and dairy products like cheese and yogurt, as well as in "nondairy" food occurring as contaminants or unlabeled additives. Milk and products thereof may be found in a large variety of processed food, including pasta, confections, margarine, pies, cookies, pudding, sausage, sauces, and soups, in which extracted milk proteins are used as emulsifiers or a foreign protein source.

Soy Allergens

Soy protein is widely used in processed foods; thus, soy is considered as a frequently occurring food allergen. Allergenic reactions may occur to small quantities of soy protein (the levels of soy consumption that may trigger an adverse reaction vary; however, they are in the low-microgram scale). Anaphylaxis has been also reported.[14] Soy may also cross-react with other allergens, including peanuts and cow's milk allergens. Major allergens from soybean include the seed storage proteins Gly m Bd, the glycinin acidic chain, and the α-subunit of β-conglycinin.[15–17] Because of the almost unlimited uses of soy (e.g., as a texturizer, emulsifier, or protein filler), it is a particularly insidious hidden allergen (e.g., in pasta, cereals, pastries, bakery products, infant food, sausages, processed meats, and hamburgers).

Sesame Seed Allergens

Sesame seeds are widely, and increasingly, used in many processed foods. A few milligrams of sesame protein are able to cause allergic symptoms, and in many cases anaphylactic reactions have been reported after inadvertent consumption of sesame.[18] White sesame seeds contain at least 10 allergenic proteins,[19] with S albumin identified as the major sesame allergen.[20] In the food industry, sesame seeds are used as whole seeds or for the production of sesame paste and oil. Sesame-containing products include salad dressings, confections, and various fast food bakery items. Sesame is also used increasingly in vegetarian food (vegetarian burgers) and gluten-free foods (e.g., bread, cakes, pastries, and biscuits) used to treat celiac disease.[8,18]

Celery as Allergen

Celery is often found in prepacked food as it is widely used in the food industry because of its aromatic flavor. Allergic reactions occur predominantly to raw celery and less frequently to cooked celery, but allergenicity of celery powder is comparable to that of raw celery. Celery-allergic patients may react to doses of allergen in the milligram range, but there are insufficient data to determine threshold levels. Cereals can be contaminated with raw celery during crop harvesting. Pasta can be contaminated with celery by the use of natural pigments obtained from spinach to give green color to the product.

RASFF Reports

It is more than obvious that clear notification and labeling for each product that may contain even minute amounts of a potential allergen for an individual is necessary. Furthermore, the necessity for the development of precise detection methods for all the allergens discussed that may be present in cereals is outlined further in the Rapid Alert System for Food and Feed (RASFF) reports. From the 24 reports for detection of allergens in cereals presented in Table 6.1 (years 2007 to 2009), the majority of the cases refer to detection of gluten (nine cases) and wheat (one case), followed by soya, milk, and egg (three cases for each allergen). There are also reports for sesame, peanut, and nuts.

METHODS FOR ALLERGEN DETECTION IN CEREALS

There are several technical approaches for the detection of allergens in cereals. The methods employed either target the allergen itself (protein or glycoprotein) or a marker (specific protein or DNA fragment) that indicates the presence of the offending food. Detection of the allergen per se is not always feasible since this

DETECTION OF ALLERGENS IN CEREALS

Table 6.1 RASFF Notifications on Food Products for the Years 2007 to 2009

	Reference	Notification Type	Control Type	Notified by	Origin	Subject	Distribution
January 18, 2007	2007.0043	Alert	Company's own check	Denmark	Sweden	Undeclared nuts in biscuits from Sweden	Denmark, Finland, Norway, Sweden
February 9, 2007	2007.0104	Alert	Official control on the market	Greece	Belgium	Undeclared soya in chocolate cookies from Belgium	Romania, Luxembourg, Greece, Germany, Slovakia, Czech Republic
April 30, 2007	2007.0303	Alert	Official control on the market	Ireland	Canada United Kingdom	Undeclared gluten (2,393 mg/kg-ppm) in gluten-free organic cereal flakes from Canada via the United Kingdom	Ireland, United Kingdom, Poland
June 22, 2007	2007.0414	Alert	Official control on the market	Ireland	United Kingdom	Undeclared gluten (401; 505 mg/kg-ppm) in gluten-free organic fruit muesli from the United Kingdom	Ireland
October 31, 2007	2007.0787	Alert	Official control on the market	United Kingdom	Japan United Kingdom Netherlands	Undeclared soya in rice crackers from the United Kingdom, raw material from Japan, via the Netherlands	United Kingdom, Ireland
March 15, 2007	2007.AQW	Information	Border rejection	Malta	Turkey	Undeclared wheat in various cakes from Turkey	
March 15, 2007	2007.AQX	Information	Border rejection	Malta	Turkey	Undeclared wheat in biscuits from Turkey	
August 13, 2007	2007.BXY	Information	Official control on the market	Austria	China Austria	Undeclared gluten (>800 mg/kg-ppm) in gluten-free buckwheat flour from Austria, raw material from China	Austria

Continued

Table 6.1 (Continued) RASFF Notifications on Food Products for the Years 2007 to 2009

	Reference	Notification Type	Control Type	Notified by	Origin	Subject	Distribution
August 23, 2007	2007.CAE	Information	Border rejection	Lithuania	Ukraine	Undeclared soya in biscuits from Ukraine	
March 18, 2008	2008.0309	Alert	Official control on the market	United Kingdom	United Kingdom	Undeclared gluten (67.6 mg/kg-ppm) in maize flour polenta from the United Kingdom	United Kingdom, Ireland
July 4, 2008	2008.0807	Alert	Official control on the market	Austria	Germany	Undeclared gluten (704, 656, 448, 402 mg/kg-ppm) in buckwheat flour from Germany	Austria
October 3, 2008	2008.1182	Alert	Official control on the market	Cyprus	United Kingdom	Undeclared gluten (64.67) in gluten-free white bread mix from the United Kingdom	Cyprus
March 9, 2009	2009.0289	Alert	Official control on the market	Austria	Austria China	Undeclared gluten (3,600 mg/kg; label only mentions possible traces of gluten) in organic buckwheat flour from Austria, with raw material from China	Austria, Hungary, South Africa
April 1, 2009	2009.0405	Alert	Company's own check	Sweden	Sweden	Undeclared milk ingredient (casein: 66, 68, 89 mg/kg-ppm) in gluten-free muffin mix from Sweden	Austria, Sweden, Germany, Finland, Netherlands, Norway
April 8, 2009	2009.0442	Alert	Official control on the market	Czech Republic	Poland	Undeclared peanut (3,603 mg/kg-ppm) in cocoa-filled rolls from Poland	Czech Republic
April 14, 2009	2009.0468	Alert	Food poisoning	Hungary	Ireland	Undeclared gluten (53.9, 76.5 mg/kg-ppm) in organic gluten-free bread mix from Ireland	Hungary

DETECTION OF ALLERGENS IN CEREALS

April 24, 2009	2009.0521	Alert	Company's own check	United Kingdom	Undeclared egg in chocolate cake from the United Kingdom	Ireland
April 24, 2009	2009.0524	Alert	Consumer complaint	United Kingdom	Undeclared nuts (>200 mg/kg-ppm) in organic puffed rice from the United Kingdom	United Kingdom, Ireland
May 4, 2009	2009.0572	Alert	Official control on the market	Cyprus	Undeclared gluten (90 mg/kg-ppm) in corn flour from Greece	Cyprus
May 19, 2009	2009.0631	Alert	Official control on the market	Denmark	Undeclared sesame in bakery product from Denmark	Denmark, Sweden
June 9, 2009	2009.0738	Alert	Official control on the market	Slovakia	Undeclared egg (11.50 mg/kg-ppm) in cocoa and hazelnut cream-filled biscuits from Turkey	Hungary, Slovakia
June 26, 2009	2009.0821	Alert	Official control on the market	Slovakia	Undeclared milk ingredient (19.10 mg/kg-ppm) in crackers with ham from Romania	Slovakia
July 9, 2009	2009.0892	Alert	Official control on the market	Slovakia	Undeclared egg (29.50 mg/kg-ppm) in wheat pasta from Italy	Slovakia, Ethiopia, Jordan, China, South Africa, Russian Federation, Kosovo, Autonomous Region of
October 7, 2009	2009.1303	Information	Company's own check	United Kingdom	Undeclared milk ingredient and soya in berry oat biscuits from the United Kingdom	Gibraltar, United Kingdom

Source: The Rapid Alert System for Food and Feed. Portal database. (http://ec.europa.eu/food/food/rapidalert)

may often be present in trace amounts, may vary in abundance between cultivars, or may be masked by the food matrix. Moreover, the sensitivity of the method utilized may influence detection. As agreed, detection limits for different food products are between 1 and 100 mg allergenic protein/kg food, depending on the respective food.[21] Protein-based methods involve immunochemical detection protocols such as the enzyme-linked immunosorbent assay (ELISA), one-dimensional sodium dodecyl sulfate polyacrylamide gel electrophoresis (SDS-PAGE) followed by immunoblotting, and less frequently two-dimensional (2D) gel electrophoresis and rocket immunoelectrophoresis (RIE). The matrix-assisted laser desorption/ionization time of flight (MALDI-TOF) mass spectrometry (MS) and biosensors are two other methods utilized to study cereal allergens at the protein level. Methods operating on the DNA level are based on the polymerase chain reaction (PCR and real-time PCR). Approaches that combine methods, like PCR-ELISA or use of biosensors in combination with ELISA, give accurate quantitative results as well.[22,23] The choice of method is mainly dependent on the food concerned (availability of specific antibodies/DNA primers and the achievable detection limit) and on the history of processing involved during food production. Protein- and DNA-based methods, respectively, have their characteristic merits and drawbacks concerning their applicability in the detection and quantification of allergens in various food products.[21] The predominant methods most frequently used for allergen detection in cereals are ELISA and PCR; thus, a short description of the basic principles of these methods and their application in allergen detection is given. However, more profound and extensive information, including technical aspects for all the methods discussed for allergen detection in cereals, can be found in other bibliographic sources.

Enzyme-Linked Immunosorbent Assay

The ELISA technique is the most frequent method used in food analysis to detect and quantify allergens due to its high precision, simple handling, and good potential for standardization. The allergenic factor itself or a specific marker protein can be detected by specific enzyme-labeled antibodies. A colorimetric reaction following the formation of this antigen/antibody-enzyme complex can lead to quantitation of the allergenic factor using a standard curve generated with purified reference standards. There are two common ELISA approaches followed: sandwich ELISA and competitive ELISA. Sandwich ELISA is the most common immunoassay used and has been developed for the detection of several food allergens. Competitive ELISA is preferred for the detection of relatively small proteins, and several methods have been described for some food allergens. Various test kits for both ELISA formats are commercially available and are also used for the detection of allergens in cereals (Table 6.2). The main differences between kits for the same food are the target (allergen per se or marker protein), the detection limit, the time of analysis required, and the costs. In general, kits are (semi)quantitative and achieve a detection limit between 1 and 10 mg/kg with an average analysis time requirement of 2–3 h. Among the various kits (around 150) for allergen detection that are available in the market, 90% have been developed since 2003. However,

DETECTION OF ALLERGENS IN CEREALS

Table 6.2 Indicative Commercially Available ELISA Test Kits for Allergen Detection in Cereals and Other Food Products

Allergenic Food	Target	Format	LOD (mg/kg)	Supplier
Wheat, rye, barley	Gliadin and glutenin	Quant. S-ELISA	1	Tepnel
	Gliadin and glutenin	Quant. S-ELISA	1	Neogen
	Gliadin	Qualit ELISA	10	Neogen
	Gliadin	Quant. S-ELISA	1.5	R-Biopharm
	Gliadin	Quant. ELISA	2.5	Elisa Systems
	Gliadin	Qual. LFA	2.5	R-Biopharm
	Gluten	Qual. LFA	10	Elisa Technologies
Egg	Ovomucoid and ovalbumin	Quant. S-ELISA	1	Elisa Systems
	Egg protein	Quant. S-ELISA	0.3	Pro-Lab Diagnostic
	Egg white protein	Quant. S-ELISA	2	R-Biopharm
	Egg protein	Quant. S-ELISA	2.5	Neogen
	Ovomucoid	Quant. S-ELISA	<0.1	Tepnel
Milk	β-Lactoglobulin and casein	Quant. S-ELISA	1	Elisa Systems
	Casein	Quant. C-ELISA	1	Tepnel
	β-Lactoglobulin	Quant. C-ELISA	2.5	Tepnel
	β-Lactoglobulin	Quant. C-ELISA	5	R-Biopharm
	β-Lactoglobulin	Quant. S-ELISA	2.5	Neogen
Sesame	2S albumin	Quant. S-ELISA	1	Elisa Systems
	Sesame protein	Quant. S-ELISA	<1	Tepnel
Soy	Soy trypsin inhibitor	Quant. S-ELISA	1	Elisa Systems
	Soy protein	Quant. S-ELISA	0.3	Tepnel

Note: C-ELISA = competitive ELISA; LFA = lateral flow assay; LOD = Limit of detection according to the manufacturer; qual. = qualitative; quant. = quantitative; S-ELISA = sandwich ELISA. Manufacturer Web sites are as follows: Elisa Systems, http://www.elisasystems.net; Neogen, http://www.neogen.com; Pro-Lab Diagnostics, http://www.pro-lab.com; r-Biopharm, http://www.r-biopharm.com; Tepnel, http://www.tepnel.com.

only four have AOAC approval (Table 6.3). Due to differences (origin of production, polyclonal/monoclonal, epitope recognition) between the antibodies used in each commercial kit for the detection of a specific allergen, as well as the type of ELISA utilized in each method, there are problems that occur in the precise quantification of the allergen. This is clearly shown in various interlaboratory cooperations (FAPAS, DLA, etc.) in which accredited laboratories participate for the verification of the reliability of their test results. In a proficiency test for hazelnut protein in 2007 with 39 participants in 18 countries, three different commercial kits (Elisa Systems, R-Biopharm, Neogen) gave extremely different assigned values (1.15, 31.6, and 21.8, respectively).

The present trend shows that lateral flow devices (LFDs) and dipstick tests for rapid screening will gain importance. LFD and dipstick tests are inexpensive, rapid, and portable; do not require instrumentation; and are extremely simple to perform. Currently, dipstick tests are only qualitative. Several products in the form of dipsticks or comparable formats for qualitative or semiquantitative detection of gliadin and gluten, casein, egg, soya, sesame, and mustard are already available from various distributors; these products have limits of detection between 1 and 25 mg of allergen per kilogram of food.[24] These tests offer a simple, rapid, and inexpensive solution for screening and on-site testing for HACCP (Hazard Analysis of Critical

Table 6.3 AOAC-Approved Allergen Detection Kits

Test Kit	Manufacturer	Analytes	Matrices
BioKits Peanut Assay Kit	Gen-Probe/Tepnel.	Peanuts	Breakfast cereal, cookies/biscuits, ice cream, milk chocolate, plain chocolate, milled nuts
Veratox® for Peanut Allergen	Neogen	Peanuts	Breakfast cereal, cookies, ice cream, milk chocolate
Ridascreen® Fast Peanut	R-Biopharm	Peanuts	Breakfast cereal, cookies, ice cream, milk chocolate
Ridascreen® Gliadin	R-Biopharm	Gliadin	Wheat, buckwheat, rice, corn, oats, syrup, sausage

Control Points) monitoring. Lateral flow tests are also used to detect environmental contamination during gluten detection.

Polymerase Chain Reaction

The PCR is an alternative method to ELISA that is routinely used for the identification and quantification (real-time PCR) of genetically modified organisms, pathogens, and food-related plant and animal species. There are also an increasing number of reports from laboratories that have started using this approach for the detection of allergens in food products. In principle, a specifically targeted DNA fragment is amplified by a thermostable polymerase in a series of repeated cycle steps. The product of the reaction (amplicon), if present, visualized by gel electrophoresis or subsequent Southern blotting and hybridization, will indicate the presence of the allergen under investigation. Ordinary PCR results are qualitative; however, incorporation of internal standards may facilitate semiquantitative measurement. Quantification of a specific allergen in a matrix may be obtained by the use of real-time PCR or the combination PCR-ELISA. For a developed analytical PCR assay, the DNA extraction and purification method utilized is crucial to obtain the maximal assay sensitivity. A sensitivity of 10 mg/kg or less has been suggested for detection of allergens in food.[10] Several PCR assays for the detection of many allergens, including wheat, soy, egg, milk, celery, and sesame in different food matrices have been published,[25–29] and many described either detection or quantification of cereal allergens in cereal-containing food or gluten-free food products.

DETECTION OF FOOD ALLERGENS AND POTENTIALLY ALLERGENIC FOOD CONSTITUENTS IN CEREAL FOOD PRODUCTS

Detection of Cereal Allergens in Cereal Food Products

Immunochemical-based methods such as ELISA and Western immunoblotting are used for detection of cereal allergens. Several challenges in the detection of gluten (secalins and hordeins as well) have to be faced, like the heterogeneity of the analyte (gliadin, peptides); cultivar-dependent variations in the composition of subgroups and subtypes of gliadins, secalins, and hordeins; lack of solubility of these proteins in buffers compatible with immunoassay formats; or effects of processing on the molecular structure and biological activity of the analyte.

The most frequent method for the analysis of gluten in food products for the determination of gluten in the milligram/kilogram range is based on ELISA. The antibodies used in such assays are mainly raised against various subgroups of gliadins (α-, γ-, ω-12, and ω-5 gliadin), which contain defined amino acid sequence motifs with apparent contribution to celiac toxicity.[4] One of the first immunoassays to receive AOAC approval for determination of food analytes was developed for determination of gluten in foods using a monoclonal antibody that recognized ω-gliadin with a detection limit of 10 mg/kg of gluten in foods. It was also the first method designed to assess the gluten content of heat-processed food.[30,31] Various protocols have been published[32] describing assays for detection of trace quantities of gluten in various food products as well as specifically detecting the toxic motifs of gliadins[33] or how to overcome the problem of cultivar-dependent variation of obtained analytical results.[34,35] Specific immunoassays to detect wheat, and not the related cereals rye and barley, were difficult to develop due to extensive sequence homology between seed storage prolamins from these species. Antibodies raised against certain discrete amino acid sequences failed to distinguish prolamins from wheat, rye, and barley due to degeneracy of these sequences.[36,37] Celiac-toxic cereals in gluten-free foods rye and barley have been found to be toxic as well; thus, detection of gliadin is not a matter of distinguishing the source. Furthermore experiments using antibodies raised against specific motifs that occur in α- and γ-gliadins and ω-secalin showed that careful selection of the antibody used in ELISAs on the basis of fine specificity to gliadin is useful for sensitive detection of gliadin in foods.[38] Another study was designed to develop a highly sensitive and specific assay to quantify low levels of wheat, barley, and rye prolamins in foods for those with celiac disease. The toxic epitope QQPFP occurs repeatedly in α-, γ-, and ω-gliadins, hordeins, and secalins. A sandwich ELISA that used a single monoclonal antibody (R5) raised against a secalin extract was able to identify gliadins, hordeins, and secalins with assay sensitivities of 0.78, 0.39, and 0.39 ng/ml, respectively, and a gluten detection limit of 3.2 mg/kg.[39] The method, together with another ELISA assay, was further tested for validation during an interlaboratory study and proved to be comparable and robust.[40]

The available commercial test kits utilize sandwich ELISA with antibodies targeting mainly the gliadin fraction, with detection sensitivity in the range of 1 to 1.5 mg/kg (Table 6.2). A kit available from both Tepnel and Neogen distributors utilizes monoclonal antibodies to ω-gliadin protein in a noncompetitive, sandwich-type ELISA. The standards provided are ready to use for accurate quantification in milligrams/kilogram. Food samples, like raw materials, processed food, cooked or uncooked food, are first extracted with a specially formulated buffer, diluted, and then tested in the assay. Wheat gliadin as well as similar proteins from durum wheat (40–60%), triticale, rye (110–130%), and barley (4–8%) can be detected. However, proteins from oats, maize, rice, and millet species are not detected.

Another commercial kit of equally high sensitivity is also supplied by Neogen. Antibodies bind gliadin (prolamins of wheat, barley, and rye) in a sandwich-type ELISA. Gliadin is extracted from samples with a 40% ethanol solution by shaking in a shaker or rotator. A subsequent dilution of the extract in phosphate saline buffer is made, and the diluted samples are added to antibody-coated wells (capture antibody) in which gliadin binds to the antibody during the incubation period. A high number of washes removes any unbound gliadin, and a second antibody, which is enzyme labeled (detector antibody), is added. The detector antibody binds to the gliadin during the second incubation period. Unbound enzyme-labeled antibody is washed away, and a one-step substrate is added. Color develops as a result of the presence of bound-labeled antibody, and a stopping reagent is added after a certain period. The color of the solution is observed, and quantification of gliadin content is made. The optical densities of the controls form a standard curve, and the sample optical densities are plotted against the curve to calculate the exact concentration of gliadin in parts per million. The manufacturers suggest that special precautions should be taken when testing for gluten. Due to the fact that this is a sensitive test, it can detect wheat that may be present in the atmosphere of the lab where testing is done (even from a lunchtime sandwich or biscuits) and will give a positive result. A recommendation for testing in a different lab where there is no chance of cross contamination (or to the extreme, in a laminar flow cabinet) and an extended 12-step washing of the wells (as opposed to the 6 times stated in the kit protocol) are suggested.

Three other types of test kits for gliadin detection are provided by R-Biopharm. Two of these test kits utilize a sandwich enzyme immunoassay for the quantitative analysis of prolamins (detection limit at 1.5 mg/kg gliadin, corresponding to 3 mg/kg gluten) from wheat (gliadin), rye (secalin), and barley (hordein) in either raw or processed foods. Furthermore, the test can be used for the detection of contaminations by prolamins from wheat (gliadin), rye (secalin), and barley (hordein) in unwrought goods such as flours (buckwheat, rice, corn, oats) and in processed foods like noodles and bakery products. In both test kits, monoclonal antibodies are used and bind the gliadin fractions from wheat and corresponding prolamins from rye and barley. The antibodies exhibit no cross-reaction with oats, corn, rice, millet, teff, buckwheat, quinoa, or amaranth. The third product uses a competitive ELISA for the quantitative analysis of peptide fragments of prolamins from wheat (gliadins), rye (secalin), and barley (hordein) in beer, starch, and starch syrup. The monoclonal antibody recognizes, among others, the toxic sequence QQPFP, which is expressed repeatedly in the prolamin molecules. The limit of detection is 922 μg peptide/g of food, and the limit of quantification is at 1,250 μg peptide/g food. There are also four LFD/dipstick assays (provided by R-Biopharm, Tepnel, ELISA Technologies, and Hallmark) for the detection of gluten traces in food. These tests provide rapid results (detection times between 5 and 15 min) with limits of detection down to 5 mg of gluten per kilogram of food tested.

Qualitative and quantitative characterization of cereal allergen proteins has been also obtained in the concept of a nutritional quality improvement project for cultivated rice by combination of 2D-PAGE followed by immunodetection. The glutelin α-polypeptides of the genus *Oryza* were qualitatively and quantitatively characterized by 2D-PAGE (composed of nonequilibrium pH gradient gel electrophoresis and higher-temperature SDS-PAGE) and sequential immunodetection using glutenin subunit-specific antibodies.[41] The development of biosensors, which exploit the antibodies raised against gliadin epitopes, provides another alternative approach with good performance for gluten detection. There are a number of references,[42–45] that reported the development of electrochemical immunosensors and advanced fluorescence biosensors capable of executing various assays in parallel with high sensitivity for gluten detection and excellent correlation with routine ELISA tests.

Non-immuno-based methods have also been developed and extensively used to characterize gluten proteins. MALDI-TOF-MS was the first epitope-independent procedure utilized to study and quantify gliadins in both processed and unprocessed gluten-containing food samples. The procedure was able to quantify gluten in these samples below the toxic levels for patients with celiac disease. Quantification showed a linear response in the range of 0.4–10 mg per 100 g and a high detection sensitivity similar to that of ELISA.[46] A number of similar studies have been made to study the gluten avenin proteins in gluten-free food samples[47] or the glutenin subunits in specific cereal cultivars or gluten-free products.[48–51] The main aspects of current and prospective applications of MS and proteomic technologies to the structural characterization of gliadins were reported by Ferranti et al.[52]

Electrophoresis has also been used separately or in combination with other methods to study cereal allergens. An improved capillary zone electrophoresis (CZE) method was used to separate and characterize high molecular weight (HMW) glutenin subunits in hexaploid triticale. The CZE method proved to be an efficient alternative to the SDS-PAGE procedure for early selection of useful genotypes with good bread-making quality.[53] A proteomic approach was also applied to study the glutenin components from *Triticum durum* flour. Proteins were first analyzed by 2D gel electrophoresis, and their identity was confirmed by nano-liquid chromatography tandem mass spectrometry analysis of tryptic peptides. The results of this approach were also supported by data resulting from measurements by MALDI-TOF analysis, which allowed detection of large tryptic peptides.[54]

PCR is another approach used extensively for gluten detection and quantification due to its sensitivity, accuracy, ease of use, and rapid application. One of the first PCR methods developed was an assay to determine wheat in gluten-free products. The assay proved sensitive for wheat (1 pg wheat DNA), and various food products were analyzed with this PCR method, although rye produced a weak signal.[1] This method was well adapted for detection of wheat in oat products with the introduction of a modified DNA extraction procedure.[55] Thereafter, various PCR assays for the detection of wheat were published.[29] A quantitative competitive PCR system to detect wheat, barley, or rye in gluten-free food and a real-time PCR for identification of wheat, rye, barley, and oats were described.[27,28] The development of independent real-time PCR assays for identification and quantification of four plant species (barley, rice, sunflower, and wheat) were also described. These assays specifically detect γ-hordein, gos9, helianthinin, and acetyl-coenzyme A (CoA) carboxylase sequences, respectively, and are able to quantify the target DNA with limits down to 10 genome copies for barley, sunflower, or wheat and approximately 100 haploid genomes for rice in real-time PCR systems.[56]

A combination of ELISA and PCR methods has been reported. In this immuno-PCR (iPCR) assay, immunological detection of gliadin by monoclonal antibody R5 conjugated with an oligonucleotide is amplified by PCR. Furthermore, if quantification is required, the iPCR is performed as real-time PCR (real-time iPCR) in one step, with the sensitivity of gliadin analysis increased more than 30-fold above the level reached by a conventional enzyme immunoassay alone.[57] PCR has been also used in breeding programs for the detection and negative selection of wheat cultivars with poor bread-making quality, demonstrating that it can be an efficient alternative to standard procedures of separation for early selection of useful wheat genotypes with good bread-making quality. In such a PCR assay, polymorphisms between the coding sequences of HMW glutenin x-type genes at the Glu-1 locus are used to amplify Glu-1B x-type-specific fragments to distinguish genotypes.[58] This approach has also been combined with capillary electrophoresis (CE) and laser-induced fluorescence (LIF) detection, resulting in fast and accurate identification of Glu-1 gene molecular markers.[59]

Detection of Other Allergens in Cereals

Egg Detection

Several ELISA test kits for the detection of egg in food products have become available. The quantitative tests are based on sandwich ELISAs involving polyclonal antibodies recognizing total egg protein, egg white protein, or a specific allergen (ovalbumin or ovomucoid), with detection limits ranging between less than 1 and 5 mg/kg for the respective test kit. A highly sensitive ELISA test involving polyclonal antibodies specific to whole egg proteins was described by Yeung et al.[60] The ELISA was applied to ice creams, noodles, pasta, and breads and showed a detection limit of 0.2 mg/kg. Another sensitive sandwich ELISA employing a capture antibody against egg white and a detection antibody specific for ovalbumin was described by Hefle et al.[61] The detection limit of this assay was 1 mg/kg when tested on various pasta products. Most recently, the development of a dipstick immunoassay for the detection of trace amounts of egg proteins in food was published by Baumgartner et al.[62] The assay involved polyclonal antibodies against egg white protein. The dipstick assay rendered qualitative results with a detection limit of 0.02 mg/kg.

Tepnel and Neogen provide a highly sensitive and specific test for the estimation of low levels of egg white protein powder or whole egg content in raw and cooked foodstuffs (including baked and pasteurized products). Egg white contains approximately 10% protein, of which nearly 80% is allergenic, with the main allergens being ovalbumin, ovotransferrin, ovomucoid, and lysozyme. Polyclonal antibodies against ovomucoid protein are used in a sandwich-type ELISA. The protein from the sample extracts binds in the first place to the antibody, which is coated on the wells, and biotinylated polyclonal antibodies to ovomucoid are subsequently utilized to bind to the captured protein to complete the reaction. The presence of the biotinylated antiovomucoid is then enhanced using avidin peroxidase (horseradish peroxidase, HRP), and the bound peroxidase enzyme activity is determined by reaction with tetramethylbenzidine (TMB) substrate.

Another sandwich ELISA test for egg allergen is provided by Neogen and is used for the quantitative analysis (provides exact concentrations in milligrams/kilogram) of egg residue in food products such as pasta, as well as other food types like salad dressing, cake mix, and ice cream. Primarily any egg residue is extracted from the sample in a phosphate-buffered saline (PBS) solution by shaking in a heated water bath. Following either centrifugation or filtration, the extracted egg residue is sampled and subsequently used in an ordinary sandwich ELISA procedure. Finally, control optical densities form a standard curve, and sample optical densities are plotted against the curve to calculate the exact concentration of egg residue in parts per million.

Elisa Systems provides an assay that detects the presence of egg white material in various food products, including cereals. The assay is rapid and reliable and provides quantitative results in the parts-per-million scale. A sandwich enzyme immunoassay for the quantitative analysis of egg in food products like noodles or baking mixtures for cakes or bread is provided by R-Biopharm. The test utilizes polyclonal antibodies against egg white proteins and is calibrated against the National Institute for Standards and Technology (NIST) RM8445 standard (whole egg powder) for ELISA and shows a limit of detection of less than 0.3 mg/kg of whole egg powder NIST RM 8445 (corresponds to 0.044 mg/kg egg white protein)

Detection of Whey Proteins and Caseins

There are numerous reports of antibodies, both polyclonal and monoclonal, being raised to both whey proteins and caseins and applied to the study of the fate of milk proteins during processing.[63,64] Immunoassays have also been developed to monitor the levels of β-lactoglobulin in modified infant formulas with reduced allergenicity. One of these[65] utilized a rabbit polyclonal antiserum to develop a two-site ELISA, employing the antiserum as detector and capture antibodies in the assay. The assay sensitivity was 0.002 ng/ml and was specific for β-lactoglobulin. Immunochemical detection methods for major milk allergens have been described but may not be appropriate for processed foods.

An indirect competitive immunoassay using polyclonal antibodies to casein is provided by Neogen and Tepnel for use for the detection of bovine casein and caseinates at low concentrations (milligrams/kilogram) in raw materials or processed foods (e.g., baby food) and uncooked and cooked foods. Food samples are extracted in a carbonate/bicarbonate extraction solution before testing in the assay. The presence of casein is an indicator of the presence of milk, milk proteins, or milk derivatives.

On the other hand, a sandwich enzyme immunoassay for the quantitative analysis of casein in various food types, including bakery goods, is provided by R-Biopharm. Monoclonal antibodies specifically detect α-, β-, and κ-caseins of cow's milk and show no cross-reactivity to either β-lactoglobulin or caseins of other animal species (sheep, goat). The assay exhibits a low limit of detection of 0.12 mg/kg casein as well as a low limit of quantification of around 0.5 mg/kg casein.

Elisa Systems offers a β-lactoglobulin residue and a casein protein ELISA test suitable for screening food products for the presence of this potential allergen caused by cross contamination with dairy products and raw materials at a level of detection below 2.5 mg/kg.

Soy Detection

Some of the first immunoassays applied to the analysis of foods were developed for the detection of soybean protein in food as an adulterant, with soybean at levels in excess of 1%. Immunoassays for detection of soybean in foods have been based on polyclonal antibodies developed to soya protein fractions rather than individually defined protein species. One of the difficulties encountered in early attempts to quantify soybean was the effect processes such as cooking had on both the extraction of soybean from cooked foods and its subsequent detection in an immunoassay. One successful strategy has been presented[66,67] and subsequently been developed as a commercial kit by Tepnel Biosystems. Other immunoassays have been reported[68,69] that showed enhanced specificity or no cross-reactivity against extracts of many common legume and other food ingredients. ELISAs were constructed with antibodies raised against the native molecule and a denatured polypeptide of glycinin and showed increased immunoreactivity and detection limit. ELISA methods were also developed using antibodies against the whole soy protein fraction and against Kunitz-type soybean trypsin inhibitor and were reported to recognize heat-treated and native soy fractions equally well. Immunoassays for detection of soybean in foods are available in kit form as quantitative ELISAs and qualitative dipstick rapid assays, primarily available from Neogen, Tepnel Biosystems, and R-Biopharm companies. The assays utilize antibodies to soy protein in a noncompetitive, sandwich-type ELISA for accurate quantification in milligrams/kilogram. Usually, food samples are extracted using a Tris/high-salt/gelatin buffer, subsequently diluted, and then tested in the assay.

Sesame Protein Detection

An immunoassay for sesame proteins was developed by Brett et al.,[70] but there were no validation data available. Currently, there are only a few sandwich ELISA test kits commercially available for the detection of sesame in food products (Table 6.2). The assays either target total soluble sesame protein or a 2S albumin; they have sensitivities of less than 0.1 and less than 1 mg/kg, respectively.

The first commercial test of its kind, provided by Tepnel, is a high-sensitivity (limit of detection < 1 mg/kg), noncompetitive, sandwich-type ELISA based on specific antibodies to sesame storage proteins. The test is intended to be used for the detection of sesame content in a wide range of raw and cooked foodstuffs. Sesame proteins from sample extracts bind to the antibody-coated wells. Biotinylated antisesame protein antibodies bind to the captured sesame sample proteins, and concentration is then determined using avidin peroxidase (HRP) reagent and TMB substrate.

As far as PCR approaches for allergen detection are concerned, Tepnel has available commercial kits for milk, soy, and peanut detection that are provided in an easy-to-use module. After sample extraction, the primer set of choice is used in a premade PCR master mix together with the DNA extract in an ordinary PCR reaction. Agarose gel electrophoresis of the amplicons then allows qualitative detection of the allergen. Two real-time PCR kits are also provided by R-Biopharm, for soy and celery qualitative detection limited to less than five copies of DNA.

REFERENCES

1. Hefle S. L., Nordlee J. A., and Taylor S. L. (1996). Allergenic foods. *Critical Reviews in Food Science and Nutrition*, 36 (Suppl.), 69–89.
2. European Commission (2007). Commission Directive 2007/68/EC of 27 November 2007 amending Annex IIIa to Directive 2000/13/EC of the European Parliament and of the Council as regards certain food ingredients. Official Journal of the European Union. L310:11.
3. Breiteneder H. (2006). Classifying food allergens. In *Detecting allergens in food*, edited by Koppelman S. J. and Hefle S. L, Taylor & Francis, Boca Raton, FL.
4. Stern M., Ciclitira P. J., van Eckert R., Feighery C., Janssen W., Mendez E., Mothes Th., Troncone R., and Wieser H. (2001). Analysis and clinical effects of gluten in coeliac disease. *European Journal of Gastroenterology and Hepatology*, 13, 741–747.
5. Neuhausen S. L., Feolo M., Camp N. J., Farnham J., Book L., and Zone J. J. (2002). Genome-wide linkage analysis for celiac disease in North American families. *American Journal of Medical Genetics*, 111, 1–9.
6. Devery J. M., Bender V., Penttila I., and Skerritt J. H. (1991). Identification of reactive synthetic gliadin peptides specific for coeliac disease. *International Archives of Allergy and Applied Immunology*, 95, 356–362.
7. Papageorgiou M., Kiskini A., Christou C., Siragakis G., and Mandala I. (2007). The case of carob (*Ceratonia siliqua*) use for developing gluten-free products—Its influence on gluten-free dough characteristics. First International Symposium on Gluten-Free Cereal Products and Beverages, September 12–14, Cork, Ireland, *Symposium Abstracts,* p. 95.
8. Papageorgiou M., Kiskini A., Giannopoulos S., Siragakis G., and Mandala I. (2008). Alternative ingredients for gluten-free products development. The case of carob (*Ceratonia siliqua*) and its effect on gluten-free dough rheologys. In *Trends in cereal science and technology: Industrial applications*, February 4–5, Thessalonki Workshop Proceedings, p. 114.
9. Resano A., Crespo E., Fernandez Benitez M., Sanz M. L., and Oehling A. (1998). Atopic dermatitis and food allergy. *Journal of Investigational Allergology and Clinical Immunology*, 8, 271–276.
10. Taylor S. and Nordlee J. (1996). Detection of food allergens. *Food Technology,* 50, 231–234.
11. Anet J., Back J. F., Baker R. S., Barnett D., Burley R. W., and Howden M. E. H. (1985). Allergens in the white and yolk of hen's egg. A study of IgE binding by egg proteins. *International Archives of Allergy Immunology*, 77, 364–371.

12. Docena G. H., Fernandez R., Chirdo F. G., and Fossati C. A. (1996). Identification of casein as the major allergenic and antigenic protein of cow's milk. *Allergy*, 51, 412–416.
13. Jedrychowski L. (1999). Reduction of the antigenicity of whey proteins by lactic acid fermentation. *Food and Agricultural Immunology*, 11, 91–99.
14. Sampson H. A., Mendelson L., and Rosen J. P. (1992). Fatal and near-fatal anaphylactic reactions to food in children and adolescents. *New England Journal of Medicine*, 327, 380–384.
15. Ogawa T., Tsuji H., Bando N., Kitamura K., Zhu Y. L., Hirano H., and Nishikawa K. (1993). Identification of the soybean allergenic protein Gly m Bd 30K, with soybean seed 34-kDa oil-body-associated protein. *Bioscience, Biotechnology and Biochemistry*, 57, 1030–1033.
16. Ogawa T., Bando N., Tsuji H., Nishikawa K., and Kitamura K. (1995). α-Subunit of β-conglycinin, an allergenic protein recognized by IgE antibodies of soybean-sensitive patients with atopic dermatitis. *Bioscience, Biotechnology and Biochemistry*, 59, 831–833.
17. Zeece M. G., Beardslee T. A., Markwell J. P., and Sarath G. (1999). Identification of an IgE-binding region in soybean acidic glycinin G1. *Food and Agricultural Immunology*, 11, 83–90.
18. Pajno G. B., Passalacqua G., Magazzu G., Barberio G., Vita D., and Canonica G. W. (2000). Anaphylaxis to sesame. *Allergy*, 55, 199–201.
19. Beyer K., Bardina L., Grishina G., and Sampson H. A. (2002). Identification of sesame seed allergens by 2-dimensional proteomics and Edman sequencing: seed storage proteins as common food allergens. *Journal of Allergy and Clinical Immunology*, 110, 154–159.
20. Wolff N., Cogan U., Admon A., Dalal I., Katz Y., Hodos N., Karin N., and Yannai S. (2003). Allergy to sesame in humans is associated primarily with IgE antibody to a 14 kDa 2S albumin precursor. *Food and Chemical Toxicology*, 41, 1165–1174.
21. Koch P., Schäppi G. F., Poms R. E., Wüthrich B., Anklam E., and Battaglia R. (2003). Comparison of commercially available ELISA kits with human sera-based detection methods for peanut allergens in foods. *Food Additives & Contaminants*, 20, 797–803.
22. Bremer M., Siragakis G., Haasnoot V., and Smiths N. (2004). Biosensor immunoassay for the detection of hazelnut allergen in olive oil. In *Proccedings Abstract of the 9th International Symposium on Immunological, Chemical and Clinical Problems of Food Allergy*. Budapest, Hungary., p. 39.
23. Yman I. M., Eriksson A., Johansson M. A., and Hellenäs K. E. (2006). Food allergen detection with biosensor immunoassays. *Journal of the AOAC International*, 89, 856–861.
24. Schubert-Ullrich P., Rudolf J., Ansari P., Galler B., Führer M., Molinelli A., and Baumgartner S. (2009). Commercialized rapid immunoanalytical tests for determination of allergenic food proteins: an overview. *Analytical and Bioanalytical Chemistry*, 395, 69–81.
25. Allmann M., Candrian U., Höfelein C., and Luthy J. (1993). Polymerase chain reaction (PCR): a possible alternative to immunochemical methods assuring safety and quality of food. *Zeitschrift für Lebensmittel-Untersuchung und -Forschung*, 196, 248–251.
26. Jankiewicz A., Hübner P., Bögl K. W., Dehne L. I., Vieths S., Baltes W., and Lüthy J. (1997). Celery allergy: PCR as a tool for the detection of trace amounts of celery in processed foods. In *Proceedings of Euro Food Chem IX*, Interlaken, Switzerland, September 24–26.

27. Dahinden I., von Büren M., and Lüthy J. (2001). A quantitative competitive PCR system to detect contamination of wheat, barley or rye in gluten-free food for coeliac patients. *European Food Research and Technology*, 212, 228–233.
28. Sandberg M., Lundberg L., Ferm M., and Malmeheden Yman I. (2003). Real time PCR for the detection and discrimination of cereal contamination in gluten free foods. *European Food Research and Technology*, 217, 344–349.
29. Poms R. E., Klein C. L., and Anklam E. (2004). Methods for allergen analysis in food: a review. *Food Additives and Contaminants*, 21, 1–31.
30. Skerritt J. H., and Hill A. S. (1991). Enzyme immunoassay for determination of gluten in foods: collaborative study. *Journal of the Association of Official Analytical Chemists*, 74, 257–264.
31. Skerritt J. H. and Hill A. S. (1991). Self-management of dietary compliance in coeliac disease: rapid detection of gluten using a simple ELISA home test. *Journal of the Association of Official Analytical Chemists*, 74, 257–264.
32. Denery-Papini S., Nicolas Y., and Popineau Y. (1999). Efficiency and limitations of immunochemical assays for the testing of gluten-free foods. *Journal of Cereal Science*, 30, 121–123.
33. Ellis H. J., Doyle A. P., Day, P., and Ciclitira, P. J. (1998). Coeliac disease: measurement of gluten using a monoclonal antibody to a coeliac toxic peptide of A-gliadin. *Gut*, 43, 190–195.
34. Troncone R., Vitale M., Donatiello A., Farris E., Rossi G., and Auricchio S. (1986). A sandwich enzyme immunoassay for wheat gluten. *Journal of Immunological Methods*, 92, 21–23.
35. Chirdo F. G., Fossati C. A., and Anon M. C. (1995). Optimization of a competitive ELISA with polyclonal antibodies for quantitation of prolamines in food. *Food Agricultural Immunology*, 7, 333–343.
36. Brett G. M., Mills E. N. C., Goodfellow B. J., Fido R., Tatham A. S., Shewry P. R. and Morgan M. R. A. (1999). Epitope mapping studies of broad specificity monoclonal antibodies to cereal prolamins. *Journal of Cereal Science*, 29, 117–128.
37. Skerritt J. H., Hill A. S., and Andrews J. L. (2000). Antigenicity of wheat prolamins: detailed epitope analysis using a panel of monoclonal antibodies. *Journal of Cereal Science*, 32, 259–279.
38. Sánchez D., Tucková L., Burkhard M., Plicka J., Mothes T., Hoffmanová I., and Tlaskalová-Hogenová H. (2007). Specificity analysis of anti-gliadin mouse monoclonal antibodies used for detection of gliadin in food for gluten-free diet. *Journal of Agricultural Food Chemistry*, 4;55(7), 2627–2632.
39. Valdés I., García E., Llorente M., and Méndez E. (2003). Innovative approach to low-level gluten determination in foods using a novel sandwich enzyme-linked immunosorbent assay protocol. *European Journal of Gastroenterology and Hepatology*, 15, 465–474.
40. Méndez E., Vela C., Immer U., and Janssen FW. (2005). Report of a collaborative trial to investigate the performance of the R5 enzyme linked immunoassay to determine gliadin in gluten-free food. *European Journal of Gastroenterology and Hepatology*, 17, 1053–1063.
41. Khan N., Katsube-Tanaka T., Iida S., Yamaguchi T., Nakano J., and Tsujimoto H. (2008). Identification and variation of glutelin alpha polypeptides in the genus *Oryza* assessed by two-dimensional electrophoresis and step-by-step immunodetection. *Journal of Agricultural Food Chemistry*, 56, 4955–4961.

42. Varriale A., Rossi M., Staiano M., Terpetschnig E., Barbieri B., Rossi M., and D'Auria S. (2007). Fluorescence correlation spectroscopy assay for gliadin in food. *Analytical Chemistry*, 79, 4687–4689.
43. Sánchez-Martínez M. L., Aguilar-Caballos M. P., and Gómez-Hens A. (2007). Long-wavelength fluorescence polarization immunoassay: determination of amikacin on solid surface and gliadins in solution. *Analytical Chemistry*, 79, 7424–7430.
44. Nassef H. M., Bermudo Redondo M. C., Ciclitira P. J., Ellis H. J., Fragoso A., and O'Sullivan C. K. (2008). Electrochemical immunosensor for detection of celiac disease toxic gliadin in foodstuff. *Analytical Chemistry*, 80, 9265–9271.
45. Mairal T., Frese I., Llaudet E., Redondo C. B., Katakis I., von Germar F., Drese K., and O' Sullivan C. K. (2009). Microfluorimeter with disposable polymer chip for detection of coeliac disease toxic gliadin. *Lab on a Chip*, 21;9(24), 3535–3642.
46. Camafeita E., Alfonso P., Mothes T., and Méndez E. (1997). Matrix-assisted laser desorption/ionization time-of-flight mass spectrometric micro-analysis: the first non-immunological alternative attempt to quantify gluten gliadins in food samples. *Journal of Mass Spectrometry*, 32, 940–947.
47. Camafeita E. and Méndez E. (1998). Screening of gluten avenins in foods by matrix-assisted laser desorption/ionization time-of-flight mass spectrometry. *Journal of Mass Spectrometry*, 33, 1023–1028.
48. Cozzolino R., Di Giorgi S., Fisichella S., Garozzo D., Lafiandra D., and Palermo A. (2001). Matrix-assisted laser desorption/ionization mass spectrometric peptide mapping of high molecular weight glutenin subunits 1Bx7 and 1Dy10 in Cheyenne cultivar. *Rapid Communication in Mass Spectrometry*, 15, 778–787.
49. Cozzolino R., Di Giorgi S., Fisichella S., Garozzo D., Lafiandra D., and Palermo A. (2001). Proteomics of gluten: mapping of subunit 1 Ax2* in Cheyenne cultivar by matrix-assisted laser desorption/ionization. *Rapid Communication in Mass Spectrometry*, 15, 1129–1135.
50. Hernando A., Valdes I., and Méndez E. (2003). New strategy for the determination of gliadins in maize- or rice-based foods matrix-assisted laser desorption/ionization time-of-flight mass spectrometry: fractionation of gliadins from maize or rice prolamins by acidic treatment. *Journal of Mass Spectrometry*, 38, 862–871.
51. Muccilli V., Cunsolo V., Saletti R., Foti S., Masci S., and Lafiandra D. (2005). Characterization of B- and C-type low molecular weight glutenin subunits by electrospray ionization mass spectrometry and matrix-assisted laser desorption/ionization mass spectrometry. *Proteomics*, 5, 719–728.
52. Ferranti P., Mamone G., Picariello G., and Addeo F. (2007). Mass spectrometry analysis of gliadins in celiac disease. *Journal of Mass Spectrometry*, 42, 1531–1548.
53. Salmanowicz B. P. (2008). Detection of high molecular weight glutenin subunits in triticale (x Triticosecale Wittm.). cultivars by capillary zone electrophoresis. *Journal of Agricultural Food Chemistry*, 56, 9355–9361.
54. Mamone G., De Caro S., Di Luccia A., Addeo F., and Ferranti P. (2009). Proteomic-based analytical approach for the characterization of glutenin subunits in durum wheat. *Journal of Mass Spectrometry*, 44, 1709–1723.
55. Köppel E., Stadler M., and Lüthy J. (1998). Detection of wheat contamination in oats by polymerase chain reaction (PCR) and enzyme-linked immunosorbent assay (ELISA). *Zeitschrift für Lebensmittel-Untersuchung und -Forschung*, 206, 399–403.
56. Hernández M., Esteve T., and Pla M. (2005). Real-time polymerase chain reaction based assays for quantitative detection of barley, rice, sunflower, and wheat. *Journal of Agricultural Food Chemistry*, 7;53(18), 7003–7009.

57. Henterich N., Osman A. A., Méndez E., and Mothes T. (2003). Assay of gliadin by real-time immunopolymerase chain reaction. *Nahrung*, 47, 345–348.
58. Schwarz G., Felsenstein F. G., and Wenzel G. (2004). Development and validation of a PCR-based marker assay for negative selection of the HMW glutenin allele Glu-B1–1d (Bx-6) in wheat. *TAG. Theoretical and applied genetics. Theoretische und angewandte Genetik*, 109, 1064–1069.
59. Salmanowicz B. P. and Moczulski M. (2004). Multiplex polymerase chain reaction analysis of Glu-1 high-molecular-mass glutenin genes from wheat by capillary electrophoresis with laser-induced fluorescence detection. *Journal of Chromatography A*, 2;1032(1–2), 313–318.
60. Yeung J. M., Newsome W. H., and Abbott M. A. (2000). Determination of egg proteins in food products by enzyme immunoassay. *Journal of the Association of Official Analytical Chemists International*, 83, 139–143.
61. Hefle S. L., Jeanniton E., and Taylor S. L. (2001). Development of a sandwich enzyme-linked immunosorbent assay for the detection of egg residues in processed foods. *Journal of Food Protection*, 64, 1812–1816.
62. Baumgartner S., Steiner I., Kloiber S., Hirmann D., Krska R., and Yeung J. (2002). Towards the development of a dipstick immunoassay for the detection of trace amounts of egg proteins in food. *European Food Research and Technology*, 214, 168–170.
63. Kuzmanoff K. M. and Beattie C. W. (1991). Isolation of monoclonal antibodies monospecific for bovine β-lactoglobulin. *Journal of Dairy Science*, 74, 3731–3740.
64. Jeanson S., Dupont D., Grattard N., and Rolet-Répécaud O. (1999). Characterisation of the heat treatment undergone by milk using two inhibition ELISAs for quantification of native and heat denatured α-lactalbumin. *Journal of Agricultural Food Chemistry*, 47, 2249–2254.
65. Makinen-Kiljunen S. and Palosuo T. (1991). A sensitive enzyme-linked immunosorbent assay for determination of bovine β-lactoglobulin in infant feeding formulas and in human milk. *Allergy*, 47, 347–352.
66. Hitchcock C. H. S., Bailey F. J., Crimes A. A., Dean A. G., and Davis P. J. (1981). Determination of soya proteins in food using an enzyme-linked immunosorbent assay procedure. *Journal of the Science of Food and Agriculture*, 32, 157–165.
67. Rittenberg J. H., Adams A., Palmer J., and Allen J. C. (1987). Improved enzyme-linked immunosorbent assay for determination of soy protein in meat products. *Journal of the Association of Official Analytical Chemists International*, 70, 582–587.
68. Yatsumoto K., Sudo M., and Suzuki T. (1990). Quantitation of soya protein by enzyme-linked immunosorbent assay of its characteristic peptide. *Journal of the Science of Food and Agriculture*, 50, 377–389.
69. Yeung J. M. and Collins P. G. (1996). Determination of soy proteins in food products by enzyme immunoassay. *Food Technology and Biotechnology*, 35, 209–214.
70. Brett G. M., Bull V. J., and Morgan M. R. A. (1998). Identification of hidden allergens within foods. *Allergy*, 53 (Suppl 46), 109–110.

CHAPTER 7

Fish, Crustaceans, and Mollusks

Poi-Wah Lee and Steve L. Taylor

CONTENTS

Introduction 178
Allergenic Properties of Fish 178
    Allergic Reactions to Fish 178
    Cross-Reactivity among Fish Species 178
    Threshold 179
    Fish Allergens 179
Allergenic Properties of Crustaceans 183
    Allergic Reactions to Crustaceans 183
    Cross-Reactivity among Crustacean Species 183
    Threshold 184
    Crustacean Allergens 184
Allergenic Properties of Mollusks 186
    Allergic Reactions to Mollusks 186
    Cross-Reactivity Involving Molluscan Species 186
    Threshold 187
    Molluscan Allergens 187
Detection and Quantification Methods 189
    Sample Extraction 190
    Fish Assays 191
    Crustacean Assays 193
    Mollusk Assays 195
References 195

INTRODUCTION

This chapter presents a concise overview of the allergenic properties of seafoods: fish, crustaceans, and mollusks. In addition, the analytical techniques for detecting and quantifying the allergenic protein residues derived from fish, crustaceans, and mollusks in foods are discussed. Several detection methods for fish residues have been published, but they are not well developed yet, and problems still exist regarding the specificity of the antibodies for detecting the allergenic fish residues regardless of the fish species. A few methods exist for detecting the major tropomyosin allergen found in crustacean shellfish and have proven useful for detecting crustacean residues in foods. No published methods exist for the detection of residues of mollusks. Laws in the United States and the European Union mandated the listing of fish and crustacean shellfish on food ingredient labels; the European Union has recently included molluscan shellfish on this list of allergens to be declared. Therefore, there is a growing need for the development of reliable, rapid, and practical methods for routine analysis of undeclared allergenic seafood residues in foods.

ALLERGENIC PROPERTIES OF FISH

Allergic Reactions to Fish

Fish are capable of inducing the hypersensitivity reactions mediated by immunoglobulin (Ig) E through ingestion, direct contact, and inhalation of fish odors and fumes generated during cooking.[1-6] The symptoms usually occur within 30 min after ingesting fish and are comprised of skin, respiratory, and gastrointestinal symptoms.[7,8] Life-threatening and fatal anaphylaxis due to the ingestion of fish can also occur in some cases. Yunginger et al.[9] reported an adult who died of an anaphylactic reaction to fish due to the ingestion of French fries prepared in oil contaminated with fish. Of 32 food allergy-related casualties documented between 1994 and 1999, one case of a fatal anaphylactic reaction to fish was described.[10] Unlike cow's milk and egg allergy, which are commonly outgrown, fish allergies often persist throughout life once sensitized,[11,12,13] although studies performed by Kajosaari[14] and Solensky[15] reported that children and adults can sometimes develop tolerance to fish. Fish are considered to be among the most commonly allergenic foods on a worldwide basis.[16,17] The prevalence of fish allergy is not precisely known but was estimated at 0.4% of the population in the United States on the basis of a random digit-dial telephone survey.[18]

Cross-Reactivity among Fish Species

Serological cross-reactivity between various fish species has been reported. DeMartino et al.[19] found, in a group of 20 cod-allergic children, that all study children showed positive skin tests to 1 or more of 17 fish species. Nevertheless, these children were not uniformly sensitive to all the fish species tested; in fact, a higher frequency of positive skin tests to eel, bass, dentex, sole, and tuna was observed.

In a study conducted by Hansen et al.,[20] all eight clinically codfish-allergic adults demonstrated significant cross-reactivity to cod, mackerel, plaice, and herring as assessed by several tests: the skin prick test, histamine release test, radioallergosorbent test (RAST), and sodium dodecyl sulfate polyacrylamide gel electrophoresis (SDS-PAGE) with immunoblotting. Sten et al.[21] examined whether codfish-allergic patients exhibited cross-reactivity to ocean pout, eelpout, and eel that were rarely consumed in the Scandinavian diet. All 18 patients had specific IgE to all four species of fish, and 17/18 patients reacted to all fish species in the skin prick test. A cross-reactivity study in Norway demonstrated that 9/10 of the fish-allergic patients had positive skin tests to the native parvalbumins from cod, salmon, and pollock. Of the 7 patients who were skin tested with herring, wolfish, tuna, and mackerel, all patients reacted strongly to the herring and wolfish, whereas 6/7 patients reacted weakly or were unresponsive to tuna and mackerel. The skin prick test results were supported by the in vitro tests of fish-specific IgE antibodies.[22]

Despite the extensive serological cross-reactivity among fish species, several studies demonstrated that the fish-allergic patients are able to consume one or more fish species without experiencing any adverse reactions. An early study by Aas[23] demonstrated that, among 61 cod-allergic children, 34 reacted to all fish, but 27 tolerated one or more fish species. Besides, salmon extracts elicited positive skin tests in children who could safely consume salmon. A prospective study by Bernhisel-Broadbent et al.[24] revealed that 26 of the negative oral fish challenges corresponded to positive skin prick tests. Through the use of immunoblotting and enzyme-linked immunosorbent assay (ELISA) inhibition assays, serum-specific IgE showed reactivity to fish that the patients were able to clinically tolerate, as confirmed by oral challenges. These studies concluded that the serological and in vitro diagnostic tests of the cross-reactivity among fish species do not necessarily correlate to the clinical reactivity. However, Helbling et al.[25] observed high correlation between the skin prick test and responses to oral challenges. In this study, cross-reactivity among various fish species of taxonomically distinct orders was shown to be clinically relevant. Therefore, fish-allergic individuals should avoid all fish species until proven that the species is safe to be consumed by oral food challenge studies.[25]

Threshold

Fish are known to induce severe IgE-mediated allergic reactions at low doses of exposure. The lowest provoking doses for fish evaluated in a double-blind, placebo-controlled food challenge (DBPCFC) test of 14 fish-allergic patients was estimated at 5 mg of either cod or herring.[26] However, the threshold dose for fish remains to be elucidated since low-dose challenges have only been conducted on small numbers of patients and with only a few species of fish.[26]

Fish Allergens

Parvalbumin (Gad c 1) has been identified as a pan-allergen present in most species of fish and frog and is responsible for the observed cross-reactivity.[27–29] This allergen was capable of sensitizing fish-allergic patients to multiple fish species, in some cases resulting in positive skin tests to certain fish species that the patients had never consumed.[20-22,30] It was estimated that individuals who were allergic to a fish species carry a 50% risk of reacting to the second species.[31] Parvalbumins are small, acidic, and water-soluble sarcoplasmic proteins (10–13 kDa), but the ability of cod parvalbumin to form dimers (24 kDa) that still possess IgE-binding capacity has been reported.[32] Parvalbumins are classified under the EF-hand superfamily, a group of proteins with a highly conserved helix-loop-helix structural motif that binds to divalent cations (e.g., calcium and magnesium) with varying affinities.[33] According to the crystal structure of carp parvalbumin that was solved by x-ray crystallography, the parvalbumin was comprised of three domains: AB, CD, and EF.[34] Each domain consists of a central loop flanked by two amphipathic α-helices of 12 contiguous residues from which the oxygen ligands for calcium are derived.[35,36] Both the CD and EF domains possess the calcium-binding properties; the AB domain lacks the ability to bind calcium, although it has structure similar to the CD and EF regions.[34] The exact functions of parvalbumins remain obscure; nevertheless, the consensus view of their functions in muscle include acting as calcium buffers in cytosol and promoting relaxation following muscle contraction by sequestering the intracellular calcium.[37]

Parvalbumins can be divided into two distinct phylogenetic lineages, α and β. The α-parvalbumin has a pI greater than 5 and contains an additional residue in the C-terminal helix, whereas β-parvalbumin has a pI lower than 4.5.[38] Moreover, both α- and β-forms of parvalbumins differ in at least 11 residues, in which cysteine at position 18 and aspartic acid at position 61 are typically found in β-parvalbumins.[39] All vertebrates, including human, express parvalbumin in varying levels in the skeletal muscles. Lower vertebrates, such as fish, contain higher quantities of parvalbumin in the muscles than higher vertebrates.[39] The concentration of parvalbumins in the fish skeletal muscles also varies with the muscle types. White muscle typically contains more parvalbumin than dark muscle. Lim et al.[40] reported that parvalbumin was found in the white muscle of tuna (*Thunnus tonggol*) but was absent in the dark muscle. The allergenicity of the white and dark fish muscles is largely associated with the parvalbumin content. Kobayashi et al.[41] showed that dark muscle was less allergenic than white muscle due to the lower content of parvalbumin in dark muscle. Some fish species have been shown to express from two to five parvalbumin isotypes that possess different affinity for calcium and magnesium.[42,43] Complementary DNA (cDNA) cloning revealed that two distinct parvalbumin isotypes exist in Atlantic salmon, carp, Atlantic codfish, and Alaska pollack.[44-47] No studies have examined the importance of the cross-reactive properties and allergenicity of these parvalbumin isotypes to fish-allergic individuals.

Gad c 1 was the first major cod (*Gadus callarias*) allergen identified and purified.[48] Subsequent studies have isolated the homologous allergens from Atlantic salmon (*Salmo salar*), horse mackerel (*Trachurus japonicus*), Japanese eel (*Anguilla japonica*), bigeye tuna (*Thunnus obesus*), carp (*Cyprinus carpio*), cod (*Gadus morhua*), mackerel (*Scomber japonicus, S. australasicus, S. scombrus*), and Alaska pollack (*Theragra chalcogramma*).[44-47,49-53] These allergens were either purified by combinations of gel filtration, anion exchange, and high-performance liquid chromatographic techniques or isolated by the cDNA cloning method. In these studies, the isolated parvalbumins were confirmed to represent the major allergens in fish due to their ability to bind serum-specific IgE from fish-allergic subjects.

Gad c 1 is a stable allergen. Studies have shown that the allergenicity of Gad c 1 was not significantly affected by extreme pH, heat denaturation, and chemical modifications, suggesting that the allergenic activity of Gad c 1 is primarily dependent on the primary structure rather than on the molecular conformation.[54] However, the contribution of steric conformation on the allergenicity of fish parvalbumin is not negligible. Several studies have demonstrated that the depletion of calcium from carp and frog parvalbumins significantly reduced the IgE binding to these parvalbumins.[29,45,55] According to the circular dichroism analysis, the loss of IgE reactivity was associated with the change in conformation of the calcium-depleted parvalbumins.[55] These findings were further supported by the production of hypoallergenic mutants of the carp and Pacific mackerel parvalbumin using site-directed mutagenesis to replace the two aspartic acid residues in each of the calcium-binding domains with alanine residues. As a result, both mutants no longer had the ability to bind calcium and showed a significant reduction in the IgE reactivity compared to their wild-type counterpart.[56,57]

The elucidation of IgE-binding epitopes is essential for better understanding the interaction between allergens and components of the immune system. Early studies by Elaysed and Apold[58] identified several IgE-binding epitopes based on the immunological reactivity of the limited trypsin-hydrolyzed peptide fragments and the synthetic peptides of Gad c 1 with the serum IgE from fish-allergic patients. Five different fragments corresponding to the residues 13–32 (AB domain), 33–44 (axis joining AB and CD domains), 49–64 (calcium-binding loop of CD domain), 65–74 (axis joining CD and EF domains), and 88–96 (calcium-binding loop of EF domain) of Gad c 1 were assumed to contain IgE-binding epitopes.[58] Using the computational matching of mimitopes onto the molecular surface of the natural carp parvalbumin, three epitope regions were identified. Two of the epitopes were found in regions connecting the AB and CD domain and the CD and EF domain, while the third epitope was located in the calcium-binding region of the EF domain.[59] A study by Yoshida et al.[60] identified region 21–40 in Pacific mackerel parvalbumin as the major IgE-binding epitope by the epitope mapping of 10 overlapping 20-mer peptides; region 21–40 appeared to be specific to mackerel parvalbumin.

In addition to the major fish parvalbumin allergens, a higher molecular weight allergen was found in the myostromal protein fraction of the bigeye tuna muscle by Hamada et al.[61] The allergen has been identified as collagen based on the results of SDS-PAGE, immunoblotting, and amino acid analysis. In this study, the serum IgE from fish-allergic patients recognized three protein bands, including two protein bands of 120 kDa and a band of 240 kDa, which corresponded to the α-chain and β-chain (dimer of α-chain) of collagen, respectively.[61] Although cross-reactivity among collagens from various fish species is common, there is a lack of cross-reactivity between collagens from fish and other animals.[62]

Fish gelatin is comprised of collagen that is derived from the fish skins and bones and is commonly used as a stabilizer in pharmaceutical and food products.[8] Several studies have investigated the potential allergenicity of fish gelatin. Sakaguchi et al.[63] showed that patients with fish allergy and bovine gelatin allergy had specific IgE antibodies reacting to fish gelatin, specifically to the α_1- and α_2-chains of the tunafish type I collagen. In addition, cross-reactivity among gelatins from various fish species, including tuna, saurel, salmon, mackerel, and cod, was evident.[63] André et al.[64] reported that 3 of the 100 sera from fish-sensitive individuals showed reactivity in immunoblotting to tuna flesh, tuna skin, and gelatin prepared from tuna skin, but no cross-reactivity was observed between bovine/porcine and fish gelatin. Nevertheless, further investigation showed that the 3 subjects did not have any clinical reactivity to the tuna skin gelatin, and they did not react to the tuna skin gelatin in the skin prick test or to 5 g of tuna gelatin in a food challenge test.[64] However, a later DBPCFC trial revealed that 1 of 30 clinically codfish-allergic individuals experienced a mild subjective reaction after ingesting a cumulative dose of 7.61 g of fish gelatin derived from codfish skins.[65] Hansen et al.[65] concluded with a 95% certainty that 90% of fish-allergic consumers would not react to the ingestion of a 3.61-g cumulative dose of fish gelatin. Based on these reports, the potential risk of fish gelatin in eliciting an adverse reaction among fish-allergic individuals remains speculative.

There is also evidence of other minor allergens besides collagen in fish. Dory et al.[66] demonstrated the presence of seven IgE-binding and possibly allergenic proteins of 12, 22, 30, 45, 60, 67, 104, and 130 kDa in pre-rigor mortis cod extracts using the pooled sera from 12 cod-allergic individuals. Higher relative content of the IgE-reactive bands was observed when the codfish was stored for a longer period of time.[66] Galland et al.[67] purified a 41-kDa protein from the crude extracts of raw cod. The purified protein was considered an allergen due to its ability to bind IgE antibodies from the pooled sera of cod-allergic individuals.[67] Besides, the IgE from the pooled sera also recognized five other allergenic proteins having a molecular mass of 13, 22, 28, 49, and 60 kDa in the crude cod extracts.[67] Subsequent study identified that the 41-kDa protein was homologous to the aldehyde phosphate dehydrogenase.[68] Moreover, the 41-kDa protein was recognized by a monoclonal antiparvalbumin antibody, which is probably attributed to the low similarity of the 41-kDa protein to the acidic residues of the calcium-binding domains in parvalbumin.[68] Lim et al.[69] reported that sera from 2 of the 10 individuals with allergies to tropical fish showed IgE binding to proteins of 29 and 54 kDa in addition to the 12-kDa parvalbumin in cod, threadfin, pomfret, and tengirri. One of the codfish-allergic European subjects also reacted to the protein bands of 12 and 29 kDa in cod, pomfret, and tengirri.[69]

While the majority of the studies demonstrated that the fish-allergic subjects primarily reacted with a fish protein identified as parvalbumin, this is not always the case. Kelso et al.[70] and James et al.[27] reported two subjects with monospecific allergy who showed IgE reactivity to only a protein band at 25 kDa in swordfish and 40 kDa in tuna. A research group in India compared the allergen profiles of two Indian fish: hilsa and pomfret.[71] The IgE immunoblotting revealed that the sera from 10 fish-allergic patients reacted to protein bands ranging from 29 to 94 kDa and 32 to 97 kDa in the raw muscle extracts of hilsa and pomfret, respectively.[71] The patients' sera also bound to a common protein of 50 kDa in both fish extracts, but none of the sera showed binding to the low molecular weight allergen (i.e., parvalbumin), suggesting that the epitopes in the proteins of these Indian fish are species specific.[71] However, no further studies were done to purify and characterize these potential allergens. Later study investigating the IgE-binding properties of four thermally treated Indian fish revealed that frying and boiling of the fish muscle abolished the binding of IgE antibodies to the allergenic proteins in hilsa and pomfret, whereas the allergenic proteins in bhetki and Indian mackerel were thermally stable.[72]

ALLERGENIC PROPERTIES OF CRUSTACEANS

Allergic Reactions to Crustaceans

Crustacean shellfish can induce IgE-mediated hypersensitivity reactions through ingestion, direct contact, and inhalation of shellfish cooking vapors.[73] Typically, symptoms ensue within 30 min after ingesting crustacean species and are comprised of skin, respiratory, and gastrointestinal symptoms.[74,75] Life-threatening and fatal anaphylaxis cases have been reported occasionally.[76,77] Unlike some other IgE-mediated food allergies, sensitization to crustacean shellfish often occurs later in life rather than in infancy, but this is probably because exposure tends also to occur later in life. Once sensitized, crustacean shellfish allergy is thought to be persistent, although clinical research on this topic has been scant. Allergies to crustacean shellfish are considered among the most common food allergies on a worldwide basis.[16] In a random digit-dial telephone survey conducted in the United States of almost 15,000 individuals, crustacean shellfish allergy was identified as the most common food allergy, with an estimated prevalence of 1.9% of the population.[18] In a more recent Food Safety Survey conducted in the United States among 4,400 individuals, the prevalence of shellfish allergy was estimated at 1.9% and 1.3%, respectively, among respondents with self-reported and self-reported, physician-diagnosed food allergy.[78] Allergies to crustacean shellfish are also reported to be high in certain Asian countries.[79,80]

Cross-Reactivity among Crustacean Species

Crustacean shellfish belong to the Anthropoda phylum. Crustacean shellfish include shrimp, prawns, crab, lobster, crayfish, and barnacles. The majority of individuals with allergies to crustacean shellfish appear to be allergic to all crustacean species, including shrimp, crab, and lobster.[81] However, some individuals appear to be reactive only to specific species.[81,82] In a study from Thailand, specific allergy to a saltwater shrimp species (*Penaeus monodon*) occurred in 17.6% of 68 allergic children with a history of shrimp allergy, while specific allergy to a freshwater shrimp species (*Macrobrachium rosenbergii*) occurred in 23.5% of children in this group.[75]

Most edible crustaceans belong to the order Decapoda within the class Malacostraca, including shrimp, prawn, lobster, and crab. However, barnacles are also crustacea but belong to the class Maxillopoda. Barnacles are consumed in certain parts of the world and have also been identified as allergenic.[83–85] Some barnacle-allergic individuals reportedly cross-react to ingestion of other crustacean species, while others are tolerant.[83]

Since crustaceans are invertebrates, sensitization to other invertebrate species such as dust mites may also lead to sensitization to shrimp.[86] Immunotherapy treatment for dust mite allergy has, on occasion, led to the development of shrimp allergy.[87,88] Two of five barnacle-allergic individuals were cross-reactive with dust mites.[83]

Threshold

Little research has been conducted on the minimal eliciting doses for crustacean shellfish among sensitized individuals. In clinical challenge studies conducted on a limited number of subjects, the minimal dose of shrimp needed to elicit an allergic response was two to four shrimps.[74]

Crustacean Allergens

Crustacean shellfish appear to contain multiple allergenic proteins.[89] However, tropomyosin is viewed as a particularly important major allergen and a pan-allergen responsible for most of the widespread cross-reactivity observed between various crustacean shellfish species.[79,85,90–92] Tropomyosin is a protein found in all muscle tissues that is involved in regulating the contraction of skeletal muscle.[89] The structure and biological role of tropomyosin in muscle contraction are relatively well understood.[89] Tropomyosin is heat stable and can be found in the cooking water after preparation of shrimp.[91] Tropomyosin binds IgE from the sera of more than 80% of all shrimp-allergic individuals and inhibits IgE reactivity to shrimp whole body extract, indications that tropomyosin is a major shrimp allergen responsible for most of the allergenic activity of shrimp.[91] Tropomyosins have now been identified as allergens from a large number of crustacean shellfish species (Table 7.1). In addition, tropomyosins are now recognized as a pan-allergen among a wider range of invertebrate species, including arachnids (house dust mites), insects (e.g., cockroaches), nematodes, and molluscan shellfish (see further discussion).[89,93] While tropomyosin also exists in the muscle tissues of vertebrate species, the vertebrate tropomyosins appear to be nonallergenic.[94] The amino acid sequences of vertebrate tropomyosins share only 53–57% identity with Met e 1, a known shrimp allergen.[95] The low degree of sequence identity likely explains the lack of allergic cross-reactivity among vertebrate and invertebrate tropomyosins.[96] Five IgE-binding epitopes were identified in Pen a 1 using 46 synthetic overlapping 15-mer peptides: region 1, 43–57; region 2, 85–105; region 3, 133–148; region 4, 187–202; region 5, 247–284.[97,98] These epitopes are positioned at regular intervals of approximately 42 amino acids, suggesting a relationship with the coiled-coil structure of tropomyosin.[89]

In addition to tropomyosin, other allergens have been identified and characterized in crustacean shellfish. Arginine kinase (Pen m 2) was originally identified from the black tiger shrimp (*Penaeus monodon*) but was shown to react with IgE from the sera of only about 27% (5 of 18) of shrimp-allergic subjects.[82] Arginine kinase was also subsequently identified as an allergen from the white Pacific shrimp,

FISH, CRUSTACEANS, AND MOLLUSKS

Table 7.1 Tropomyosin Allergens Identified in Crustacean Shellfish

Crustacean Species	Allergen Identifier	References
Indian white shrimp, *Penaeus indicus*	Pen i 1	90
Brown shrimp, *Penaeus aztecus*	Pen a 1	91
Greasyback or sand shrimp, *Metapenaeus enis*	Met e 1	163
Neptune or Taiwan shrimp, *Parapenaeus fissurus*	Par f 1	164
Common shrimp, *Cragon cragon*		165
Northern red shrimp, *Pandalus borealis*		166
White shrimp, *Penaeus setiferous*		86
Black tiger shrimp, *Penaeus monodon*	Pen m 1	101, 167
Karuma prawn, *Penaeus japonicus*		167
Pink shrimp, *Pandalus eous*		167
White leg Pacific shrimp, *Litopenaeus vannamei*	Lit v 1	100
Freshwater prawn, *Macrobrachium rosenbergii*		75
Indian spiny lobster, *Paniluris homarus*		168
American lobster, *Homarus americanus*	Hom a 1	169
Spiny lobster, *Paniluris stimpsoni*		170
European lobster, *Homarus gammarus*		171
Mud crab, *Scylla serrata*		168
Common crab, *Charybdis feriatus*	Cha f 1	171
Rock crab, *Cancer pagurus*		166
King crab, *Paralithodes camtschaticus*		167
Snow crab, *Chionoecetes opilio*		167
Horsehair crab, *Erimacrus isenbeckii*		167
Sand swimming crab, species uncertain		172
Acorn barnacle, *Balanus rostratus*		85
Goose barnacle, *Capitulum mitella*		85

Litopenaeus vannamei, Lit v 2.[99] Furthermore, common IgE-binding epitopes are present in the arginine kinases of other invertebrate species, suggesting that this may be another invertebrate pan-allergen.[82] Myosin light chain (MLC), a 20-kDa shrimp protein, was identified as an allergen (Lit v 3) from *Litopenaeus vannamei* that was able to bind to IgE from the sera of 21 of 38 (55%) shrimp-allergic subjects.[100] A highly similar allergen exists in cockroach (Bla g 8). Sarcoplasmic calcium-binding protein (SCP), another 20-kDa shrimp protein, was identified as an allergen from the black tiger shrimp (*Penaeus monodon*) that was able to bind to IgE from the sera of 8 of 16 (50%) shrimp-allergic subjects.[101] Some evidence of cross-reactivity was found with similar proteins in kuruma shrimp, American lobster, and pink shrimp but not in two species of crab.[101] SCP was later also confirmed as a shrimp allergen from *Litopenaeus vannamei* (Lit v 4) that was able to bind to IgE from the sera of 31 of 52 (60%) shrimp-allergic subjects.[102] SCP does not appear to be another invertebrate pan-allergen as inhibition of IgE binding was only observed with extracts of other crustaceans, crab and lobster.[102] The biological function of SCP is unknown, but it may function in a manner similar to parvalbumin, the major fish allergen.[102] Curiously, parvalbumin, SCP, and MLC are all EF-hand, calcium-binding proteins, although the degree of sequence identity between SCP and cod parvalbumin (Gad m 1) is only 12%.[102]

ALLERGENIC PROPERTIES OF MOLLUSKS

Allergic Reactions to Mollusks

Molluscan shellfish allergy has been less thoroughly investigated than either fish or crustacean shellfish allergy. However, allergies to all types of molluscan shellfish are well documented.[96] Molluscan shellfish are known to induce IgE-mediated hypersensitivity reactions through ingestion, direct contact, and inhalation of shellfish cooking vapors.[96] Typically, the onset of symptoms occurs within 30 min of consumption and can involve skin, respiratory, and gastrointestinal symptoms.[96] Life-threatening or fatal anaphylaxis cases have only been reported for snails, limpets, and oysters,[76,103–106] but the potential likely exists with other molluscan shellfish. Like the crustacean shellfish, sensitization to mollusks often occurs later in life. Once sensitized, molluscan shellfish allergy is thought to be persistent,[96] although clinical research on this topic has been scant. Allergies to molluscan shellfish have not been considered among the most common food allergies on a worldwide basis.[16] However, subsequently, Canada and the European Union have added molluscan shellfish to their lists of commonly allergenic foods.[96] In a random digit-dial telephone survey conducted in the United States of almost 15,000 individuals, molluscan shellfish allergy was estimated to occur in 0.4% of the population.[18] As noted, a more recent Food Safety Survey conducted in the United States among 4,482 individuals revealed that the prevalence of shellfish allergy was an estimated 1.9% and 1.3%, respectively, among respondents with self-reported and self-reported, physician-diagnosed food allergy[78]; however, not all of the respondents in the survey conducted by these investigators were able to distinguish between crustacean and molluscan shellfish. In a questionnaire survey in France, the self-reported prevalence of shellfish allergy among 2,716 school children was 0.15%.[107] In a survey of patients presenting at 17 allergy clinics in 15 Baltic cities in Europe, 6.2% indicated allergies to clams, 3.2% to oysters, and 1.4% to snails.[108] In more restricted studies of clinical populations of allergic subjects, allergies to molluscan shellfish were identified for squid, oysters, clams, and mussels in 33, 12, 10, and 10, respectively, among 142 food-sensitized Spanish patients,[109] in 2.8% of 355 Spanish children,[110] and in 7 and 5, respectively, of 305 Japanese pediatric patients to cuttlefish and octopus.[111]

Cross-Reactivity Involving Molluscan Species

Molluscan shellfish belong to a distinctly different phylum (Mollusca) than the crustacean shellfish. The Mollusca phylum is divided into eight classes, including three classes—Gastropoda, Bivalvia, and Cephalopoda—that are important sources of human food. Edible gastropods include snails, whelks, abalone, conches, and limpets. Edible bivalves include clams, cockles, scallops, mussels, and oysters. Edible cephalopods include squid, octopus, and cuttlefish. With this diversity, cross-reactivity is a complex and incompletely understood issue. Certainly, some individuals with molluscan shellfish allergy may be allergic to all species of molluscan shellfish, although this has not been well documented. The possibility is even stronger that cross-reactivity will occur among species within a particular class, such as gastropods or bivalves. Clinically, prudence would suggest counseling patients with molluscan shellfish allergy to avoid ingestion of all molluscan shellfish.[96] Clinical evidence of cross-reactivity among molluscan shellfish species seems limited and variable, but this could be due to the relatively small number of subjects who have been investigated. However, the results also suggest considerable individual variability. Among South African patients with abalone allergy, clinical evidence was found of extensive cross-reactivity with other mollusks.[112] Vuitton et al.[113] noted that four of seven snail-allergic patients were reactive to both terrestrial and marine snails. In contrast, no evidence of cross-reactivity between squid and octopus was found in a small group of Spanish patients, even though both species are cephalopods.[114]

Although admittedly a telephone survey is reliant on the accuracy of self-reports, Sicherer et al.[115] interviewed 67 mollusk-allergic individuals about allergies to four bivalves (clam, mussel, scallop, oyster) and found that 51% indicated allergy to only one species, 19% to two species, 5% to three species, and 22% to all four species. Among 70 patients in Hong Kong with histories of mollusk allergies, skin tests were performed against clam, oyster, scallop, abalone, and limpet extracts. Cross-sensitization probabilities ranged between 33% and 67% among the bivalves and between 54% and 79% among the gastropods. Even greater individual variability was found in the probability of cross-reactions between gastropods and bivalves.[106] Cross-reactions can also occur between mollusks and crustaceans.[106,110,116] Furthermore, evidence also exists of cross-reactivity between mollusks and either dust mites or insects, especially between snails and dust mites,[87,88] but also between limpet and dust mites[117] and mussels and dust mites.[118]

Threshold

Regarding the threshold, no information exists on the minimal eliciting doses for residues of molluscan shellfish among allergic individuals. However, total avoidance is counseled.

Molluscan Allergens

Molluscan shellfish also appear to contain multiple allergenic proteins.[96] However, tropomyosin is the only well-characterized allergen that exists in molluscan shellfish.[96,119] Tropomyosin is an important, major allergen from molluscan shellfish. IgE-binding tropomyosins have been identified in numerous molluscan shellfish species (Table 7.2). In most of these species, tropomyosin is the major IgE-binding protein. However, in snails, tropomyosin is a minor allergen.[120] Although

Table 7.2 Tropomyosin Allergens Identified in Molluscan Shellfish

Molluscan Species	References
Gastropod	
Abalone	112, 119, 124, 168, 173
Fan shell	174
Snail	120
Turban shell	119, 123
Whelk	119, 168, 175
Bivalves	
Clam	119, 168, 176
Cockle	119
Mussel	124
Oyster	119, 121, 122, 117, 178
Scallop	124, 160, 179
Cephalopods	
Cuttlefish	92, 168
Octopus	92, 168, 180
Squid	92, 168, 181

tropomyosin is identified as a major allergen in crustacean shellfish also, cross-reactivity observed between various molluscan and crustacean shellfish species is not universal.[96] In an extensive study of tropomyosins from gastropods and bivalves, Emoto et al.[119] showed that molluscan tropomyosins share relatively modest degrees of amino acid sequence identities (about 60%) with crustacean tropomyosins. Some of the IgE-binding epitopes identified in brown shrimp tropomyosin are conserved among molluscan shellfish species, but others are not.[119]

Thus, individual cross-reactivity to molluscan as well as crustacean shellfish is likely dependent on the nature of the IgE-binding epitopes for the particular individual. The amino acid sequences of molluscan tropomyosins are more highly conserved within the various classes of molluscan shellfish.[96,119] Thus, cross-reactions may be more likely to occur within particular classes of molluscan shellfish species rather than between mollusks and crustaceans or even between various classes of mollusks.[96] Only a few epitopes have been clinically well defined among molluscan tropomyosins. Identical IgE-binding epitopes, with the amino acid sequence IQLLEEDMERSEER, have been identified in two oyster allergens, Cra g 1 and Cra g 2, which are probably tropomyosin isoforms.[121,122] The IgE-binding epitope of *Turbo cornutus*, a turban shell gastropod, is different and is located within the carboxy-terminal region of tropomyosin,[123] which is highly conserved between molluscan and crustacean shellfish species.[124]

Molluscan shellfish likely contain other allergens beyond tropomyosin.[96] Variable levels of evidence exist for other IgE-binding proteins in several gastropods (snail, pen shell, turban shell, fan shell, whelk, abalone, and limpet); bivalves (oyster, scallop, and razor clam); and cephalopods (squid, octopus, and cuttlefish).[96] However, most of these nontropomyosin allergens remain unidentified, and their clinical significance remains to be demonstrated.[96] The identities of several of these other allergens have been proposed, including hemocyanin from grand keyhole limpet,[104,105] myosin heavy chain from snail,[125] and amylase from limpet.[117] A 49-kDa allergen of unknown identity was identified from a species of abalone, *Haliotis midae*,[112] and designated as Hal m 1 by the International Union of Immunological Societies (IUIS). But, this allergen has not been confirmed to exist in other species of abalone, and tropomyosin appears to be the major allergen in other species of abalone, *Haliotis diversicolor* and *H. discus*.[119,124]

DETECTION AND QUANTIFICATION METHODS

The presence of undeclared seafood allergens in food products can pose a serious health risk among sensitized individuals; consequently, reliable quantification methods for detecting trace amounts of allergenic seafood residues in different complex food matrices are vital to ensure that the food manufacturers comply with labeling regulations and to protect consumers. This review primarily focuses on the ELISA, which is the principal protein-based technique that is most commonly described in the literature.

ELISA has found application in the food industry because it offers high specificity and sensitivity in quantifying a small amount of analyte within a complex food matrix without extensive sample preparation.[126] The fundamental requirements in ELISA development involve the generation of appropriate antibodies with the desired properties of affinity and specificity to particular proteins in foods. Two types of antibodies can be produced: polyclonal and monoclonal. A monoclonal antibody preparation gives rise to individual antibodies of identical structure and reactivity that are specific for a single epitope.[127] This antibody is often derived from mouse cells by fusing antibody-producing B cells with a myeloma cell to generate hybrid cells, known as *hybridomas*, which secrete large quantities of monoclonal antibodies indefinitely.[127] Monoclonal antibodies have been produced to specific seafood allergens. Examples include carp parvalbumin-specific and shrimp tropomyosin-specific monoclonal antibodies.[128,129] A polyclonal antibody is a heterogeneous mixture of antibodies possessing the ability to recognize multiple epitopes on the antigen.[127] Polyclonal antibody can be produced from a wide range of vertebrate species, such as rabbits, sheep, goats, or horses.[126] Polyclonal antisera have also been produced that are specific to certain seafood allergens. Examples include the polyclonal anticod parvalbumin and antiprawn tropomyosin antibody produced by rabbits.[130,131] For the purpose of detecting allergenic residues in processed foods, polyclonal antibody offers superior properties when compared to monoclonal antibody. As the processing of foods can lead to extensive changes in the conformation of proteins, such changes can reduce or abolish the antibody recognition of certain specific antigenic epitopes. Thus, polyclonal antibodies, directed against multiple epitopes, are more likely to recognize the modified proteins.[132]

Immunogen, a substance that is used to immunize animals for antibody production, is composed of either a purified allergen or crude extracts of an allergenic source that is occasionally heat treated. In general, the target analytes in the ELISA can be classified into two major categories. Some ELISAs are capable of specifically detecting for the presence of allergens in foods, such as an ELISA that detects fish parvalbumin and crustacean tropomyosin in foods, while other ELISAs were developed to detect a mixture of proteins, which were usually obtained from the crude extracts of an allergenic food, such as an ELISA for soluble fish proteins.[133]

Sample Extraction

The extraction efficiency of an analyte from various food matrices is one of the key issues in determining the applicability of an assay. Ideally, the extraction procedures should completely separate and extract the analyte from any food matrices into the liquid phase of the extraction medium.[134] However, the complexity of food matrices and the processing treatments often have a negative impact on the extraction efficiency. Food matrices contain fats, carbohydrates, proteins, minerals, and other minor components that intermingle to form a complex mixture. The interaction between these components and the target proteins in the food matrices may adversely affect the extraction efficiency. For example, the high lipid content in chocolate can lower the protein solubility, thus decreasing the extraction efficiency.[135] Cocoa contains polyphenolic substances (tannins) that can hinder the extraction of allergenic residues.[134] Food processing is another important factor that greatly influences extraction efficiency because various processing treatments, such as high-heat, high-pressure, proteolytic, acidic, and alkaline treatments can result in aggregation, denaturation, or hydrolysis of target proteins in foods.[136,137] Such changes in protein structures can hamper the extractability of the soluble proteins.[138] As an example, the roasting of peanuts may decrease the extractability of the target proteins because the proteins are less soluble in the aqueous solutions.[139] Consequently, the limitations of the extraction procedures have to be addressed when validating the performance of an assay.

No standardized procedures exist for extracting the allergenic food residues prior to detection by the ELISA. The extraction procedures often have to be customized for the analyte of interest and manipulated, if necessary, to accommodate for the complexity of each food matrix. Before extraction begins, the representative food samples containing the allergenic residues have to be ground to a fine powder or homogeneous mixture.[134] Generally, buffers with low ionic strength and neutral to slightly basic pH, such as phosphate-buffered saline and tris-buffered saline, among others, are used to extract the allergenic residues. These aqueous buffers are applicable for extracting parvalbumin from fish and tropomyosin from crustacean and molluscan shellfish because these muscle proteins are water soluble. Extraction additives, such as fish gelatin, skim milk powder, bovine serum albumin, and other proteins can be added to the buffers to improve the extractability of the target proteins,[134] but these extraction additives should not cross-react with the antibodies used in the ELISA. Moreover, studies have shown that the addition of surfactant (SDS) and reducing agent (β-mercaptoethanol) improved the extraction of insoluble proteins from processed foods.[140] Seiki et al.[141] developed a crustacean ELISA by incorporating the surfactant and reducing agent in the sample extraction procedures. However, these approaches have not been evaluated with the fish or molluscan shellfish allergen detection systems. The physical conditions for extraction, including time, temperature, and the amount of extraction buffers added to the samples, may vary according to the assays. The optimized extraction procedures should specifically maximize the extraction recovery of target proteins but minimize the extraction of other interfering substances that will possibly lead to high background in the ELISA due to nonspecific binding. After the extraction is completed, the extracts are centrifuged and the supernatant collected for analysis in the ELISA.

Fish Assays

The detection of allergenic fish residues in foods is of particular interest for labeling purposes and the safeguarding of fish-allergic consumers. Several fish authentication methods employing electrophoretic techniques, immunoassays, polymerase chain reaction (PCR) methodology, and matrix-assisted laser desorption/ionization-time of flight-mass spectrometry (MALDI-TOF-MS) are currently available. Electrophoretic techniques, with isoelectric focusing being the most frequently used method, separate the sarcoplasmic proteins by their electrical charge differences and identify the fish species based on the species-specific banding patterns of the whole proteins or parvalbumins.[142,143] Immunoassays like ELISA, on the other hand, use either monoclonal or polyclonal antibodies against the soluble muscle proteins of specific fish species with no cross-reactivity to unrelated fish species to discriminate between the different species of fish.[144-147] PCR-based methods involve amplification of the DNA regions of interest that are universal or species specific, followed by the analysis of the PCR fragments for species recognition using various methods, including electrophoretic techniques, DNA sequencing, restriction fragment length polymorphism (RFLP), single-stranded conformational polymorphism (SSCP), and many others.[148-150] MALDI-TOF-MS identifies fish species according to the parvalbumin isoform patterns displayed by two-dimensional electrophoresis in conjunction with the unique MALDI-TOF mass fingerprints of the peptides generated by the trypsin hydrolysis of the parvalbumin isoforms.[151]

The fish authentication techniques are extremely specific for detecting single or multiple fish species. In addition, they are qualitative methods that are validated to identify the fish species among various seafood and meat samples instead of as components of formulated and processed foods. Hence, they have limited application in detecting and quantifying the allergenic protein residues derived from irrelevant fish species in foods. To utilize these authentication methods, the food manufacturers need to have advance knowledge about the particular fish species that may contaminate the processing plant facility or the finished food products, but this kind of situation seldom occurs in reality.

Research into the development of methods intended to detect allergenic residues from a wide range of fish species in foods has been published. Fæste and Plassen[131] developed a sandwich ELISA for the quantification of fish in foods using polyclonal anticod parvalbumin antibody as the capture and detector antibody. The ELISA had a limit of detection of 0.01 mg parvalbumin/kg food, which was equivalent to 5 mg fish/kg food. However, the detection of fish parvalbumin was inconsistent for different fish species. Among the 32 fish species tested, the ELISA showed the greatest recovery rates (>50%) for fish that are most commonly consumed, such as cod, tilapia, salmon, carp, mackerel, and pollock. Nevertheless, several freshwater fish, including Nile perch, European eel, sturgeon, northern pike, and a cartilaginous fish, the spiny dogfish, showed a recovery rate lower than 1%. A similar observation was made by Chen et al.[152] with respect to the variable immunoreactivity of the commercially available mouse monoclonal antifrog parvalbumin antibody against the raw extracts from several fish species.

Gajewski and Hsieh et al.[153] developed a monoclonal antibody against the crude extracts of the cooked catfish muscle proteins. The comparisons of their antibody with the commercially available mouse monoclonal antifrog parvalbumin antibody showed further evidence of the variable specificity of both antibodies against the cooked extracts from different fish species. The quantitative variation of the ELISA when detecting various species of fish might be attributed to the variable amount of parvalbumin present in the fish extracts and differences in the binding affinity of the antibody to the antigen.[152]

Hence, the utilization of the antiparvalbumin antibody that has equal specificity to parvalbumin from different species of fish is considered to be more advantageous for the quantification of fish residues in foods. Although monoclonal antibody had also been produced against carp and bluefin tuna parvalbumin,[128,154] the cross-reactivity of these antibodies with various species of fish is largely unknown. An alternative to the antiparvalbumin antibodies is to develop antibodies that recognize specific fish proteins or peptides that are highly conserved across all fish species but do not show cross-reactivity with other nonfish species.

In addition to the ELISA-based methods, surface plasmon resonance (SPR) biosensor and PCR-based techniques for the detection of fish parvalbumin have been described. Lu et al.[155] first reported a rapid SPR biosensor for the detection and quantification of the fish allergen parvalbumin. The detection limit for parvalbumin was determined at 3.55 µg/L based on the kinetic analysis of the interaction between the purified carp parvalbumin and the monoclonal antibody against the bluefin tuna parvalbumin (MAb EG8). Moreover, the SPR biosensor analysis of the sardine fish cake and dried skipjack tuna revealed that MAb EG8 bound to a common epitope on the fish parvalbumin from different food sources. Although this assay showed a potential for use in fish parvalbumin detection and quantification, the applicability of this assay, including the detection of parvalbumin derived from additional fish species, and the quantification of fish parvalbumin in complex food matrices remained to be elucidated.

In 2007, Choi and Hong[156] published a PCR method using primers that targeted specifically the gene of mackerel parvalbumin. However, the use of this method is limited to the detection of allergenic residues derived from mackerel but not other fish species in foods. Sun et al.[150] later developed a real-time PCR method using a probe and primers that reacted specifically to the fish parvalbumin gene. The developed real-time PCR successfully amplified the DNA in 28 of the 30 fish species, with the exception of golden threadfin bream and yellowfin tuna. The sensitivity of the assay was reported at 5 pg of purified fish DNA, and cross-reactivity with 13 non-fish species was not observed. As reported by the authors, more research is required to verify the applicability of the method for additional fish species and to correlate the DNA copy numbers with the actual amount of allergenic fish residues present in foods.

All of the analytical methods published so far, regardless of protein-based or DNA-based methods for detecting allergenic fish residues, had a similar shortcoming: the inability of the existing methods to detect the undeclared fish residues derived from all species of fish in foods. Therefore, the development of methods for detecting fish allergens remains an area for more research and improvement.

Crustacean Assays

Due to the high consumption of crustacean species and the widespread use of these species in processed foods, the development of rapid and sensitive methods for detecting undeclared allergenic crustacean residues in foods has become a necessity. The first ELISA for the quantification of crustacean tropomyosin was developed by Jeoung et al.[129] In this study, tropomyosin (Pen a 1) that was purified from the crude extract of brown shrimp (*Penaeus aztecus*) was used to produce the Pen a 1-specific monoclonal antibodies. A sandwich-type ELISA was then developed using two monoclonal antibodies with different Pen a 1 epitope specificities as the capture and detector antibodies. The optimized ELISA could detect Pen a 1 at a concentration range of 4–125 ng/ml. It was observed that the ELISA was also capable of detecting Pen a 1-like proteins in crab and lobster extracts. The authors recommended the use of the developed ELISA for measuring and standardizing the Pen a 1 content in the commercial shrimp extracts used for diagnosis and immunotherapy. Even though the authors made a suggestion in regard to the detection of shrimp contamination in foods using the assay, no further studies were done to verify such potential application.

For the detection of crustaceans in both raw and cooked foods, Fuller et al.[130] described a sandwich ELISA using rabbit polyclonal antibodies raised against the purified tropomyosin from Western King prawns (*Penaeus latisulcatus*). The detection limit of the assay was reported at 1 ppm of prawn and lobster, with no cross-reactivity observed with molluscan shellfish (mussel and oyster), fish, poultry, and meat. Eight food samples were spiked with prawn extract at 7.5 ppm and were either unprocessed or cooked before testing in the ELISA. The observed recoveries for the raw and cooked food samples spiked with prawn extracts were 74–140% and 41–143%, respectively.

Werner et al.[157] developed a sandwich ELISA for the detection of crustacean tropomyosin in foods. The assay was constructed based on the affinity-purified polyclonal antibodies against the partially purified tropomyosin from shrimp (*Pandalus borealis*). The detection limit for the assay was 1 ppm (micrograms of tropomyosin/gram of food), and cross-reactivity was observed with the other crustaceans (lobster, prawn, and crab) and cockroach. Five different representative food samples that were spiked with various levels of tropomyosin (1, 10, and 100 μg/g of food samples) and detected in the developed ELISA showed recovery rates of 63–120%. The assay demonstrated reasonably good reproducibility and repeatability in detecting foods containing tropomyosins at different concentrations.

A sandwich ELISA for the detection of crustacean protein in processed foods was also described by Seiki et al.[141] Tropomyosin purified from the black tiger prawn (*Penaeus monodon*) was used to produce the antitropomyosin monoclonal and polyclonal antibodies for the ELISA. To minimize the effects of food matrices, purified porcine tropomyosin was added to the diluents used for diluting the food sample extracts prior to analysis by the ELISA. The assay was reported to have a detection limit of 1 ppm (milligrams tropomyosin/kilogram of food sample). Moreover, the assay showed high reactivity to the decapoda group in crustaceans, including prawn, shrimp, lobster, and crab, although the reactivity varied depending on the tropomyosin contents in the crustacean extracts. No cross-reactivity was observed with the cephalopoda, bivalvia, and gastropoda groups in mollusks.

In contrast to the above-mentioned ELISA, Seiki et al.[141] validated the utility of their ELISA for specific food matrices by using model processed foods that were produced under conditions that closely resembled the pilot plant or industrial manufacturing process. Three model processed foods (i.e., fish meat sausage, freeze-dried egg soup, and chicken meatball) containing crustacean protein showed mean recoveries of 85–141%. In addition, crustacean residues were detected in 15 commercial food products, with shrimp or crab declared on the food labels using the developed ELISA.

Currently, four companies offer commercial test kits for the detection of crustacean residues in foods. The Australia-based company ELISA SYSTEMS Proprietary Limited (http://www.elisas.com.au/) offers the ELISA SYSTEMS Crustacean Residue ELISA kit to screen food products for the presence of tropomyosin residues from several species of crustaceans, including shrimp, prawn, crayfish, crab, and lobster. The kit utilizes polyclonal antibodies against shrimp tropomyosin in a sandwich ELISA format. The limit of quantification for the assay was reported at 0.05 ppm of tropomyosin.

Another U.K.-based company, Tepnel Life Sciences (http://www.tepnel.com/) offers the Biokits Shellfish Assay kit for the detection and quantification of shellfish residues in foods, either cooked or uncooked. The kit was developed using polyclonal antibodies against the crustacean tropomyosin in a sandwich-type ELISA. The sensitivity of the kit is reported at 0.1 ppm. The kit shows higher specificity to the crustaceans, including crab, lobster, brown shrimp, tiger prawn, langoustine, and crayfish, but also a low level of reactivity to certain mollusks, including oyster, mussel, and squid.

In addition, two ELISA kits for detection of crustacean protein are available in Japan: Nissui Pharmaceutical Company Limited (the N kits) and Maruha Nichiro Holdings Incorporated (the M kit). Both the M and N kits use polyclonal and monoclonal antibodies to tropomyosin of the black tiger prawn (*Penaeus monodon*) with a crustacean protein solution as the calibrator. The limit of quantitation in both cases is about 0.3 mg/kg. These two ELISA kits performed well in interlaboratory evaluations with crustacean protein solutions incorporated into several different model processed foods.[158]

A SPR has also been developed for the detection of crab tropomyosin.[159] In this case, IgY antibodies were raised against purified crab tropomyosin.

Mollusk Assays

To date, no method for the detection of mollusk residues in foods has been published or commercialized. Although ELISA assays are currently available for the detection of crustacean tropomyosin, the majority of the ELISAs lack the ability to detect the molluscan tropomyosin. Monoclonal antibody against the molluscan tropomyosin has been described in the literature. Lu et al.[160] developed monoclonal antibody against Japanese abalone (*Haliotis discus*) that showed reactivity to tropomyosins from abalone, crustaceans, and chicken, but not to other mollusks. The same group of researchers later published the development of monoclonal antibodies against the American lobster (*Homarus americanus*) that showed specificity to bivalve (oyster), cephalopod (squid and octopus), and gastropod (whelk and abalone) groups in the mollusk, in addition to the crustacean tropomyosins.[161] These monoclonal antibodies could potentially be used to develop assays for detecting mollusk allergens in foods. As the Directive 2006/142/EC has amended the Annex IIIa Directive 2000/13/EC to include mollusk as one of the allergens required for labeling on the ingredient list in the European Union, a specific and sensitive method is needed for the detection of undeclared mollusk residues.[162] This method not only allows the food industry to implement effective allergen control strategies and to comply with the labeling regulations but also provides the regulatory agencies with an analytical tool to investigate consumer complaints and to evaluate the adherence of the food industry to the ingredient labeling laws and regulations.

REFERENCES

1. Göransson, K. 1981. Contact urticaria to fish. *Contact Derm.* 7:282–283.
2. Halkier-Sørensen, L. and K. Thestrup-Pedersen. 1988. Skin temperature and skin symptoms among workers in the fish processing industry. *Contact Derm.* 19:206–209.
3. Halkier-Sørensen, L. and K. Thestrup-Pedersen. 1989. Skin irritancy from fish is related to its postmortem age. *Contact Derm.* 21:172–178.
4. Crespo, J. F., C. Pascual, C. Dominguez, I. Ojeda, F. M. Muñoz, and M. M. Esteban. 1995. Allergic reactions associated with airborne fish particles in IgE-mediated fish hypersensitive patients. *Allergy.* 50:257–261.
5. Domínguez, C., I. Ojeda, J. F. Crespo, C. Pascual, A. Ojeda, and M. Martín-Esteban. 1996. Allergic reactions following skin contact with fish. *Allergy Asthma Proc.* 17:83–87.
6. Rodríguez, J., M. Reaño, R. Vives, et al. 1997. Occupational asthma caused by fish inhalation. *Allergy.* 52:866–869.

7. Helbling, A., M. L. McCants, J. J. Musmand, H. J. Schwartz, and S. B. Lehrer. 1996. Immunopathogenesis of fish allergy: identification of fish-allergic adults by skin test and radioallergosorbent test. *Ann Allergy Asthma Immunol.* 77:48–54.
8. Taylor, S. L., J. L. Kabourek, and S. L. Hefle. 2004. Fish allergy: fish and products thereof. *J Food Sci.* 69:175–180.
9. Yunginger, J. W., K. G. Sweeney, W. Q. Sturner, et al. 1988. Fatal food-induced anaphylaxis. *JAMA.* 260:1450–1452.
10. Bock, S. A., A. Muñoz-Furlong, and H. A. Sampson. 2001. Fatalities due to anaphylactic reactions to foods. *J Allergy Clin Immunol.* 107:191–193.
11. Dannaeus, A., and M. Inganäs. 1981. A follow-up study of children with food allergy. Clinical course in relation to serum IgE- and IgG-antibody levels to milk, egg and fish. *Clin Allergy.* 11:533–539.
12. Priftis, K. N., D. Mermeri, A. Papadopoulou, M. Papadopoulos, A. Fretzayas, and E. Lagona. 2008. Asthma symptoms and bronchial reactivity in school children sensitized to food allergens in infancy. *J Asthma.* 45:590–595.
13. Bock, S. A. 1982. The natural history of food hypersensitivity. *J Allergy Clin Immunol.* 69:173–177.
14. Kajosaari, M. 1982. Food allergy in Finnish children aged 1 to 6 years. *Acta Paediatr Scand.* 71:815–819.
15. Solensky, R. 2003. Resolution of fish allergy: a case report. *Ann Allergy Asthma Immunol.* 91:411–412.
16. Codex Alimentarius Commission. 1999. *Report of the twenty-third session of the Codex Alimentarius Commission*, Alinorm 99/37. Rome, Italy: Food and Agriculture Organization of the United Nations/World Health Organization.
17. Bousquet, J., B. Bjorksten, C. A. F. M. Bruijnzeel-Koomen, et al. 1998. Scientific criteria and the selection of allergenic foods for labeling. *Allergy.* 53:3–21.
18. Sicherer, S. H., A. Muñoz-Furlong, and H. A. Sampson. 2001. Prevalence of seafood allergy in the United States determined by a random telephone survey. *J Allergy Clin Immunol.* 114:159–165.
19. De Martino, M., E. Novembre, L. Galli, et al. 1990. Allergy to different fish species in cod-allergic children: In vivo and in vitro studies. *J Allergy Clin Immunol.* 86:909–914.
20. Hansen, T. K., C. Bindslev-Jensen, P. S. Skov, and L. K. Poulsen. 1997. Codfish allergy in adults: IgE cross-reactivity among fish species. *Ann Allergy Asthma Immunol.* 78:187–194.
21. Sten, E., T. K. Hansen, P. S. Skov, et al. 2004. Cross-reactivity to eel, eelpout and ocean pout in codfish-allergic patients. *Allergy.* 59:1173–1180.
22. Van Do, T, S. Elsayed, E. Florvaag, I. Hordvik, and C. Endresen. 2005. Allergy to fish parvalbumins: studies on the cross-reactivity of allergens from 9 commonly consumed fish. *J Allergy Clin Immunol.* 116:1314–1320.
23. Aas, K. 1966. Studies of hypersensitivity of fish—allergological and serological differentiation between various species of fish. *Int Arch Allergy Appl Immunol.* 30:257–267.
24. Bernhisel-Broadbent, J., S. M. Scanlon, and H. A. Sampson. 1992. Fish hypersensitivity. I. In vitro and oral challenge results in fish-allergic patients. *J Allergy Clin Immunol.* 89:730–737.
25. Helbling, A., R. Haydel, M. L. McCants, J. J. Musmand, J. El-Dahr, and S. B. Lehrer. 1999. Fish allergy: is cross-reactivity among fish species relevant? Double-blind placebo-controlled food challenge studies of fish allergic adults. *Ann Allergy Asthma Immunol.* 83:517–523.

26. Taylor, S. L., S. L. Hefle, C. Bindslev-Jensen, et al. 2002. Factors affecting the determination of threshold doses for allergenic foods: how much is too much? *J Allergy Clin Immunol.* 109:24–30.
27. James, J. M., R. M. Helm, A. W. Burks, and S. B. Lehrer. 1997. Comparison of pediatric and adult IgE antibody binding to fish proteins. *Ann Allergy Asthma Immunol.* 79:131–137.
28. Bernhisel-Broadbent, J., S. M. Scanlon, and H. A. Sampson. 1992. Fish hypersensitivity. II. Clinical relevance of altered fish allergenicity caused by various preparation methods. *J Allergy Clin Immunol.* 90:622–629.
29. Hilger, C., L. Thill, F. Grigioni, et al. 2004. IgE antibodies of fish allergic patients cross-react with frog parvalbumin. *Allergy.* 59:653–660.
30. Tuft, L. and G. I. Blumstein. 1946. Studies in food allergy. V. Antigenic relationship among members of fish family. *J Allergy.* 17:329–339.
31. Wild, L. G. and S. B. Lehrer. 2005. Fish and shellfish allergy. *Curr Allergy Asthma Rep.* 5:74–79.
32. Das Dores, S., C. Chopin, C. Villaume, J, Fleurence, and J.-L. Guéant. 2002. A new oligomeric parvalbumin allergen of Atlantic cod (Gad m I) encoded by a gene distinct from that of Gad c I. *Allergy.* 57(Suppl. 72):79–83.
33. Nakayama, S. and R. H. Kretsinger. 1994. Evolution of the EF-hand family of proteins. *Annu Rev Biophys Biomol Struct.* 23:473–507.
34. Kretsinger, R. H. and C. E. Nockolds. 1973. Carp muscle calcium-binding protein. II. Structure determination and general description. *J Biol Chem.* 248:3313–3326.
35. Strynadka, N. C. J. and M. N. G. James. 1989. Crystal structures of the helix-loop-helix calcium-binding proteins. *Annu Rev Biochem.* 58:951–998.
36. Permyakov, S. E., A. G. Bakunts, A. I. Denesyuk, E. L. Knyazeva, V. N. Uversky, and E. A. Permyakov. 2008. Apo-parvalbumin as an intrinsically disordered protein. *Proteins.* 15:822–836.
37. Erickson, J. R., and T. S. Moerland. 2006. Functional characterization of parvalbumin from the Arctic cod (*Boreogadus saida*): similarity in calcium affinity among parvalbumins from polar teleosts. *Comp Biochem Physiol Part A Mol Integr Physiol.* 143:228–233.
38. Goodman, M. and J-F. Pechére. 1977. The evolution of muscular parvalbumins investigated by the maximum parsimony method. *J Mol Evol.* 29:131–158.
39. Permyakov, E. A. 2006. *Parvalbumin.* New York: Nova Science.
40. Lim, D. L., K. H. Neo, D. L. Goh, L. P. Shek, and B. W. Lee. 2005. Missing parvalbumin: implications in diagnostic testing for tuna allergy. *J Allergy Clin Immunol.* 115:874–875.
41. Kobayashi, A., H. Tanaka, Y. Hamada, S. Ishizaki, Y. Nagashima, and K. Shiomi. 2006. Comparison of allergenicity and allergens between fish white and dark muscles. *Allergy.* 61:357–363.
42. Huriaux, F., P. Vandewalle, and B. Focant. 2002. Immunological study of muscle parvalbumin isotypes in three African catfish during development. *Comp Biochem Physiol B, Biochem Mol Biol.* 132:579–584.
43. Wilmert, J. L., N. M. Madhoun, and D. J. Coughlin. 2006. Parvalbumin correlates with relaxation rate in the swimming muscle of sheepshead and kingfish. *J Exp Biol.* 209:227–237.
44. Lindstrøm, C. D-V., T. Van Do, I. Hordvik, C. Endresen, and S. Elsayed. 1996. Cloning of two distinct cDNAs encoding parvalbumin, the major allergen of Atlantic salmon (*Salmo salar*). *Scand J Immunol.* 44:335–344.

45. Swoboda, I., A. Bugajska-Schretter, P. Verdino, et al. 2002. Recombinant carp parvalbumin, the major cross-reactivity fish allergen: a tool for diagnosis and therapy of fish allergy. *J Immunol.* 168:4576–4584.
46. Van Do, T., I. Hordvik, C. Endresen, and S. Elsayed. 2003. The major allergen (parvalbumin) of codfish is encoded by at least two isotypic genes: cDNA cloning, expression and antibody binding of the recombinant allergens. *Mol Immunol.* 39:595–602.
47. Van Do, T., I. Hordvik, C. Endresen, and S. Elsayed. 2005. Characterization of parvalbumin, the major allergen in Alaska pollack and comparison with codfish allergen M. *Mol Immunol.* 42:345–353.
48. Elsayed, S., and K. Aas. 1971. Isolation of purified allergens (cod) by isoelectric focusing. *Int Arch Allergy Appl Immunol.* 40:428–438.
49. Shiomi, K., S. Hayashi, M. Ishikawa, K. Shimakura, and Y. Nagashima. 1998. Identification of parvalbumin as an allergen in horse mackerel. *Fish Sci.* 64:300–304.
50. Shiomi, K., Y. Hamada, K. Sekiguchi, K. Shimakura, and Y. Nagashima. 1999. Two classes of allergens, parvalbumins and higher molecular weight substances, in Japanese eel and bigeye tuna. *Fish Sci.* 65:943–948.
51. Van Do, T., I. Hordvik, C. Endresen, and S. Elsayed. 1999. Expression and analysis of recombinant salmon parvalbumin, the major allergen in Atlantic salmon (*Salmo salar*). *Scand J. Immunol.* 50:619–625.
52. Hamada, Y., H. Tanaka, S. Ishizaki, M. Ishida, Y. Nagashima, and K. Shiomi. 2003. Purification, reactivity with IgE and cDNA cloning of parvalbumin as the major allergen of mackerel. *Food Chem Toxicol.* 41:1149–1156.
53. Hamada, Y., H. Tanaka, A. Sato, S. Ishizaki, Y. Nagashima, and K. Shiomi. 2004. Expression and evaluation of IgE-binding capacity of recombinant Pacific mackerel parvalbumin. *Allergol Int.* 53:271–278.
54. Elsayed, S. and K. Aas. 1971. Characterization of a major allergen (cod). Observations on effect of denaturation on the allergenic activity. *J Allergy.* 47:283–291.
55. Bugajska-Schretter, A., M. Grote, L. Vangelista, et al. 2000. Purification, biochemical, and immunological characterization of a major food allergen: different immunoglobulin E recognition of the apo- and calcium-bound forms of carp parvalbumin. *Gut.* 46:661–669.
56. Swoboda, I., A. Bugajska-Schretter, B. Linhart, et al. 2007. A recombinant hypoallergenic parvalbumin mutant for immunotherapy of IgE-mediated fish allergy. *J Immunol.* 178:6290–6296.
57. Tomura, S., S. Ishizaki, Y. Nagashima, and K. Shiomi. 2008. Reduction in the IgE reactivity of Pacific mackerel parvalbumin by mutations at Ca^{2+}-binding sites. *Fish Sci.* 74:411–417.
58. Elsayed, S. and J. Apold. 1983. Immunochemical analysis of cod fish Allergen M: locations of the immunoglobulin binding sites as demonstrated by the native and synthetic peptides. *Allergy.* 38:449–459.
59. Untersmayr, E., K. Szalai, A. B. Riemer, et al. 2006. Mimitopes identify conformational epitopes on parvalbumin, the major fish allergen. *Mol Immunol.* 43:1454–1461.
60. Yoshida, S., A. Ichimura, and K. Shiomi. 2008. Elucidation of a major IgE epitopes of Pacific mackerel parvalbumin. *Food Chem.* 111:857–861.
61. Hamada, Y., Y. Nagashima, and K. Shiomi. 2001. Identification of collagen as a new fish allergen. *Biosci Biotechnol Biochem.* 65:285–291.
62. Hamada, Y., Y. Nagashima, K. Shiomi, et al. 2003. Reactivity of IgE in fish-allergic patients to fish muscle collagen. *Allergol Int.* 52:139–147.

63. Sakaguchi, M., M. Toda, T. Ebihara, et al. 2000. IgE antibody to fish gelatin (type I collagen) in patients with fish allergy. *J Allergy Clin Immunol.* 106:579–584.
64. André, F., S. Cavagna, and C. André. 2003. Gelatin prepared from tuna skin: a risk factor for fish allergy or sensitization? *Int Arch Allergy Immunol.* 130:17–24.
65. Hansen, T. K., L. K. Poulsen, P. S. Skov, et al. 2004. A randomized, double-blinded, placebo-controlled oral challenge study to evaluate the allergenicity of commercial, food-grade fish gelatin. *Food Chem Toxicol.* 42:2037–2044.
66. Dory, D., C. Chopin, L. Aimone-Gastin, et al. 1998. Recognition of an extensive range of IgE-reactive proteins in cod extract. *Allergy.* 53:42–50.
67. Galland, A. V., D. Dory, L. Pons, et al. 1998. Purification of a 41 kDa cod-allergenic protein. *J Chromatogr B Biomed Sci Appl.* 706:63–71.
68. Das Dores, S., C. Chopin, A. Romano, et al. 2002. IgE-binding and cross-reactivity of a new 41 kDa allergen of codfish. *Allergy.* 57(Suppl. 72):84–87.
69. Lim, D. L-C., K. H. Neo, F. C. Yi, et al. 2008. Parvalbumin—the major tropical fish allergen. *Pediatr Allergy Immunol.* 19:399–407.
70. Kelso, J. M., R. T. Jones, and J. W. Yunginger. 1996. Monospecific allergy to swordfish. *Ann Allergy Asthma Immunol.* 77:227–228.
71. Das, A., P. Chakraborti, U. Chatterjee, G. Mondal, and B. P. Chatterjee. 2005. Identification of allergens in Indian fishes: Hilsa and Pomfret exemplified by ELISA and immunoblotting. *Indian J Exp Biol.* 43:1170–1175.
72. Chatterjee, U., G. Mondal, P. Chakraborti, H. K. Patra, and B. P. Chatterjee. 2006. Changes in the allergenicity during different preparations of pomfret, hilsa, bhetki and mackerel fish as illustrated by enzyme-linked immunosorbent assay and immunoblotting. *Int Arch Allergy Immunol.* 141:1–10.
73. Hefle, S. L., R. K. Bush, and S. L. Taylor. 2007. Seafood allergies. In: *Wilderness medicine*, 5th edition, ed. P. S. Auerbach, Mosby/Elsevier, Philadelphia, pp. 1559–1566.
74. Daul, C. B., J. E. Morgan, J. Hughes, and S. B. Lehrer. 1988. Provocation challenge studies in shrimp-sensitive individuals. *J Allergy Clin Immunol.* 81:1180–1186.
75. Jirapongsananuruk, O., C. Sirpramong, P. Pacharn, et al. 2008. Specific allergy to *Penaeus monodon* (seawater shrimp) or *Macrobrachium rosenbergii* (freshwater shrimp) in shrimp-allergic children. *Clin Exp Allergy.* 38:1038–1047.
76. Pumphrey, R. S. H. 2004. Fatal anaphylaxis in the U.K., 1992–2001. *Novartis Found Symp.* 257:116–128.
77. Steensma, D. P. 2003. The kiss of death: a severe allergic reaction to shellfish induced by a good-night kiss. *Mayo Clinic Proc.* 78:221–222.
78. Vierk, K. A., K. M. Koehler, S. B. Fein, and D. A. Street. 2007. Prevalence of self-reported food allergy in American adults and use of food labels. *J Allergy Clin Immunol.* 119:1504–1510.
79. Lopata, A. L. and S. B. Lehrer. 2009. New insights into seafood allergy. *Curr Opin.ion Allergy Clin Immunol.* 9:270–277.
80. Chiang, W. C., M. I, Kidon, W. K. Liew, A. Goh, J. P. L. Tang, and O. M. Chay. 2007. The changing face of food hypersensitivity in an Asian community. *Clin Exp Allergy* 37:1055–1061.
81. Waring, N. P., C. B. Daul, R. D. deShazo, M. L. McCants, and S. B. Lehrer. 1985. Hypersensitivity reactions to ingested crustaceans: clinical evaluation and diagnostic studies in shrimp-sensitive subjects. *J Allergy Clin Immunol.* 76:440–445.
82. Yu, C.-J., Y.-F. Lin, B.-L. Chiang, and L.-P. Chow. 2003. Proteomics and immunological analysis of a novel shrimp allergen, Pen m 2. *J Immunol.* 170:445–453.

83. Marinho, S., M. Morais-Almeida, A. Gaspar, et al. 2006. Barnacle allergy: allergen characterization and cross-reactivity with mites. *J Investig Allergol Clin Immunol.* 16:117–122.
84. Moreno Escobosa, M. C., L. E. Alonso, A. A. Sanchez, et al. 2002. Barnacle hypersensitivity. *Allergol Immunopathol (Madrid).* 30:100–103.
85. Suma, Y., S. Ishizaki, Y. Nagashima, Y. Lu, H. Ushio, and K. Shiomi. 2007. Comparative analysis of barnacle tropomyosin: divergence from decapods tropomyosins and role as a potential allergen. *Comp Biochem Physiol B.* 147:230–236.
86. Fernandes, J., A. Reshef, L. Patton, R. Ayuso, G. Reese, and S. B. Lehrer. 2003. Immunoglobulin E antibody reactivity to the major shrimp allergen, tropomyosin, in unexposed Orthodox Jews. *Clin Exp Allergy.* 33:956–961.
87. Van Ree, R., L. Anonicelli, J. H. Akkerdaas, et al. 1996. Asthma after consumption of snails in house dust mit allergic patients: a case of IgE cross reactivity. *Allergy.* 51:387–393.
88. Pajno, G. B., S. La Gutta, G. Barberio, G. W. Canonica, and G. Passalacqua. 2002. Harmful effect of immunotherapy on children with combined snail and mite allergy. *J Allergy Clin Immunol.* 109:627–629.
89. Jeong, K. Y., C.-S. Hong, and T.-S. Yong. 2006. Allergenic tropomyosins and their cross-reactivities. *Protein Peptide Lett.* 13:835–845.
90. Shanti, K. N., B. M. Martin, S. Nagpal, D. D. Metcalfe, and P. V. Rao. 1993. Identification of tropomyosin as the major shrimp allergen and characterization of its IgE-binding epitopes. *J Immunol.* 151:5354–5363.
91. Daul, C. B., M. Slattery, G. Reese, and S. B. Lehrer. 1994. Identification of the major brown shrimp (*Penaeus aztecus*) allergen as the muscle protein tropomyosin. *Int Arch Allergy Immunol.* 105:49–55.
92. Motoyama, K., S. Ishizaki, Y. Nagashima, and K. Shiomi. 2006. Cephalopod tropomyosins: identification as major allergens and molecular cloning. *Food Chem Toxicol.* 44:1997–2002.
93. Reese, G., R. Ayuso, and S. B. Lehrer. 1999. Tropomyosin: an invertebrate pan-allergen. *Int Arch Allergy Immunol.* 119:247–258.
94. Ayuso, R., S. B. Lehrer, L. Tanaka, et al. 1999. IgE antibody response to vertebrate meat proteins including tropomyosin. *Ann Allergy Asthma Immunol.* 83:399–405.
95. Goodman, R. E., A. Silvanovich, R. E. Hileman, G. A. Bannon, E. A. Rice, and J. D. Astwood. 2002. Bioinformatic methods for identifying known or potential allergens in the safety assessment of genetically modified crops. *Commun Toxicol.* 8:251–269.
96. Taylor, S. L. 2008. Molluscan shellfish allergy. *Adv Food Nutr Res.* 54:139–177.
97. Ayuso, R., S. B. Lehrer, and G. Reese. 2002. Identification of continuous, allergenic regions of the major shrimp allergen Pen a 1 (tropomyosin). *Int Arch Allergy Immunol.* 127:27–37.
98. Reese, G., R. Ayuso, T. Carle, and S. B. Lehrer. 1999. IgE-binding epitopes of shrimp tropomyosin, the major allergen Pen a 1. *Int Arch Allergy Immunol.* 118:300–301.
99. Garcia-Orozco, K. D., E. Aispuro-Hernandez, G. Yepiz-Plascencia, A. M. Calderon de la Barca, and R. R. Sotelo-Mundo. 2007. Molecular characterization of arginine kinase, an allergen from the shrimp, *Litopenaeus vannamei. Int Arch Allergy Immunol.* 144:23–28.
100. Ayuso, R., G. Grishina, L. Bardina, et al. 2008. Myosin light chain is a novel shrimp allergen, Lit v 3. *J Allergy Clin Immunol.* 122:795–802.

101. Shiomi, K., Y. Sato, S. Hamamoto, H. Mita, and K. Shimakura. 2008. Sacroplasmic calcium-binding protein: identification as a new allergen of the black tiger shrimp *Penaeus monodon*. *Int Arch Allergy Immunol.* 146:91–98.
102. Ayuso, R., G. Grishina, M. D. Ibanez, et al. 2009. Sarcoplasmic calcium-binding protein is an EF-hand-type protein identified as a new shrimp allergen. *J Allergy Clin Immunol.* 124:114–120.
103. Gonzalez Galan, I., J. M. Garcia Menaya, G. Jimenez Ferrera, and G. Gonzalez Mateos. 2002. Anaphylactic shock to oysters and white fish with generalized urticaria to prawns and white fish. *Allergol Immunopathol.* 30:300–303.
104. Morikawa, A., M. Kato, K. Tokuyama, T. Kuroume, M. Minoshima, and S. Iwata. 1990. Anaphylaxis to grand keyhole limpet (abalone-like shellfish) and abalone. *Ann Allergy.* 65:415–417.
105. Maeda, S., A. Morikawa, M. Kato, et al. 1991. Eleven cases of anaphylaxis caused by grand keyhole limpet (abalone-like shellfish). *Arerugi.* 40:1415–1420.
106. Wu, A. Y. and G. A. Williams. 2004. Clinical characteristics and pattern of skin test reactivities in shellfish allergy patients in Hong Kong. *Allergy Asthma Proc.* 25:237–241.
107. Rance, F., X. Grandmollet, and H. Grandjean. 2005. Prevalence and main characteristics of schoolchildren diagnosed with food allergies in France. *Clin Exp Allergy.* 35:167–172.
108. Eriksson, N. E., C. Moller, S. Werner, J. Magnusson, U. Bengtsson, and M. Zolubus. 2004. Self-reported food hypersensitivity in Sweden, Denmark, Estonia, Lithuania, and Russia. *J Investig Allergol Clin Immunol.* 14:70–79.
109. Castillo, R., J. Delgado, J. Quiralte, C. Blanco, and T. Carillo. 1996. Food hypersensitivity among adult patients: epidemiological and clinical aspects. *Allergol Immunopathol.* 24:93–7.
110. Crespo, J. F., C. Pascual, A. W. Burks, R. M. Helm, and M. M. Esteban. 1995. Frequency of food allergy in a pediatric population in Spain. *Pediatr Allergy Immunol.* 6:39–43.
111. Ebisawa, M., K. Ikematsu, T. Imai, and H. Tachimoto. 2003. Food allergy in Japan. *Allergy Clin Immunol Int.* 15:214–217.
112. Lopata, A. L., C. Zinn, and P. C. Potter. 1997. Characteristics of hypersensitivity reactions and identification of a unique 49 Kd IgE-binding protein (Hal-m-1) in abalone (*Haliotis midae*). *J Allergy Clin Immunol.* 100:642–648.
113. Vuitton, D. A., F. Rance, M. L. Paquin, et al. 1998. Cross-reactivity between terrestrial snails (*Helix* species) and house-dust mite (*Dermatophagoides pteronyssinus*). I. In vivo study. *Allergy.* 53:144–150.
114. Carrillo, T., F. R. de Castro, M. Cuevas, J. Caminero, and P. Carbrera. 1991. Allergy to limpet. *Allergy.* 46:515–519.
115. Sicherer, S. H., A. Muñoz-Furlong, and H. A. Sampson. 2004. Prevalence of seafood allergy in the United States determined by a random telephone survey. *J Allergy Clin Immunol.* 114:159–165.
116. Laffond, Y. E. 1996. Reacciones alergicas por molluscos y crustaceos. *Allergol Immunol. (Madrid).* 24(Suppl. 1):36–44.
117. Azofra, J. and M. Lombardero. 2003. Limpet anaphylaxis: cross-reactivity between limpet and house-dust mite *Dermatophagoides pteronyssinus. Allergy.* 58:1146–1149.
118. DeMaat-Bleeker, F., J. H. Akkerdaas, R. van Ree, and R. C. Aalberse. 1995. Vineyard snail allergy possibly induced by sensitivity to house dust mite. *Ann Allergy.* 50:438–440.
119. Emoto, A., S. Ishizaki, and K. Shiomi. 2009. Tropomyosins in gastropods and bivalves: identification as major allergens and amino acid sequence features. *Food Chem.* 114:634–641.

120. Asturias, J. A., E. Eraso, M. C. Arilla, et al. 2002. Cloning, isolation, and IgE-binding properties of *Helix aspersa* (brown garden snail) tropomyosin. *Int Arch Allergy Immunol.* 128:90–96.
121. Ishikawa, M., M. Ishida, K. Shimakura, Y. Nagashima, and K. Shiomi. 1998. Tropomyosin, the major oyster *Crassotrea gigas* allergen and its IgE-binding epitopes. *J Food Sci.* 63:44–47.
122. Ishikawa, M., Y. Nagashima, and K. Shiomi. 1998. Identification of the oyster allergen Cra g 2 as tropomyosin. *Fish Sci.* 64:854–855.
123. Ishikawa, M., M. Ishida, K. Shimakura, Y. Nagashima, and K. Shiomi. 1998. Purification and IgE-binding properties of a major allergen in the gastropod *Turbo cornutus*. *Biosci Biotechnol Biochem.* 62:1337–1343.
124. Chu, K. H., S. H. Wong, and P. S. C. Leung. 2000. Tropomyosin is the major mollusk allergen: reverse transcriptase polymerase chain reaction, expression and IgE reactivity. *Marine Biotechnol.* 2:499–509.
125. Martins, L. M. L., G. Peltre, C. J. da Costa Faro, E. M. Vieira Pires, and F. F. de Cruz Inacio. 2005. The *Helix aspersa* (brown garden snail) allergen repertoire. *Int Arch Allergy Immunol.* 136:7–15.
126. Hefle, S. L. 1995. Immunoassay fundamentals. *Food Technol.* 49:102–107.
127. Goldsby, R. A., T. J. Kindt, B. A. Osborne, and J. Kuby. 2003. *Immunology*, 5th edition. New York: Freeman.
128. Celio, M. R., W. Baier, L. Schärer, P. A. De Viragh, and C. H. Gerday. 1988. Monoclonal antibodies directed against the calcium binding protein parvalbumin. *Cell Calcium.* 9:81–86.
129. Jeoung, B.-J., G. Reese, P. Hauck, J. B. Oliver, C. B. Daul, and S. B. Lehrer. 1997. Quantification of the major brown shrimp allergen Pen a 1 (tropomyosin) by a monoclonal antibody-based sandwich ELISA. *J Allergy Clin Immunol.* 100:229–234.
130. Fuller, H. R., P. R. Goodwin, and G. E. Morris. 2006. An enzyme-linked immunosorbent assay (ELISA) for the major crustacean allergen, tropomyosin, in food. *Food Agric Immunol.* 17:43–52.
131. Fæste, C. K. and C. Plassen. 2008. Quantitative sandwich ELISA for the determination of fish in foods. *J Immunol. Methods.* 329:45–55.
132. Davis, P. J. and S. C. Williams. 1998. Protein modification by thermal processing. *Allergy.* 53:S102–S105.
133. Taylor, S. L., J. A. Nordlee, L. M. Niemann, and D. M. Lambrecht. 2009. Allergen immunoassays—considerations for use of naturally incurred standards. *Anal Bioanal Chem.* 395:1618–2642.
134. Immer, U. 2006. Factors affecting the effectiveness of allergen detection. In *Detecting allergens in foods*, ed. S. J. Koppelman and S. L. Hefle, Woodhead, Cambridge, UK, pp. 330–347.
135. Wen, H.-W., W. Borejsza-Wysocki, T. R. DeCory, A. J. Baeumner, and R. A. Durst. 2005. A novel extraction method for peanut allergic proteins in chocolate and their detection by a liposome-based flow assay. *Eur Food Res Technol.* 221:564–569.
136. Li-Chan, E. C. Y. 2004. Properties of proteins in food systems: an introduction. In *Proteins in food processing*, ed. R. Y. Yada, CRC Press, Boca Raton, FL, pp. 2–26.
137. Sathe, S. K., S. S. Teuber, and K. H. Roux. 2005. Effects of food processing on the stability of food allergens. *Biotechnol Adv.* 23:423–429.
138. Van Hengel A. J. 2007. Food allergen detection methods and the challenge to protect food allergic consumers. *Anal Bioanal Chem.* 389:111–118.

139. Poms, R. E. and E. Anklam. 2004. Effects of chemical, physical, and technological processes on the nature of food allergens. *J AOAC Int.* 87:1466–1474.
140. Watanabe, Y., K. Aburatani, T. Mizumura, et al. 2005. Novel ELISA for the detection of raw and processed egg using extraction buffer containing a surfactant and a reducing agent. *J Immunol Methods.* 300:115–123.
141. Seiki, K., H. Oda, H. Yoshioka, et al. 2007. A reliable and sensitive immunoassay for the determination of crustacean protein in processed foods. *J Agric Food Chem.* 55:9345–9350.
142. Esteve-Romero, J. S., I. M. Yman, A. Bossi, and P. G. Righetti. 1996. Fish species identification by isoelectric focusing of parvalbumins in immobilized pH gradients. *Electrophoresis.* 17:1380–1385.
143. Civera, T. 2003. Species identification and safety of fish products. *Vet Res Commun.* 27:481–489.
144. Huang, T.-S., M. R. Marshall, K.-J. Kao, W. S. Otwell, and C.-I. Wei. 1995. Development of monoclonal antibodies for red snapper (*Lutjanus campechanus*) identification using enzyme-linked immunosorbent assay. *J Agric Food Chem.* 43:2301–2307.
145. Carrera, E., R. Martín, T. García, I. González, B. Sanz, and P. E. Hernández. 1996. Development of an enzyme-linked immunosorbent assay for the identification of smoked salmon (*Salmo salar*), trout (*Oncorhynchus mykiss*) and bream (*Brama raii*). *J Food Prot.* 59:521–524.
146. Asensio, L., I. González, M. A. Rodríguez, P.E. Hernández, T. García, and R. Martín. 2003. Development of a monoclonal antibody for grouper (*Epinephelus marginatus*) and wreck fish (*Polyprion americanus*) authentication using an indirect ELISA. *J Food Sci.* 68:1900–1903.
147. Asensio, L., L. Samaniego, M. A. Pavón, I. González, T. García, and R. Martín. 2008. Detection of grouper mislabeling in the fish market by an immunostick colorimetric ELISA assay. *Food Agric Immunol.* 19:141–147.
148. Gil, L. A. 2007. PCR-based methods for fish and fishery products authentication. *Trends Food Sci Technol.* 18:558–566.
149. Rasmussen, R. S. and M. T. Morrissey. 2008. DNA-based methods for the identification of commercial fish and seafood species. *Compr Rev Food Sci Food Saf.* 7:280–295.
150. Sun, M., C. Liang, H. Gao, C. Lin, and M. Deng. 2009. Detection of parvalbumin, a common fish allergen gene in food, by real-time polymerase chain reaction. *J AOAC Int.* 92:234–240.
151. Carrera, M., B. Cañas, C. Piñeiro, J. Vázquez, and J. M. Gallardo. 2006. Identification of commercial hake and grenadier species by proteomic analysis of parvalbumin fraction. *Proteomics.* 6:5278–5287.
152. Chen, L., S. L. Hefle, S. L. Taylor, I. Swoboda, and R. E. Goodman. 2006. Detecting fish parvalbumin with commercial mouse monoclonal anti-frog parvalbumin IgG. *J Agric Food Chem.* 54:5577–5582.
153. Gajewski, K. G. and Y-H. P. Hsieh. 2009. Monoclonal antibody specific to a major fish allergen: parvalbumin. *J Food Prot.* 72:818–825.
154. Kawase, S., H. Ushio, T. Ohshima, H. Yamanaka, and H. Fukuda. 2001. Preparation of monoclonal antibodies against tuna parvalbuin. *Fish Sci.* 67:559–561.
155. Lu, Y., T. Ohshima, and H. Ushio. 2008. Rapid detection of fish major allergen parvalbumin by surface plasmon resonance biosensor. *J Food Sci.* 69:C652–C658.
156. Choi, K. Y. and K. W. Hong. 2007. Genomic DNA sequence of mackerel parvalbumin and a PCR test for rapid detection of allergenic mackerel ingredients in food. *Food Sci Biotechnol.* 16:67–70.

157. Werner, M. T., C. K. Fæste, and E. Egaas. 2007. Quantitative sandwich ELISA for the detection of tropomyosin from crustaceans in foods. *J Agric Food Chem.* 55:8025–8032.
158. Sakai, S., R. Matsuda, R. Adachi, et al. 2008. Interlaboratory evaluation of two enzyme-linked immunosorbent assay kits for the determination of crustacean protein in processed foods. *J AOAC Int.* 91:123–129.
159. Yman, I. M., A. Eriksson, M. A. Johansson, and K.-E. Hellenas. 2006. Food allergen detection with biosensor immunoassays. *J AOAC Int.* 89:856–861.
160. Lu, Y., T. Ohshima, H. Ushio, and K. Shiomi. 2004. Preparation and characterization of monoclonal antibody against abalone allergen tropomyosin. *Hybrid Hybridomics* 23:357–361.
161. Lu, Y., T. Ohshima, H. Ushio, Y. Hamada, and K. Shiomi. 2007. Immunological characteristics of monoclonal antibodies against shellfish major allergen tropomyosin. *Food Chem.* 100:1093–1099.
162. European Commission. 2006. Commission Directive 2006/142/EC of 22 December 2006 amending Annex IIIa of Directive 2000/13/EC of the European Parliament and of the Council listing the ingredients which must under all circumstances appear on the labeling of foodstuffs. *Off. J. Eur. Union.* L 368:110–111.
163. Leung, P. S. C., K. H. Chu, W. K. Chow, et al. 1994. Cloning, expression, and primary structure of *Metapenaeus ensis* tropomyosin, the major heat-stable shrimp allergen. *J Allergy Clin Immunol.* 94:882–890.
164. Lin, R. Y., H. D. Shen, and S. H. Han. 1993. Identification and characterization of a 30-Kd major allergen from *Parapenaeus fissures*. *J Allergy Clin Immunol.* 92:837–845.
165. Witteman, A. M., J. H. Akkerdaas, J. van Leeuwen, J. S. van der Zee, and R. C. Aalberse. 1994. Identification of a cross-reactive allergen (presumably tropomyosin) in shrimp, mites and insects. *Int Arch Allergy Immunol.* 105:56–61.
166. DeWitt, A. M., L. Mattson, I. Lauer, G. Reese, and J. Lidholm. 2004. Recombinant tropomyosin from *Penaeus aztecus* (rPen a 1) for measurement of specific immunoglobulin E antibodies relevant in food allergy to crustaceans and other invertebrates. *Mol Nutr Food Res.* 48:370–379.
167. Motoyama, K., Y. Suma, S. Ishizaki, Y. Nagashima, and K. Shiomi. 2007. Molecular cloning of tropomyosins identified as allergens in six species of crustaceans. *J Agric Food Chem.* 55:985–991.
168. Leung, P. S. C., W. K. Chow, S. Duffey, H. S. Kwan, M. E. Gershwin, and K. H. Chu. 1996. IgE reactivity against a cross-reactive allergen in crustacea and mollusca: evidence for tropomyosin as the common allergen. *J Allergy Clin Immunol.* 98:954–961.
169. Mykles, D. L., J. L. Cotton, H. Taniguchi, K. Sano, and Y. Maeda. 1998. Cloning of tropomyosins from lobster (*Homarus americanus*) striated muscles: fast and slow isoforms may be generated from the same transcript. *J Muscle Res Cell Motil.* 19:105–115.
170. Leung, P. S. C., Y. C. Chen, D. L. Mykles, W. K. Chow, C. P. Li, and K. H. Chu. 1998. Molecular characterization of the lobster muscle protein tropomyosin as a seafood allergen. *Mol Mar Biol Biotechnol.* 7:12–20.
171. Leung, P. S. C., Y. C. Chen, M. E. Gershwin, S. H. Wong, H. S. Kwan, and K. H. Chu. 1998. Identification and molecular characterization of *Charybdis feriatus* tropomyosin, the major crab allergen. *J Allergy Clin Immunol.* 102:847–852.
172. Hua, Z. Q., X.-Z. Wang, L.-J. Chen, L. I. Wen, and Y.-P. Liu. 2007. Purification, identification and characterization of the major allergen from Linnaeus. *Chin J Immunol.* 23:256–259.

173. Choi, J. H., S. Yoon, Y. J. Suh, et al. 2003. Measurement of specific IgE to abalone (*Haliotis discus hannai*) and identification of IgE-binding components. *Korean J Asthma Allergy Clin Immunol.* 23:349–357.
174. Leung, P. S. C. and K. H. Chu. 1998. Molecular and immunological characterization of shellfish allergens. *Front Biosci.* 3:306–312.
175. Lee, B.-J. and H.-S. Park. 2004. Common whelk (*Buccinum undatum*) allergy: identification of IgE-binding components and effects of heating and digestive enzymes. *J Korean Med Sci.* 19:703–799.
176. Jiménez, M., F. Pineda, I. Sánchez, I. Orozco, and C. Senent. 2005. Allergy due to *Ensis macha. Allergy.* 60:1090–1091.
177. Ishikawa, M., K. Shimakura, Y. Nagashima, and K. Shiomi. 1997. Isolation and properties of allergenic proteins in the oyster *Crassostrea gigas. Fish Sci.* 63:610–614.
178. Leung, P. S. C. and K. H. Chu. 2001. cDNA cloning and molecular identification of the major oyster allergen from the Pacific oyster *Crassostrea gigas. Clin Exp Allergy.* 31:1287–1294.
179. Nakamura, A., K. Watanabe, T. Ojima, D. H. Ahn, and H. Saeki. 2005. Effect of Maillard reaction on allergenicity of scallop tropomyosin. *J Agric Food Chem.* 53:7559–7564.
180. Ishikawa, M., F. Suzuki, M. Ishida, Y. Nagashima, and K. Shiomi. 2001. Identification of tropomyosin as a major allergen in the octopus *Octopus vulgaris* and elucidation of its IgE-binding epitopes. *Fish Sci.* 67:934–942.
181. Miyazawa, H., H. Fukamachi, Y. Inagaki, et al. 1996. Identification of the first major allergen of a squid (*Todarodes pacificus*). *J Allergy Clin Immunol.* 98:948–953.

Index

2D-PAGE detection, 166
2S albumins, 33, 51
7S globulins, 35, 81
11S globulins, 35, 81

A

Adverse reactions, 5
Albumins, isolation via aqueous buffers, 50
AllAllergy database, 32
Allergen Database, 32
Allergen Database for Food Safety, 32
Allergen databases, 31–32
Allergen isolation
    legumes, 50–51
    lupin, 51–52
    peanut, 51
    soybean, 51
Allergen nomenclature, 32–33
Allergen properties, 31
    allergen databases, 31–32
    lupin allergens, 45–48
    nomenclature, 32–33
    peanut allergens, 36–40
    protein families with legume allergens, 33–36
    soybean allergens, 40–41, 44–45
Allergen sequences, Internet-based, 32
Allergen structures, Internet-based, 32
Allergen testing, rationale, 13–14
Allergenic foods
    analysis, 7
    detection methods, 8–9
    labeling requirements, 6
    major, 4–5
    managing to protect consumers, 3–4
Allergenic proteins, 2
AllergenOnline database, 32, 39, 41
Allergens, 2. *See also* Food allergens
Allergome database, 32, 39, 46
    peanut allergens in, 36
AllerMatch database, 32
AllFam database, 31, 32
Almond
    commercial test kits, 119
    DNA detection methods, 92
    known single allergens, 82
    potential and limitations of published methods, 102–103
    protein-based detection techniques, 84–85
Almond major protein (AMP), 102
Alpha-amylase/protease inhibitors, 156

Alpha-amylase/trypsin inhibitors, 156
Alpha-lactalbumin, 129
    capillary electrophoresis detection, 135
    liquid-liquid extraction method, 134
Alpha-livetin, 138, 139, 142, 157
Alpha-parvalbumin, 180
Amino acid sequence homologues, 181
    lupin allergens, 47
    peanut allergens, 38–39
    soybean allergens, 42–44
Analytical methods, 5–7. *See also* Separation and analysis methods
    challenges, 8
    legume allergens, 53–54
    validation of, 8
Anaphylactic reactions, 14
    to crustaceans, 183
    to fish, 178
    to mollusks, 186
    to soy allergens, 157
    to tree nuts, sesame seeds, mustard, celery, 78
Anxiety, due to food allergies, 3
AOAC-approved allergen detection kits, 164
Apovitellenin, 138, 139
Arginine kinase, 184–185
Array technology, 102
Association of Analytical Communities (AOAC) Presidential Task Force, 24
Australia
    allergenic foods regulated by, 6
    labeling requirements, 14, 80
Austria, RASFF notifications, 159, 160
Awareness, of food allergy, 1

B

Barley, 165, 166
    allergens in, 155, 156
    CMb inhibitor in, 156
    commercial test kits, 163
Basophile histamine release assay, 53
Bean, 31
Belgium, RASFF notifications, 159
Benchmark dose (BMD), 18, 19
Bet v 1-related proteins, 35, 40, 81
    soybean allergens in, 42
Beta-casein, 137
Beta-lactoglobulin, 129, 131, 133, 136
    detection of, 144
    thermostability, 133
Beta-parvalbumin, 180

INDEX

Big 8, 7, 41
Bioinformatic analysis, 22
Biosensor assay, 53, 101, 162, 167
 for cow's milk proteins, 137
 for hazelnut detection, 87, 88
 for peanut analysis, 57
 for sesame allergen detection, 89
 for soybean analysis, 60
Bird-egg syndrome, 138
Bivalvia, 186
 tropomyosin allergens in, 188
Bovine gelatin allergy, 182
Bovine serum albumin, 129
Brazil nut
 allergic reactions, 78
 DNA detection methods, 92
 known single allergens, 82
 ligation-dependent probe amplification detection, 92
 potential and limitations of published methods, 103–104
 protein-based detection techniques, 85
Breakfast cereals, egg contamination, 157
British Standards Institution 2010, 24
Buckwheat allergy, 6

C

Canada
 allergen labeling, 80
 allergenic foods regulated by, 6
 gluten labeling, 5
 labeling requirements, 14
 RASFF notifications, 159
Capillary electrophoresis, 102, 134, 167
 separating milk proteins with, 135
Caseins, 129, 130
 detecting with sandwich ELISA, 135
 detection in cereals, 169–170
 thermostability, 133
Cashew nut
 DNA detection methods, 92–93
 known single allergens, 82
 potential and limitations of published methods, 104–106
 protein-based detection techniques, 86
 real-time PCR detection, 92
Celery, 78
 allergen labeling by country, 79–80, 80–81
 allergenic properties, 81, 83
 allergens in, 77–78
 commercial test kits for allergen detection, 118–119
 detection and quantification, 100–102

 detection in cereals, 155
 DNA detection methods, 92–97
 known single allergens, 82
 labeling requirements, 154
 potential and limitations of published methods, 116–118
 in processed foods, 158
 protein-based detection techniques, 91
 sample preparation, 99–100
Celery allergens, 5, 6, 9, 17
 methodology aspects, 83, 98
 thresholds and symptoms of allergic reactions, 78–81
Celiac disease, 13, 156
 and cereal-based allergens, 155–156
Cell-based release assay, for soybean analysis, 60
Cephalopoda, 186
 tropomyosin allergens in, 188
Cereal allergens
 detection, 153
 detection in cereal food products, 164–168
 detection methods, 158, 162
Cereal allergies, 6, 9
 gluten-containing, 8
 labeling requirements, 15
Cereals
 as allergens, 155–156
 egg allergens in, 156–157, 168–169
 milk allergens in, 157
 sesame protein detection in, 170–171
 soy detection in, 170
 whey proteins and caseins in, 169–170
Chestnut, known single allergens, 82
Chickpeas, 31
Children
 emotional stress due to allergy, 3
 food allergy prevalence, 1, 14
China, RASFF notifications, 159, 160
Chocolate manufacture, contamination risks, 20
Chromatography detection, 54
 for lupin, 54, 62
 for peanut analysis, 58
 for soybean analysis, 61
Class A pollen coat proteins, 35
CMb inhibitor, 156
Cod
 allergies to, 178–179
 DBPCFC tests, 179
Codex Alimentarius Commission, 5
 allergenic foods regulated by, 6
 Standard for Gluten Free Products, 154, 156
Codex Committee on Food Labeling, 5
Codex guidelines, 14
Collagen, as fish allergen, 181

Commercial test kits, 162, 166, 171
   for allergen detection, 118–119
   AOAC-approved, 164
   for cereal-based allergens, 163, 165
   for crustacean protein detection, 194
   for egg allergen detection, 144–145
   ELISA-based, 163
   for sesame detection, 170
Competitive ELISA, 101, 104, 162
   for almond allergen detection, 84
   for Brazil nut allergen detection, 85, 103
   for cow's milk protein detection, 136
   for hazelnut allergen detection, 87, 88
   for mustard allergen detection, 90
   for pecan allergen detection, 89, 110
   for sesame detection, 115
Competitive PCR detection, 167
Conalbumin, 137, 139
Confections, milk allergens in, 157
Consumer protection, against allergenic foods, 3–4
Contaminants, challenges for immunological methods, 23
Cookies, milk contamination, 157
Cooking procedures, adverse effects on ELISAs, 24
Cow's milk allergens, 129, 131, 133, 157, 169
   casseins, 130
   cross-reactivity with milk of other species, 157
   detection, 135–137
   distinguishing from milk of other species, 135
   isolation of, 134–135
   properties, 130
   whey proteins, 130
Cow's milk allergy, 17
   prevalence, 132
Creams, egg contamination, 157
Cross-contact, 17
   legislation in Japan and Switzerland, 17
   minimizing, 20
Cross-contamination, 6, 107
   avoidance with ELISA testing, 107
Cross-linking, of milk proteins, 133, 134
Cross-reactivity, 4
   among crustacean species, 183–184
   among fish species, 178, 182
   among molluscan species, 186–187, 188
   in celery detection, 117
   with commercial test kits, 118
   between cow's milk proteins and other species, 131
   of ELISA testing, 118
   in hazelnut allergen detection, 108
   between hen's eggs and eggs of other species, 156
   of invertebrate-species allergens, 184
   involving parvalbumin, 179–180
   to lupin and other legume allergens, 46
   with milks of various species, 157
   within mollusk classes, 187
   in mustard testing, 116
   in pecan allergen detection, 110
   in pistachio detection, 110
   in PR10 proteins, 35
   of SCP, 185
   and sequence homology, 33
   between soy and other allergens, 157
   in walnut allergen detection, 112
Crustacean allergens, 184–186
   arginine kinase, 184, 185
   detection and quantification methods, 189–195
   ELISA test kits for, 194
   labeling requirements, 178
   persistence of, 183
   sarcoplasmic calcium-binding protein (SCP), 185
   tropomyosin type, 184, 185
Crustaceans, 6, 8, 177–178. *See also* Shellfish allergy
   allergenic properties, 183–186
   allergic reactions to, 183
   assays, 193–195
   cross-reactivity among species, 183–184
   labeling requirements, 15, 154
   threshold of allergenicity, 184
Cupin protein family, 34–35, 81
   peanut allergens in, 38
   soybean allergens in, 42
Cysteine protease inhibitors, in soybeans, 43

D

D-Gallactose-binding lectin, in peanut allergens, 39
Dairy products, labeling requirements, 154
Dark chocolate, peanut allergens in, 23
Dedicated utensils, 20
Defensin protein family, 41
   soybean allergens in, 42
Delayed hypersensitivity, 2
Denmark, RASFF notifications, 161
Derogations. *See* EU derogations
Detection limit, 162
Detection methods, 13
   for allergenic foods, 8–9

AOAC-approved kits, 164
  for cereal-based allergens, 158–164
  DNA methods, 21
  ELISA, 162–163
  ELISA commercial test kits, 163
  for fish, crustacean, and molluscan allergens, 189–195
  general characteristics, 23
  immunoassay methods, 22
  legume allergens, 55, 58
  lupin allergens, 58
  mass spectrometry, 22–23
  method application, validation, and standardization, 23–24
  milk allergens, 135–137
  past, present, future, 20
  peanut allergens, 55, 56–58
  polymerase chain reaction, 164
  protein-based methods, 84–91
  sample extraction, 190–191
  soybean allergens, 58
Dietetic foods, 14
Dipstick detection methods, 22, 23, 163, 166
  for egg allergens, 145
DNA detection methods, 21, 98
  comparison with protein-based methods, 120
  egg detection challenges, 23
  for fish assays, 191
  for legume allergens, 52–53
  for tree nuts, sesame, mustard, celery, 92–97
Dot blot, 53
  for Brazil nut allergen detection, 85
  for multiplex tree nut assays, 113
  for peanut analysis, 56
  for soybean analysis, 59
Double-blind placebo-controlled food challenge (DBPCFC), 18, 78, 131
  fish, 179
Dressings, egg contamination, 157
Dust mites
  cross-reactivity to mollusk species, 187
  homology to crustacean allergens, 184

E

Egg allergens, 129
  allergenicity-reducing techniques, 141
  in cereals, 155, 168–169
  commercial test kits, 163
  detection, 143–145
  hen's egg allergens, 137, 138, 141
  isolation of, 141–143
  labeling requirements, 154
  prevalence, 140
  in processed food, 156–157
  properties, 139
Egg allergy, 5, 6, 9, 17
  labeling requirements, 15
  NIST reference materials, 24
Egg white
  allergens in, 139
  detection in cereals, 169
  detection through pH change, 142, 143
  thermostability of allergens, 138
Egg yolk, allergens in, 138, 139
Electrophoretic techniques, in fish assays, 191
Electrospray ionization tandem MS (ESI-MS-MS), 23
Elimination diets, 5
ELISA testing, 8, 100, 106, 120, 162, 165. *See also* Competitive ELISA; Sandwich ELISA
  96-well plate format, 22
  adverse effects of cooking procedures, 24
  for cashew detection, 104, 105
  for celery detection, 118
  for cereal-based allergens, 162–163
  commercial test kits, 163, 194
  correlation with PCR tests, 121
  for cow's milk allergens, 133, 136
  in crustacean assays, 193
  for egg allergen detection, 145, 168
  for fish, crustacean, and molluscan allergens, 189
  for fish assays, 191, 194
  general characteristics, 23
  for hazelnut allergen detection, 107
  for hen's egg detection, 143
  for multiple tree nuts, 114
  for mustard detection, 115
  for peanut allergens, 55
  for pecan detection, 109
  quantitative, 144
  for soy detection, 170
Enzyme-allergosorbent test (EAST), 53
  for lupin analysis, 62
  for peanut analysis, 57
  for soybean analysis, 60
Enzyme immunoasays (EIAs), 53
  for lupin analysis, 62
  for multiple tree nuts, 113
  for peanut analysis, 56–57
  for soybean analysis, 59–60
Enzyme-linked immunosorbent assay (ELISA) methods, 8, 22, 83. *See also* ELISA testing
EU derogations, 14, 15–16, 18
Eukaryotic aspartyl proteases, 36

European Commission
    allergens working group, 24
    derogations, 15–16
    Directive 2000/13/EC, 5
    Directive 2003/89/EC, 3, 5
    Directive 2006/142/EC, 195
    Directive 2007/68/EC, 3, 154
    General Food Law, 17
    mollusk labeling, 195
    Regulation EC No 41/2009, 155
European Committee for Standardization (CEN), 24
European Food Safety Authority (EFSA), 14
European Joint Research Centre (JRC), 55
European Union
    allergenic foods regulated by, 6
    inclusion of molluscan shellfish by, 178
    labeling requirements, 14, 154–155
    mandatory declarations, 9
    Rapid Alert System for Food and Feed (RASFF), 7
    Regulation 178/2002/EC, 17
Extractability, factors affecting, 49

F

Fenugreek, 31
Fish
    allergenic properties, 178–183
    allergic reactions to, 178
    assays, 191–193
    cross-reactivity among species, 178–179
    persistence of allergies to, 178
Fish allergens, 5, 6, 8, 9, 17, 177–178, 179–183
    and bovine gelatin allergy, 182
    collagen, 181
    detection and quantification methods, 189–195
    Gad c 1, 180–181
    in hilsa and pomfret, 182–183
    labeling requirements, 15, 154, 178
    lifelong, 2
    miscellaneous proteins, 182
    parvalbumin, 179–181
Fish assays, 191–193
Fluorescence polarization-based immunoassay, 53
Food Allergen Labeling and Consumer Protection Act (FALCPA), 4, 5, 14, 80
Food allergens, 154
    in cereals, 153
    detection of, 13
    labeling requirements, 14, 17, 154–155
    in legumes, 31
    major, 4–5
    managing in food production, 19–20
    in peanut, soybean, lupin, 23–25
    rationale for testing, 13–14
    sample extraction and cleanup, 48–52
    in tree nuts, sesame seeds, mustard, celery, 77–78
Food allergy
    analytical methods and instrumentation, 4–7
    growing awareness of, 1–2
    improved diagnosis, 1
    incidence, 1
    method performance, 8
    prevalence, 1
Food avoidance, 14
Food challenges, 5, 18
Food matrix complexity, 23
    with egg contamination, 157
    and fish allergen extraction, 190
    masking of allergens by, 162
    and preparation of total legume extracts, 49
Food production, managing allergens in, 19–20
Food safety, 2, 4

G

Gad c 1, 180
    thermostability, 181
Gamma-caseins, 131
Gastropods, 186
    cross-reactions among, 187
    tropomyosin allergens in, 188
Genetically modified organisms, 164
Genomic assays, for lupin, 54
Germany, RASFF notifications, 160
Gliadins, 156, 165
    commercial test kits, 166
    toxic motifs, 165
Globulins
    isolation from lupin, 52
    isolation via saline solutions, 50
    separation of, 51
Glutelin, 166
Gluten allergens
    in cereals, 155
    non-immuno-based methods, 167
Gluten allergy, 8
    differentiation methods, 9
Gluten free foods, 14
    Codex Alimentarius standards, 154
    labeling requirements, 154–155
    threshold of content, 155
Gluten intolerance, 156
Gluten labeling, 5, 154

Glutenins, 156
Glycinin protein family, soybean allergens in, 42
Good manufacturing practices (GMPs), 6
Greece, RASFF notifications, 161
Groundnuts, 36. *See also* Peanuts

H

Hazard Analysis of Critical Control Points ((HACCP), 163–164
Hazelnut
    commercial test kits, 119
    DNA detection methods, 93–94
    potential and limitations of published methods, 106–109
    protein-based detection techniques, 86–89
Hazelnut allergy, 78
Heat stability
    of fish allergens, 183
    of Gad c 1 fish allergen, 181
    of protein allergens, 154
    of storage proteins, 81
    of tropomyosin, 184
Hidden allergens, 80
High molecular mass (HMM) glutenins, 156
High molecular weight (HMW) glutenin, 167
High-performance liquid chromatographic (HPLC) analysis, 102, 134
    of fish allergens, 180–181
Histamine-containing foods, 13
Hong Kong, allergen labeling, 81
Hypersensitivity reactions
    delayed, 2
    immediate, 2

I

IgE antibodies, 2, 13
    analytical detection of, 6
    to fish, 178, 181, 182, 183
IgE-mediated allergic responses, 13
Immediate hypersensitivity, 2, 13
Immune reactions, 13
    T-cell-mediated, 2
Immuno-PCR (iPCR) assays, 168
Immunoassay methods, 20, 22, 165, 166
    drawbacks, 23–24
    in fish assays, 191
    for legume allergens, 52
    for soy detection, 170
    for whey and casein, 169
Immunoblot detection, 98, 164
    for almond allergens, 84
    of fish allergens, 181

for hazelnut detection, 87, 108
for soybean analysis, 59
Immunochemical assays
    for egg allergen detection, 143
    for lupin, 53
immunodiffusion methods, 53
    for peanut analysis, 56
Immunoglobulin, 129
Immunoprecipitation techniques, 98, 106
Incurred standards, 55
Infant formulas, labeling requirements, 155
Infants, food allergy prevalence, 1, 14
Informall database, 32
Informed choices, 3
Instrumentation, 5–7
International Immunogenetics Information System, 32
International Union of Immunological Societies (IUIS), 32, 81, 189. *See also* IUIS Allergen Nomenclature Sub-Committee list
Internet, allergen information, 32
Invertebrate species, cross-reactivity of allergens, 184
Ireland, RASFF notifications, 160
Isoallergens, 33
Isoforms, 33
Italy, RASFF notifications, 161
IUIS Allergen Nomenclature Sub-Committee list, 32

J

Japan
    allergen labeling, 81
    allergenic foods regulated by, 6
    cross-contact legislation, 17
    RASFF notifications, 159

K

Kunitz-type soybean trypsin inhibitors (STIs), 35, 43, 170

L

Labeling requirements, 3, 6, 14, 17, 154–155
    13 most common allergenic foods, 3
    for celery, 79–80
    for mustard, 79–80
    for prepackaged foods, 15–16
    for sesame seeds, 79–80
    for tree nuts, 79–80
Laboratory studies, 5

Lactoferrin, 129
Lactose, labeling requirements, 154
Lactose intolerance, 13
Lateral flow device (LFD) tests, 118, 163, 166
Lecithin, egg contamination, 157
Legal requirements, 14, 17. *See also* Labeling requirements
Legume allergens
  analysis methods, 53–54
  protein families containing, 33–36
Legume lectins, 35
  in peanuts, 40
  in soybeans, 43
Legume plants, with pods, 30
Legume seed extraction, 49
Legume seeds, 31
Legumin-type proteins, 81
Lentils, 31
  allergies in Mediterranean area and India, 31
Lichee nut, known single allergens, 82
Ligation-dependent probe amplification
  for almond allergen detection, 92
  for Brazil nut detection, 92
  for cashew allergen detection, 93
  for hazelnut allergen detection, 94
  for macadamia allergen detection, 94
  for multiple tree nuts, 114
  for pecan allergen detection, 94
  for pistachio allergen detection, 95
  for sesame allergen detection, 96
Limits of detection (LOD), 55
  in fish assays, 192
  for whey and casein, 170
Lipid content, and extraction efficiency, 190
Lipid-transfer proteins (LPTs), peanut allergens in, 38
Liquid chromatography (LC), 23
Low-cost tests, 8
Low-dose challenges, 19
Low molecular mass (LMM) glutenins, 156
Low-water processing, 20
Lowest observed adverse effect level (LOAEL), 18, 78
Lupin, 31
  food uses, 45–46
  natural history, 45
  sample extraction/cleanup, 50
Lupin allergens, 23–25
  alpha-conglutins, 46
  and amino acid sequence homologues, 47
  beta-conglutins, 46
  database entries, 34
  delta-conglutins, 47
  detection and quantification methods, 58, 62
  isolation, 51–52
  lupin gamma-conglutins, 47
  PR-10 proteins, 47
  properties, 45–48
  separation and analysis methods, 54
Lupin allergy, 6, 9
Lupin conglutins, separation methods, 51
Lupin plants, 46
Lupin seeds, 46
Lysozyme, 137, 139, 142, 157
  detection, 143
  isolating, 141

M

Macadamia nut
  DNA detection methods, 94
  potential and limitations of published methods, 111
Mandatory labeling, 3
Margarine, milk contamination, 157
Margin of exposure (MoE) method, 18, 19
Mass spectrometry, 20, 22–23, 54, 83, 162
  advantages over PCR and ELISA, 24
  for celery allergen detection, 91
  general characteristics, 23
  for hazelnut detection, 108
  for legume allergens, 52
  for lupin analysis, 62
  for peanut analysis, 58
  peanut profiling by, 52
  sample preparation for, 99
  for soybean analysis, 61
Matrix-assisted laser desorption/ionization time of flight (MALDI-TOF), 162, 167
  in fish assays, 191
Matrix effects, 55
Matrix ruggedness, 98
Method performance, 8
Method validation, 58
Milk allergens, 129. *See also* Cow's milk allergens
  in cereals, 155
  commercial test kits, 163
  labeling requirements, 154
  in processed food, 157
  thermal processing effects, 133
Milk allergy, 5, 6, 9
  labeling requirements, 15
  NIST reference materials, 24
  outgrowing of, 2, 131
  tolerance in early childhood, 131
Minimum eliciting doses (MEDs), 18
Molluscan allergens, 187–189

detection and quantification methods, 189–195
  lack of labeling requirements, 178
  lack of published detection methods, 178
  tropomyosin type, 188
Mollusk allergy, 6, 8, 9, 177–178
  threshold, 187
Mollusks
  allergenic properties, 186–189
  allergic reactions to, 186
  assays, 195
  cross-reactivity among species, 186–187
MoniQA project, 24
Monoclonal antibodies, 189
  in fish assays, 192
  for mollusk detection, 195
Multiple allergens, 23
  detecting in single chromatographic run, 23
Multiple-reaction monitoring (MRM), 23, 83
Multiplex assays, for tree nuts, 113–114
Multivalency, 18
Mustard, 78
  allergen labeling by country, 79–80, 80–81
  allergenic properties, 81, 83
  allergens in, 77–78
  commercial test kits for allergen detection, 118–119
  detection and quantification, 100–102
  DNA detection methods, 92–97, 96
  known single allergens, 82
  labeling requirements, 154
  potential and limitations of published methods, 115–116
  protein-based detection techniques, 90
  sample preparation, 99–100
Mustard allergy, 5, 6, 9
  methodology aspects, 83, 98
  prevalence, 78
  thresholds and symptoms of allergic reactions, 78–81

N

National Center for Biotechnology Information (NCBI) database, 39
National Institute for Standards and Technology (NIST), 24
  peanut butter reference standard, 55
Netherlands, RASFF notifications, 159
New products, risk for food-allergic consumers, 3
New Zealand
  allergenic foods regulated by, 6
  labeling requirements, 14, 80
No observed adverse effect level (NOAEL), 18

Non-immuno-based methods, 167
Nonspecific lipid transfer proteins (nsLTPs), 33
  in peanut allergens, 40
Nucleic acid detection
  sample preparation for, 99–100
  for tree nuts, sesame seeds, mustard, celery, 101–102
Nutritional characteristics, peanuts, 30–31

O

Oats, allergens in, 155, 156
Oleosins, 35
  in peanut allergens, 39, 40
  in soybean allergens, 43
Ovalbumin, 137, 138, 139, 142, 157
  detection, 143
  immunochemical identification and quantification, 143
  isolating, 141
Ovomucin, 142
Ovomucoid, 137, 138, 157, 168
  detection, 143
  ELISA detection, 144
  isolating, 141
Ovotransferrin, 142, 157

P

Papain-like proteins, 35
PARNUTS, 14
Parvalbumin, 179–181, 182, 186
  SPR and PCR detection techniques, 192, 193
Pasta
  celery contamination, 158
  egg contamination in, 157
  milk contamination, 157
Pathogenesis-related proteins (PR-10), 38. *See also* PR10 proteins
PCR detection methods
  advantages over immunological detection, 21
  for Brazil nut detection, 104
  for cashew detection, 105
  for celery, 117
  for cereal-based allergens, 164
  comparison with ELISA, 120
  for cow's milk proteins, 137
  for fish assays, 191
  general characterization, 23
  for gluten detection, 167
  for hazelnut detection, 93, 108
  for lupin analysis, 62
  for parvalbumin, 192–193
  for peanut allergens, 55, 58

for pistachio allergen detection, 95
sample preparation steps, 100
for sesame allergens, 171
shortcomings, 24
for soybean allergens, 54, 61
for walnut detection, 112
PCR-ELISA detection, 102, 162, 164
for gluten proteins, 168
for hazelnut, 93, 109
PCR inhibitors, avoiding, 100
Pea, 31
Peanut allergens, 23–25
and amino acid sequence homologues, 38–39
Ara h 1, 23, 36
Ara h 2, 36–37
Ara h 3, 37
Ara h 4, 37
Ara h 5, 37
Ara h 6, 40
Ara h 7, 40
Ara h 8, 40
Ara h 9, 40
Ara h 10, 40
Ara h 11, 40
Ara h agglutinin, 40
Ara oleosin 18 kDa, 40
database entries, 34
detection and quantification methods, 55
geographic prevalence, 31
isolation, 51
labeling requirements, 154
properties, 36–40
separation and analysis methods, 54
Peanut allergy, 5, 6, 9, 17
doubled prevalence, 1
labeling requirements, 15
lifelong, 2
prevalence, 36
Peanut plants, 37
Peanut pods, 37
Peanut seeds, 37
Peanuts, 31
LFD tests for, 118
natural history, 30
nutritional characteristics, 30–31
sample extraction/cleanup, 50
Pecan nut
DNA detection methods, 94
known single allergens, 82
potential and limitations of published methods, 109–110
protein-based detection techniques, 89
Pfam protein family database, 31, 32

Phosphate-buffered saline (PBS) buffer, 50, 99, 169, 190
Phosvitin, 138, 139
Pies, milk contamination in, 157
Pistachio nuts
DNA detection methods, 95
known single allergens, 82
potential and limitations of published methods, 110–111
Poland, RASFF notifications, 160
Pollen-fruit-vegetable syndrome, 35
Pollinosis-associated proteins, 35
Polyacrylamide gel electrophoresis, 53
Polyclonal antibodies (Pabs), 22, 170, 189
Polyclonal antisera, 22
Polymerase chain reaction (PCR) methods, 20, 21, 98. *See also* PCR detection methods
commercial test kits, 21
in fish assays, 191
for legume allergens, 52
Polypeptide fragments, 17–18
Powdered food factories, 20
PR10 proteins, 35, 83
in lupin allergens, 47, 48
peanut allergens in, 38
Preadolescence, food allergy risks, 3
Precautionary labeling, 4
Prepackaged foods, allergen labeling requirements, 15–16
Processed foods
celery allergens in, 158
crustacean protein detection in, 194
egg allergens in, 156–157
milk allergens in, 157
RASFF reports, 158
sesame seed allergens in, 158
soy allergens in, 157–158
Processed meat products, egg contamination, 157
Product liability legislation, 7
Product safety legislation, 7
Profilin protein family, 33–34, 81, 83
peanut allergens in, 38
Prolamin protein family, 33, 81, 165
cereals containing, 156
isolation via alcohol-water mixtures, 50
peanut allergens in, 38
QQPFP sequence, 166
soybean allergens in, 42, 43
Protall database, 32
Protein allergens, 17–18
in cereals, 155–156
heat resistance, 154

peanut, 38–39
in tree nuts, sesame seeds, mustard seeds, celery, 81
Protein-based detection techniques, 21, 98
for almond, 84–85
for Brazil nut, 85
for cashew, 86
for celery, 91
comparison with DNA-based published methods, 120
for hazelnut, 86–89
for legume allergens, 52
for mustard, 90
for pecan, 89
sample preparation methods, 99
for sesame, 89–90
for tree nuts, sesame, mustard, celery, 84–91
for walnut, 89
Protein detection, 100–101
Protein families
legume allergens, 33–36
peanut allergens, 38–39
soybean allergens, 42–44
Provitamin A, egg contamination, 157
Public health awareness, 1
Puddings, milk contamination, 157

Q

QQPFP sequence, 166
Quantification methods
for fish, crustacean, and molluscan allergens, 190–191
legume allergens, 55, 58
Quantitative test kits, 162

R

Radioallergosorbent test (RAST), 53
for lupin analysis, 62
for peanut analysis, 57
for soybean analysis, 60
Radioimmunoassay (RIA), 22
Rapid Alert System for Food and Feed (RASFF), 7, 158. *See also* RASFF reports
RASFF reports, 158, 159–161. *See also* Rapid Alert System for Food and Feed (RASFF)
Real-time PCR (RT-PCR), 21, 98, 164
for almond allergen detection, 92, 103
for Brazil nut detection, 92
for cashew allergen detection, 92–93, 105
for celery allergen detection, 97, 117
in celery detection, 118
commercial test kits, 171
for cow's milk detection, 136
false positives with, 106
in fish assays, 193
for gluten detection, 167, 168
for hazelnut detection, 109
in macadamia detection, 111
for macadamia nut detection, 94
for multiple tree nuts, 114
for mustard allergen detection, 96, 116
for pecan allergen detection, 94, 110
for pistachio allergen detection, 111
quantitative tests, 121
sensitivity compared with ELISA, 98
for sesame allergen detection, 95, 115
for walnut allergen detection, 95, 113
Reference materials
lack of, 8
need for development, 24
Reference materials incurred (RMIs), 24
Restriction fragment length polymorphism (RFLP), 191
Reversed-phase high-performance liquid chromatography (RP-HPLC), 51, 134, 142
Rice, as allergen, 155
Risk-taking, among adolescents, 3
Rocket immunoelectrophoresis, 53
for peanut analysis, 56
Romania, RASFF notifications, 161
Root celery allergy, 17
Runner peanuts, 36
Rye, 165, 166
allergens in, 156
commercial test kits, 163

S

S albumin, 158
Safe foods. *See also* Food safety
pressure to provide to children, 3
Sample extraction/cleanup, 48–49
for fish, crustacean, and molluscan allergens, 190–191
isolation of individual allergens, 50–52
lupin, 50
peanut extracts, 50
soybean extracts, 50
total legume extracts, 49–50
Sample homogenization/solubilization, 49
Sample preparation
for nucleic acid detection, 99–100

INDEX 217

for PCR testing, 120
for protein detection, 99
Sandwich ELISA, 100, 101, 102, 103, 135, 162, 165, 192
   for almond allergen detection, 84
   for Brazil nut allergen detection, 85, 103
   for cashew allergen detection, 86
   for celery allergen detection, 91, 118
   commercial test kits, 119, 166
   for cow's milk detection, 136
   in crustacean assays, 193, 194
   for egg allergen detection, 169
   for hazelnut allergen detection, 86, 87, 106, 107, 108
   for hen's egg protein detection, 144
   for mustard allergen detection, 90
   in mustard detection, 116
   for sesame detection, 170
   for walnut allergen detection, 89
   in walnut detection, 111, 112
   for whey and casein detection, 169
Sarcoplasmic calcium-binding protein (SCP), 186
   cross-reactivity of, 185
Sauces, milk contamination, 157
Sausage, milk contamination, 157
SDS gels
   for soybean analysis, 59
   total lupin extract, 48
   total peanut extract, 39
   total soybean extract, 44
Seafood allergens, 178. *See also* Crustacean allergens; Fish allergens
   undeclared, 189
Seed allergies, 9
Sensitivity
   in celery detection, 117, 118
   of egg detection methods, 168
   of ELISA detection methods, 98
   of gliadin detection, 165
   in pistachio allergen detection, 111
Sensitization, 2, 18
   to cow's milk, 133
   to fish, 183
   within legume families, 33
   to mollusk species, 187
   to soy, 41
Separation and analysis methods
   lupin allergens, 54
   peanut, soybean, lupin, 52, 54
   peanut allergens, 54
   soybean allergens, 54
Sequence identity, 32, 33, 98
   and cross-reactivity potential, 33
   in profilins, 34
   between SCP and parvalbumin, 186
Sesame seed allergy, 5, 6, 9
   methodology aspects, 83, 98
   prevalence, 78
Sesame seeds, 78
   allergen labeling by country, 79–80, 80–81
   allergenic properties, 81, 83
   allergens in, 77–78
   commercial test kits for allergen detection, 118–119, 163
   detection and quantification, 100–102
   detection in cereals, 155, 170–171
   DNA detection methods, 92–97, 95–96
   known single allergens, 82
   labeling requirements, 154
   potential and limitations of published methods, 114–115
   in processed foods, 158
   protein-based detection techniques, 89–90
   sample preparation, 99–100
   thresholds and symptoms of allergic reactions, 78–81
Shellfish allergy, 5, 6, 17
Single-stranded conformational polymorphism (SSCP), 191
Small and medium enterprises (SMEs), 19
Small proteins, competitive ELISA for detection of, 162
Sodium dodecyl sulfate polyacrylamide gel electrophoresis (SDS-PAGE), 142, 181
Soups, egg contamination, 157
Soybean allergens, 23–25
   and amino acid sequence homologues, 42–44
   commercial test kits, 163
   database entries, 34
   detection and quantification methods, 58, 59–61
   detection in cereals, 155, 170
   Gly m 2, 41
   Gly m 2S, 44
   Gly m 3, 41
   Gly m 4, 41
   Gly m 5, 41
   Gly m 6, 44
   Gly m agglutinin, 45
   Gly m Bd30K, 44
   Gly m CPI, 45
   Gly m EAP, 45
   Gly m LTP, 45
   Gly m oleosin, 45
   Gly T1, 45

isolation, 51
labeling requirements, 154
in processed foods, 157–158
properties, 40–41, 44–45
separation and analysis methods, 54
Soybean allergy, 5, 6, 9, 17
labeling requirements, 15
Soybean pods, 49
Soybean trypsin inhibitors (STIs), 35
Soybeans, 31
food and product uses, 41
natural history, 40–41
sample extraction/cleanup, 50
Spanish peanuts, 36
Specificity
in celery detection, 117
of fish authentication techniques, 191
of PCR detection methods, 98, 102
in pistachio detection, 111
Specificity issues, 22
Spiked standards, 55
Standardization issues, 24
Storage proteins, 81, 156
in cereals, 156
Stress, due to food allergies, 3
Structural Classification of Proteins (SCOP) database, 81
Structural Database of Allergen Proteins, 32
Sulfite allergens, 5, 6
labeling requirements, 16, 154
Sulfur dioxide allergens, 6
Surface plasmon resonance (SPR) techniques
for crab tropomyosin detection, 195
in fish assays, 192
Surfactant, in extraction process, 191
Sweden, RASFF notifications, 159, 160
Switzerland, cross-contact legislation, 17
SYBR Green detection
for hazelnut, 109
for sesame seeds, 115

T

T-cell-mediated immune reactions, 2
Tennessee red/white peanuts, 36
Test kit performance studies, 55
Tetrameric CM16 inhibitor, 156
Threshold, 18
of mollusk allergy, 187
Time of analysis, 162
Total legume extracts
peanut, 50
sample extraction/cleanup, 49

Tree nut allergy, 5, 6, 8, 9, 17
labeling requirements, 16
methodology aspects, 83, 98
prevalence, 78
Tree nuts, 78
allergen labeling by country, 79–80, 80–81
allergenic properties, 81, 83
allergens in, 77–78
commercial test kits for allergen detection, 118–119
detection and quantification, 100–102
DNA detection methods, 92–97
EU mandatory labeling, 80
known single allergens, 82
labeling requirements, 154
multiplex assays, 113–114
potential and limitations of published methods, 102–118
sample preparation, 99–100
thresholds and symptoms of allergic reactions, 78–81
Trigger reactions, 18
Tris-HCl, 50, 99
Tropomyosin allergens, 184, 187
in crustaceans, 185
detection methods, 178
in molluscan species, 188
Tuna
cross-reactivity with cod, 178
parvalbumin content, 180
Turkey, RASFF notifications, 159, 161
Two-site ELISA, 169

U

Ukraine, RASFF notifications, 160
Undeclared allergenic ingredients, 6, 7
UniProt database, 32, 39
United Kingdom, RASFF notifications, 159, 160, 161
United States
allergenic foods regulated by, 6
labeling requirements, 14

V

Valencia peanuts, 36
Variants, 33
Very low gluten, 14
labeling requirements, 155
Vicilin, 81
Virginia peanuts, 36

INDEX

W

Walnut
  DNA detection methods, 95
  potential and limitations of published methods, 111–113
  protein-based detection techniques, 89
Western blot detection
  for cow's milk proteins, 137
  for pecan, 109
Wet-based cleaning procedures, 20
Wheat allergens, 155, 156, 165
  commercial test kits, 163
Wheat allergy, 5, 17
Whey proteins, 129, 130
  detection in cereals, 169–170
  Western blot detection, 137

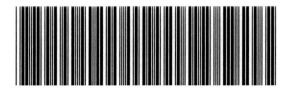